Stilianos E. Kountakis

Brent A. Senior

Wolfgang Draf

Editors

The Frontal Sinus

Stilianos E. Kountakis

Brent A. Senior

Wolfgang Draf

Editors

The Frontal Sinus

With 144 Figures, 73 in Color
and 40 Tables

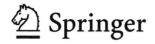 Springer

Stilianos E. Kountakis, MD, PhD
Professor and Vice Chair
Chief, Rhinology-Sinus Surgery
Medical College of Georgia
1120 15th St, Ste BP-4632
Augusta, GA 30912-4060, USA

Brent A. Senior, MD
Assoc. Prof., Chief, Rhinology, Allergy, and Sinus Surgery
Dept. of Otolaryngology/Head and Neck Surgery
Univ. of North Carolina at Chapel Hill
Chapel Hill, NC 27599--7070, USA

Wolfgang Draf, MD, PhD, FRCS (Ed)
Professor and Chairman
Dept. of ENT-Diseases, Head-, Neck and Facial Plastic Surgery
Communication Disorders, Klinikum Fulda gAG
Pacelliallee 4, D 36043 Fulda, Germany

Library of Congress Control Number: 2005924448

ISBN-10 3-540-21143-8 Springer Berlin Heidelberg New York
ISBN-13 978-3-540-21143-3 Springer Berlin Heidelberg New York

Springer is a part of Springer Science+Business Media
springeronline.com
© Springer-Verlag Berlin Heidelberg 2005
Printed in Germany

Editor: Marion Philipp, Heidelberg, Germany
Desk Editor: Martina Himberger, Heidelberg, Germany
Production: ProEdit GmbH, 69126 Heidelberg, Germany
Cover: Frido-Steinen-Broo, EStudio, Calamar, Spain
Typesetting: K. Detzner, 67346 Speyer, Germany

Printed on acid-free paper   21/3151 ML   5 4 3 2 1 0

Dedications and Acknowledgements

- Dedicated to the memory of my mother, Eftihia E. Kountakis, who with her nurturing devotion inspired my pursue of a medical career, and to my loving wife Eleni and children Eftihia, Emmanuel and Nikoleta, who bring meaning to my life.
  Many thanks to my assistant Aprell Edwards for her long hours of hard work during this project.

  Stil Kountakis

- To my wife, Dana, and my children, Rebecca, Benjamin, Grace, and Anna. A part of you is in each of these pages. Soli Deo Gloria.

  Brent Senior

- To my wife Julia, and to my children Maximilian and Clara for their constant patience.
  It is a pleasure to thank my American colleagues for excellent cooperation in editing this book.

  Wolfgang Draf

Preface

Advances in instrumentation and surgical techniques continue to yield improvements in the surgical management of sinus disease. Rhinologists have developed techniques to address disease in remote areas along the anterior skull base so that many procedures previously performed using an open approach may now be performed endoscopically. Despite these advances, the complex anatomy and remote location of the frontal recess continue to pose challenges in the surgical management of frontal sinus disease. The narrow funnel-shaped aperture and important surrounding structures can predispose to complications most rhinologists hope to avoid they can do without. Because of this, it is not uncommon to hear at rhinology meetings that it is usually best for the average otolaryngologist to avoid instrumentation in this area, especially in primary surgeries. Numerous manuscripts are published describing the anatomy, diagnostic techniques, and medical and surgical management of frontal sinus disease. But as our residents and fellows survey the literature, they often wish they had a single comprehensive source of information related to the anatomy and management of frontal sinus disorders.

This project was initiated in order to fill this void and to provide a valuable source of information not only for academic institutions but also for the private practice environment. Most of the world's leading authorities in rhinology were invited to participate. Chapters in the book are arranged in a logical fashion, providing a comprehensive body of information beginning with the history of frontal sinus surgery and addressing more complex surgical concepts as the reader progresses through the text. Each chapter was written by authors that possess extensive experience on the topic and have previously published on the particular anatomical structure or issue the chapter addresses. The result is the first exhaustive frontal sinus textbook that can be used as a reference source by both academic and practicing otolaryngologists worldwide.

Stilianos Kountakis, MD, PhD
Brent A. Senior, MD
Wolfgang Draf, MD, PhD, FRCS (Ed)

Contents

List of Contributors

Robert T. Adelson, MD
Chief Resident, Dept. of Otolaryngology Head
and Neck Surgery
Univ. of Texas Southwestern Medical Ctr.
5323 Harry Hines Blvd., Dallas, TX 75390–9035
USA

Pete S. Batra, MD
(e-mail: batrap@ccf.org)
Cleveland Clinic Foundation
Head & Cleveland Clinic Foundation
Dept. of Otolaryngology
9500 Euclid Ave., Desk A71, Cleveland, OH 44195
USA

Ulrike Bockmühl, MD, PhD
(e-mail: U.Bockmuehl.HNO@klinikum-fulda.de
Assistant Professor, Dept. of Otorhinolaryngology
Head and Neck and Facial Plastic Surgery
Klinikum Fulda gAG
Teaching Hospital of the Philipps-University Marburg
Pacelliallee 4, 36043 Fulda
Germany

Roy Casiano, MD
(e-mail: rcasiano@med.miami.edu)
University of Miami
1475 NW 12th Ave, Suite 4025
Miami, FL 33136-1002
USA

Alexander G. Chiu, MD
(e-mail: Alexander.chiu@uphs.upenn.edu)
Dept. of Otorhinolaryngology-Head
and Neck Surgery
Univ. of Pennsylvania Health System
3400 Spruce St., 5 Ravdin, Philadelphia, PA 19104
USA

James M. Chow, MD
(e-mail: Jchow@lumc.edu)
Dept. of Otolaryngology-Head and Neck Surgery
Loyola University Medical Center
2160 S. First Ave., Maywood, IL 60153
USA

Martin J. Citardi, MD
(e-mail: citardm@ccf.org)
Cleveland Clinic Foundation
Head & Cleveland Clinic Foundation
Dept. of Otolaryngology
9500 Euclid Ave., Desk A71, Cleveland, OH 44195
USA

Wolfgang Draf, MD, PhD, FRCS (Ed)
(e-mail: Wdraf@aol.com)
Professor and Chairman
Dept. of ENT-Diseases
Head-, Neck and Facial Plastic Surgery
Communication Disorders, Klinikum Fulda gAG
Teaching Hospital of the Philipps-University Marburg
Pacelliallee 4, 36043 Fulda
Germany

Marc G. Dubin, MD
Georgia Nasal and Sinus Institute
4750 Waters Ave., Ste. 112, Savannah, GA 31404
USA

Carlos S.Duque, MD
(e-mail: cduque@med.miami.edu)
University of Miami
1475 NW 12th Ave
Suite 4025
Miami, FL 33136-1002
United States of America
USA

Berrylin J. Ferguson, MD
(e-mail: fergusonbj@upmc.edu)
Otolaryngology/Head and Neck Surgery
University of Pittsburgh, Pittsburgh, PA
USA

Ramon E. Figueroa, MD, FACR
(e-mail: rfiguero@mail.mcg.edu)
Professor of Radiology, Chief of Neuroradiology
Medical College of Georgia
1120 15th St., Augusta, GA 30912
USA

Christine G. Gourin, MD, FACS
(e-mail: cgourin@mcg.edu)
Dept. of Otolaryngology – Head and Neck Surgery
Medical College of Georgia
1120 15th St., BP 4117, Augusta, GA 30912
USA

Scott M. Graham, MD
(e-mail: scott-graham@uiowa.edu)
Professor, Director
Rhinology and Paranasal Sinus Clinic
Dept. of Otolaryngology – Head and Neck Surgery
University of Iowa
Iowa City, IA 52242
USA

Charles W. Gross, MD
(e-mail: cwg9u@virginia.edu)
Dept. of Otolaryngology and Head & Neck Surgery
Division of Rhinology
University of Virginia Health System
Box 800713, Charlottesville, VA 22908-0713
USA

Jack Gwaltney, MD
Depts. of Otolaryngology and Internal Medicine
University of Virginia Health System
Charlottesville, VA 22908
USA

Joseph K. Han, MD
(e-mail: jeh5h@virginia.edu)
Dept. of Otolaryngology and Head & Neck Surgery
Division of Rhinology
University of Virginia Health System
Box 800713, Charlottesville, VA 22908-0713
USA

Peter H. Hwang, MD
(e-mail: hwangp@ohsu.edu)
3181 SW Sam Jackson Pk. Rd., PV01, Dept. OTO-
HNS, Portland OR 97239
USA

Joseph B. Jacobs, MD
(e-mail: joseph.jacobs@med.nyu.edu)
New York Univ. Med. Ctr., Dept. of Otolaryngology
530 First Ave., Ste. 3C, New York, NY 10016-6402
USA

Seth J. Kanowitz, MD
(e-mail: seth.kanowitz@med.nyu.edu)
Department of Otolaryngology
New York University School of Medicine
530 First Avenue, SUite 3C
New York, New York 10016
USA

Boris I. Karanfilov, MD
(e-mail: bk@ohiosinus.com)
Ohio Sinus Institute
750 Mt. Carmel Mall, Ste. 240, Columbus, OH 43222
USA

David W. Kennedy, MD
(e-mail: kennedyd@uphs.upenn.edu)
Dept. of Otorhinolaryngology-Head
and Neck Surgery
University of Pennsylvania Health System
3400 Spruce St., 5 Ravdin, Philadelphia, PA 19104
USA

Stilianos E. Kountakis, MD, PhD
(e-mail: skountakis@mail.mcg.edu)
Dept. of Otolaryngology–Head and Neck Surgery
Medical College of Georgia
1120 15th St., Ste. BP-416, Augusta, GA 30912-4060
USA

Frederick A. Kuhn, MD, FACS
(e-mail: DocSinus@aol.com)
Georgia Nasal and Sinus Institute
4750 Waters Ave., Ste. 112, Savannah, GA 31410
USA

Andrew P. Lane, MD
(e-mail: alane3@jhmi.edu)
Director, Div. of Rhinology
Dept. of Otolaryngology – Head and Neck Surgery
Johns Hopkins Outpatient Center
6th Fl., 601 N. Caroline St., Baltimore, MD 21287
USA

Donald C. Lanza, MD
(e-mail: dclanza@sniflmd.com)
Director, Sinus & Nasal Inst. of Florida, P.A.
St. Anthony's Outpatient Ctr.
900 Carillon Pkwy., Ste. 200, St. Petersburg, FL 33716
USA

Richard A. Lebowitz, MD
(e-mail: Richard.Lebowitz@med.nyu.edu)
Asst. Prof. of Otolaryngology
New York Univ. School of Medicine, NY
USA

Bradley F. Marple, MD, FAAOA
(e-mail: bradley.marple@utsouthwestern.edu)
Associate Professor and Vice-Chairman
Dept. of Otolaryngology Head and Neck Surgery
Univ. of Texas Southwestern Medical Ctr.
5323 Harry Hines Blvd., Dallas, TX 75390–9035
USA

Ralph Metson MD
(e-mail: ralph_metson@meei.harvard.edu)
Zero Emerson Pl., Ste. 2D, Boston, MA 02114
USA

Tanya K. Meyer, MD
Dept. of Otolaryngology
and Communication Sciences
9200 W. Wisconsin Ave., Medical College
of Wisconsin
Milwaukee, WI 53226
USA

Richard R. Orlandi, MD, FACS
(e-mail: richard.orlandi@hsc.utah.edu)
Division of Otolaryngology –
Head and Neck Surgery
The University of Utah
50 N. Medical Dr., Ste. 3C120, Salt Lake City, UT 84132
USA

James Palmer, MD
(e-mail: james.palmer@uphs.upenn.edu)
Hospital University of Pennsylvania
3400 Spruce Street, 5th floor, Ravdin Building
Philadelphia, PA 19104
USA

Ankit M. Patel, MD
300 Pasteur Dr., R135, Stanford, CA 94305
USA

Hassan H. Ramadan, MD, MSc
(e-mail: hramadan@hsc.wvu.edu)
Dept. of Otolaryngology Head & Neck Surgery
West Virginia University
P.O. Box 9200, Morgantown, WV 26506–9200
USA

Douglas Reh, MD
(e-mail: dreh@ohsu.edu)
3181 SW Sam Jackson Pk Rd PV01
Dept. OTO-HNS
Portland, OR 97239
USA

John S. Rhee, MD
Div. of Facial Plastic and Reconstructive Surgery
9200 W. Wisconsin Ave, Medical College
of Wisconsin Milwaukee, WI 53226
USA

Ioana Schipor, MD
(e-mail: ioana.schipor@uphs.upenn.edu)
Hospital University of Pennsylvania
3400 Spruce Street, 5th floor, Ravdin Building
Philadelphia, PA 19104
USA

Rodney J. Schlosser, MD
(e-mail: schlossr@musc.edu)
Medical Univ. of South Carolina
Dept. of Otolaryngology
PO Box 250550
135 Rutledge Ave., Ste. 1130, Charleston, SC 29425
USA

Allen M. Seiden, MD
(e-mail: allen.seiden@uc.edu)
Prof. of Otolaryngology, Univ. of Cincinnati
College of Medicine, Dept. of Otolaryngology –
Head and Neck Surgery
 P.O. Box 670528
231 Albert Sabin Way (formerly Bethesda Ave.)
Rm. 6412 MSB, Cincinnati, Ohio 45267–0528
USA

Brent A. Senior, MD
(e-mail: Brent_Senior@med.unc.edu)
Assoc. Prof., Chief, Rhinology, Allergy,
and Sinus Surgery, Dept. of Otolaryngology/
Head and Neck Surgery
Univ. of North Carolina at Chapel Hill
Chapel Hill, NC 27599–7070
USA

Michael Sillers, MD
(e-mail: michael.sillers@ccc.uab.edu)
Assoc. Prof., Otolaryngology/Head
 and Neck Surgery, Univ. of Alabama at Birmingham
1501 5th Ave. S., Birmingham AL 35233-1614
USA

Timothy L. Smith, MD, MPH
(e-mail: TLSmith@mcw.edu)
Div. of Rhinology and Sinus Surgery
9200 W. Wisconsin Ave.
Medical College of Wisconsin, Milwaukee, WI 53226
USA

James A. Stankiewicz, MD
(e-mail: Jstank@lumc.edu)
Dept. of Otolaryngology-Head and Neck Surgery
Loyola Univ. Medical Ctr
 2160 S. First Ave., Maywood, IL 60153
USA

Joseph Sullivan, MD
(e-mail: josulliva@mail.mcg.edu)
Neuroradiology Fellow, Neuroradiology Service
Medical College of Georgia
1120 15th St., Augusta, GA 30912
 USA

David J. Terris, MD, FACS
(e-mail: dterris@mail.mcg.edu)
Dept. of Otolaryngology – Head and Neck Surgery
Medical College of Georgia
1120 15th St., BP 4117, Augusta, GA 30912
USA

Feodor Ung, MD
(e-mail: feodor.ung@dupagemd.com)
DuPage Medical Group at Lombard
1801 S. Highland Ave., Ste. 220, Lombard, IL 60148
USA

Winston C. Vaughan, MD
(e-mail: Sinusmd@aol.com)
300 Pasteur Dr., R135, Stanford, CA 94305
USA

Birgit Winther, MD
(e-mail: bw8b@virginia.edu)
Dept.s of Otolaryngology and Internal Medicine
University of Virginia Health System
PO Box 800713, Charlottesville, VA 22908
USA

Mark C. Weissler, MD, FACS
(e-mail: mark_weissler@med.unc.edu)
G0412 Neurosciences Hospital
Univ.y of North Carolina, Campus Box 7070
Chapel Hill, NC 27599–7070
USA

Bradford A. Woodworth, MD
Medical University of South Carolina
Department of Otolaryngology
PO Box 250550135 Rutledge Ave., Suite 1130
Charleston, SC 29425
USA

Chapter 1

History of Frontal Sinus Surgery

1

Hassan H. Ramadan

Core Messages

■ With over two centuries of scientific description of frontal sinus surgery, the optimal procedure remains unclear

■ Balancing concerns of eradication of disease with cosmesis and restoration of frontal sinus function has resulted in the development of numerous procedures for treatment of frontal sinus disease

■ Endoscopic approaches are now widely applied to the management of frontal sinus disease

Contents

Introduction

The first frontal sinus procedure was described in 1750 [36]. Despite more than two centuries since the description of the first procedure on the frontal sinus, the optimal procedure remains unclear. Although frontal sinus surgery makes up only a small portion of all paranasal sinus surgery, the literature is filled with publications on this subject. Ellis in 1954 stated that "surgical treatment of chronic frontal sinusitis is difficult, often unsatisfactory and sometimes disastrous. The many surgical techniques available are expressions of our uncertainty and perhaps so our failure" [11].

The ideal treatment for diseases of the frontal sinus is one that will provide complete relief of symptoms, eradicate the underlying disease process, preserve the function of the sinus, and cause the least morbidity and the least cosmetic deformity. Over the last two centuries a variety of surgical procedures have been described for the treatment of frontal sinus disease. Those procedures flip-flopped from external to intranasal to external and currently to intranasal again. The ideal procedure has not been identified yet despite 2 centuries of various techniques.

The recent advances in imaging and endoscopic techniques have resulted in the resurgence of intranasal procedures for the treatment of frontal sinus disease. Frontal sinus disease, particularly chronic frontal sinusitis, is a highly morbid and sometimes life-threatening condition because of its potential complications. Despite the fact that over the years the incidence of complications has decreased, orbital and intracranial complications, including meningitis, subdural abscess, intracerebral abscess, and osteomyelitis continue to occur.

1

Trephination Era (1750)

Frontal sinus surgery was first described in the 18th century. It is noted that as early as 1750 Runge performed an obliteration procedure of the frontal sinus [36]. The first published report in 1870 by Wells described an external and intracranial drainage procedure for a frontal sinus mucocele [44].

In 1884 Alexander Ogston described a trephination procedure through the anterior table to evacuate the frontal sinus. He then dilated the nasal frontal duct, curetted the mucosa (Fig. 1.1A,B), and established drainage with a tube that was placed in the duct [32].

At the same time Luc described a similar procedure, and two years later the Ogston-Luc procedure was established [26]. However, this technique did not gain popularity because of the high failure rate due to nasal frontal duct stenosis [7].

Radical Ablation Procedures (1895)

At the turn of the century a number of physicians were advocating a radical frontal sinus procedure. Kuhnt in 1895 described removing the anterior wall of the frontal sinus in an attempt to clear disease. The mucosa was stripped to the level of the frontal recess, and a stent was placed for temporary drainage [9]. In 1898 Riedel/Schenke described the first procedure for obliteration of the frontal sinus [34], advocating completely removing the anterior table as well as the floor of the frontal sinus with stripping of the muco-

sa. This procedure had the advantages of removing osteomyelitic bone as well as allowing for easy detection of recurrent disease. This procedure, however was plagued by the unsightly cosmetic forehead deformity. Killian in 1903 described a modification of the Riedel-Schenke procedure [22]. In an attempt to minimize the cosmetic deformity he recommended preserving a one-centimeter bar of the supraorbital rim. He also recommended an ethmoidectomy with rotation of a mucosal flap into the frontal recess with stenting to prevent stenosis. At that time Killian's technique was embraced because of the success as well as the reduced cosmetic deformity. However the Killian procedure was later abandoned because of the high incidence of late morbidity with restenosis, supraorbital rim necrosis, postoperative meningitis, and mucocele formation, as well as death.

Conservative Procedures (1905)

Because of the significant cosmetic deformity as well as the high failure rate of those ablative external procedures, an era of conservatism followed next. This era consisted of intranasal approaches to the frontal sinus as well as external frontoethmoid techniques. In 1908 Knapp [23] described an ethmoidectomy through the medial wall and entering the frontal sinus through its floor, by which he removed diseased mucosa and enlarged the nasal frontal duct. His operation however never received widespread recognition. In 1911, Schaeffer proposed an intranasal puncture technique to re-establish the drainage and ventilation of the frontal sinus [38]. Numerous complica-

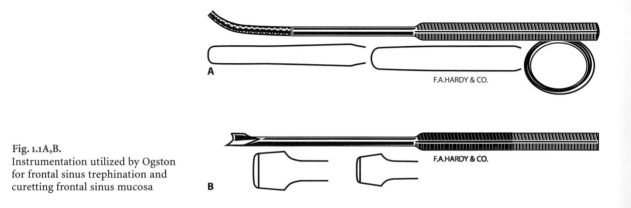

Fig. 1.1A,B.
Instrumentation utilized by Ogston for frontal sinus trephination and curetting frontal sinus mucosa

tions were encountered, however, including intracranial penetration. Between 1901 and 1908, Ingals, Halle, Good, and Wells described several intranasal procedures to the frontal sinus [14, 16, 19, 45]. Halle described a procedure in which the frontal process of the maxilla was chiseled out, and then a burr was used to remove the floor of the frontal sinus [16]. This operation was rarely used because it was associated with a high mortality rate. All of these intranasal approaches were abandoned because of the high mortality and complication rates associated with them. This increased incidence of mortality and complications was a result of the inadequate visualization of the frontal recess.

In 1914, Lothrop described a procedure to enlarge the frontal drainage pathway in a way that would prevent restenosis as well as closure as was reported with other procedures at the time [25]. The procedure described a combined intranasal ethmoidectomy and an external ethmoid approach to create a common frontal nasal communication by resecting the nasal sinus floor, the frontal sinus septum, and the superior nasal septum. Lothrop later admitted that the lack of visualization during the intranasal approach made the procedure dangerous. Further follow-up on those patients also showed that the resection of the medial orbital wall allowed the collapse of orbital soft tissue into the ethmoid area, with subsequent stenosis of the frontal drainage pathway.

External Frontoethmoidectomy (1897, 1906, 1921)

Between 1897 (Jansen [20]) and 1906 (Ritter [35]), the details of frontoethmoidectomy were described in Germany. In the Anglo-American literature, Lynch (1921) [28] in the United States and Howarth [18] in the United Kingdom popularized the principle of frontal sinus floor resection and enlargement of the frontal sinus drainage. Therefore in those countries frontoethmoidectomy was known as the Lynch and Howarth operation [17].

An incision in the medial periorbital area is used (Fig. 1.2), and the frontal process of the maxilla, as well as the lamina papyracea are removed. This allowed access to remove the frontal sinus floor and to curette the mucosa. A stent was then placed in the frontal ostium to maintain communication. The stent was left in place for approximately 10 days. The procedure however was complicated by restenosis and recurrent infections. The problem was somewhat related to the medialization of the orbital soft tissue, as described by Boyden [3], that resulted in nasal frontal narrowing with scarring and stenosis. Failure rates were reported up to 33% with the Lynch procedure.

Despite the failure of the Lynch procedure, interest in it was maintained. Sewall, Boyden, and McNaught modified the Lynch technique in an attempt to in-

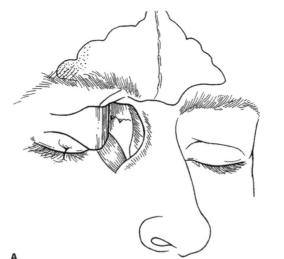
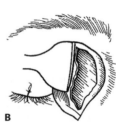

Fig. 1.2.
Lynch incision (A) with resulting access to frontal sinus and ethmoid sinuses (B)

A   B

1

crease the success rate and decrease failure and re-stenosis rates [3, 30, 40]. They described using a local mucoperiosteal flap to line and re-epithelialize the nasal frontal drainage pathway area. They also used a silicone tube to stent the frontal ostium, and they recommended leaving the stent in place for 4 weeks. Later several other authors lined the frontal drainage pathway with a mucoperiosteal flap to prevent re-stenosis and reported early success rates of about 90% [29]. Dedo, using the Sewall/Boyden technique, reported a success and patency rate of 97% at 6 year follow-up [8]. This era of utilizing modifications of the Lynch external frontoethmoidectomy continued to be the procedure of choice extending from its description in 1921 to the 1950s. Walsh in 1943, in an attempt to solve the problem of restenosis and the need for stenting, described a modification of the Lynch procedure in which the frontal drainage pathway membrane was left intact [43]. He came to those observations after he performed an experimental study on three groups of dogs. Brown, in accord with Walsh's idea, reported in 1946 a procedure to preserve the frontal drainage pathway mucosa in an attempt to reduce the failure drainage pathway and restenosis rates [5]. The problem of stenosis was significant enough that many researchers devised stents made of different materials in attempts to solve the problem [12]. Despite those modifications and stent techniques, long-term failure rates up to 30% were still reported, necessitating the continued development of better surgical procedures for the frontal sinus [29].

Osteoplastic Anterior Wall Approach to the Frontal Sinus (1958)

The osteoplastic anterior wall approach to the frontal sinus was described at the turn of the 19th century by several authors including Brieger, Schoenborn, Winkler, and later Beck and others [1, 4, 9, 39]. However, little attention was paid to this technique at the turn of the century, because of the concern about the difficulty of re-approximation of the bony flap to its original position. Osteomyelitis, infection of the bone, was also thought to be a major morbid condition of the procedure. Tato and Bergaglio in 1949 [42], and Lyman in 1950 [27] reported on obliterating the frontal sinus for frontal sinusitis with success and no cosmetic deformity.

In 1958 Goodale and Montgomery reported a series of seven patients who had an osteoplastic flap with an excellent success rate [13]. Montgomery stated that "intranasal probing and attempted enlargement or cannulization of the nasal frontal orifice are mentioned only to be condemned. Once the virginity of the nasofrontal passage has been violated, scarring and stenosis are inevitable." The osteoplastic frontal sinus procedure gained popularity in the 1960s and became the standard during that time (Fig. 1.3). A failure rate of less than 9% made this procedure popular among physicians. The use of a radiographic plate to outline the frontal sinus as described by Becker was a great advantage to safely elevate the bony flap [2].

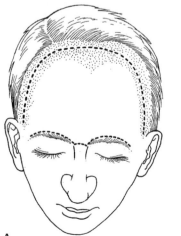
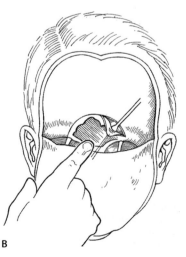

Fig. 1.3.
Osteoplastic frontal sinusotomy illustrating incision options (**A**) with resulting exposure and elevation of the anterior table of the frontal sinus (**B**)

A   B

A lot of experience accumulated with this technique, and Hardy and Montgomery reported in 1976 a 95% success rate with a median follow-up of 3 years [17]. Wide et al. in 1997 reported a 62% success rate with an additional 21% of patients achieving success after revision surgery [46].

Many otolaryngologists did not feel that the osteoplastic flap with fat obliteration was the answer to frontal sinus disease. They noted that it was an invasive procedure, which is technically difficult. It carries with it a high blood loss with potential for cosmetic deformity and poor scar formation. Many patients experience frontal neuralgias with numbness of the forehead. An additional operative site is needed for harvesting fat with potential morbidities. Long-term follow-up is necessary because of potential mucocele formation, and the presence of fat in the sinus makes it difficult to diagnose other frontal sinus problems [33].

Despite the popularity and the wide use of the osteoplastic flap, many physicians were not satisfied and did not feel that it was the ultimate procedure.

Microscopic/Endoscopic Intranasal Approaches (1991)

Earlier intranasal frontal sinus procedures had a high complication rate due to poor visualization. In 1990, Schaefer and Close reported on the use of the endoscope to treat 36 patients with frontal sinus disease. They performed endoscopic frontal sinusotomy with 12 patients reporting complete resolution of symptoms and 11 reporting improvement [37]. Draf, in 1991, reported on a series of 100 patients in which he used both a microscope and an endoscope to perform intranasal frontoethmoid surgery for frontal sinus disease. He described a concept of three procedures with a 90% success rate. He reported no complications with this endoscopic technique. All 10% of his failures had an open osteoplastic obliterative procedure. The Draf procedures were aimed at opening the frontal ostium intranasally and allowing the sinus to drain. Draf I consisted of an anterior ethmoidectomy with opening of the nasofrontal duct (NFD). Draf II in addition consists of unilateral resection of the floor of the frontal sinus; Draf III is bilateral resection of the frontal sinus floor [10].

With the advent of the endoscope, several authors have recently reported on the use of the endoscope to open the frontal sinus ostium and establish drainage of the frontal sinus. The advantages included lower morbidity rates, a shorter hospital stay, a less invasive procedure, and no external scarring [6, 15, 21, 31].

Kountakis and Gross in 2003 reported on long-term results of the modified Lothrop procedure and noted that with advancement of instrumentation and improved skills of surgeons with endoscopic procedures, success has been similar to that of the open osteoplastic approach with obliteration [24]. Stankiewicz and Wachter in 2003 reported a 90% success rate with the endoscopic approach for patients who had an osteoplastic approach and failed [41].

Conclusion

Currently, most otolaryngologists will initially perform an endoscopic procedure in most cases of chronic frontal sinusitis. An open procedure is usually reserved for patients with absent or distorted intranasal landmarks, failed endoscopic approaches, complicated frontal sinusitis, and evidence of lateral disease or posterior table erosion.

References

1. Beck, JC (1916) External frontal sinus operation. JAMA 67: 1811–1815
2. Becker D, Moore D, Lindsey W, et al (1995): Modified transnasal endoscopic Lothrop Procedure: Further considerations. Laryngoscope 105:1161
3. Boyden GL (1952) Surgical treatment of chronic frontal sinusitis. Ann Otol Rhinol Laryngol 61:558
4. Brieger (1895) Ueber chronische Eiterungen der Nebenhoehlen der Nase. Arch Ohren Nasen Kehlkopfheilk 39:213.
5. Brown, JM (1946) Frontal sinusitis. Tran Amer Laryngol, Rhinol And Otol Soc 50:314–317
6. Close LG, Lee NK, Leach JL, et al (1994) Endoscopic resection of the intranasal frontal sinus floor. Ann Otol Rhinol Laryngol 103:952–958
7. Coakley CG (1905) Frontal sinusitis: Diagnosis, treatment, and results. Trans Am Laryngol Rhinol Otol Soc 11:101
8. Dedo HH, Broberg TG, Mur AH (1998) Frontoethmoidectomy with Sewall-Bowden reconstruction: Alive and well, a 25-year experience. Am J Rhinol 12:191

1

9. Donald PJ (1995) Surgical management of frontal sinus infections. In Donald PJ, Gluckman JL, Rice DH (eds): The Sinuses. New York, Raven Press

10. Draf W (1991) Endonasal micro-endoscopic frontal sinus surgery: The Fulda concept. Oper Tech Otolaryngol Head Neck Surg 2:234

11. Ellis M (1954) The treatment of frontal sinusitis. J Laryngol Otol 68:478–490

12. Goodale, RL (1945) The use of tantalum in radical frontal sinus surgery. Ann Otol, Rhinol And Laryngol 54:757–762

13. Goodale RL, Montgomery WW (1958) Experience with osteoplastic anterior wall approach to the frontal sinus. Arch Otolaryngol 68:271

14. Goode RH (1908) An intranasal method for opening the frontal sinus establishing the largest possible drainage. Laryngoscope 18:266

15. Gross WE, Gross CW, Becker D, et al (1995) Modified transnasal endoscopic Lothrop procedure as an alternative to frontal sinus obliteration. Otolaryngol Head Neck Surg 113:427–434

16. Halle M (1906) Externe oder interne Operation der Nebenhöhleneiterungen. Berl Klin Wochenschr 43: 1369–1372, 1404–1407

17. Hardy JM, Montgomery WW (1976) Osteoplastic frontal sinusotomy: an analysis of 250 operations. Ann Otol Rhinol Laryngol 85:523–532

18. Howarth WG (1921) Operations on the frontal sinus. J Laryngol Otol 36: 417–421

19. Ingals EF (1905) New operation and instruments for draining the frontal sinus. Ann Otol Rhinol Laryngol 14:512

20. Jansen A (1894) Zur Eröffnung der Nebenhöhlen der Nase bei chronischer Eiterung. Arch Laryng Rhinol (Berl) 1: 135–157

21. Kennedy DW, Josephson JS, Zinreich SJ, et al (1989) Endoscopic sinus surgery for mucoceles: a viable alternative. Laryngoscope 99:885–895

22. Killian G (1903) Die Killianische Radicaloperation chronischer Stirnhoehleneiterungen: Weiteres kasuistisches Material and Zusammenfassung. Arch Laryngol Rhinol 13: 59.

23. Knapp A (1908) The surgical treatment of orbital complications in disease of the nasal accessory sinuses. JAMA 51: 299

24. Kountakis SE, Gross CW (2003) Long-term results of the Lothrop operation. Curr Opin Otolaryngol Head Neck Surg 11(1):37–40

25. Lothrop HA (1914) Frontal sinus suppuration. Ann Surg 59:937

26. Luc H (1893) Empyeme latent du sinus frontal duct sans cause aparante: Traitemente par l'ouverture de los frontal et la currettage du foger guerim incomplete. Arch Int Laryngol 6:216

27. Lyman EH (1950) The place of the obliterative operation in frontal sinus surgery. Laryngoscope 60:407

28. Lynch RC (1921) The technique of a radical frontal sinus operation which has given me the best results. Laryngoscope 31:1

29. May M, Schaitkin B (1995) Frontal sinus surgery: Endonasal endoscopic osteoplasty rather than external osteoplasty. Oper Tech Otolaryngol Head Neck Surg 6:184

30. McNaught RC (1936) Refinement of the external fronto ethmosphenoid operation: A new nasofrontal pedicle flap. Arch Otolaryngol 23:544

31. Metson R (1992) Endoscopic treatment of frontal sinusitis. Laryngoscope 102:712–716

32. Ogston A (1884) Trephining the frontal sinus for catarrhal diseases. Men Chron Manchester 1:235

33. Ramadan HH (2000) History of frontal sinus surgery. Arch Otolaryngol Head Neck Surg 126:98–99

34. Riedel-Schenke H: Cited by Gosdale RH (1955) The radical obliterative frontal sinus operation: A consideration of technical factors in difficult cases. Ann Otol Rhinol Laryngol 64:470

35. Ritter G (1906) II. Eine neue Methode zur Erhaltung der vorderen Stirnhöhlenwand bei Readikaloperationen chronischer Stirnhöhleneiterungen. Dtsch Med Wochenschr 32: 1294–1296

36. Runge: Cited by Stevenson RS, Guthrie D: (1949) A history of otolaryngology. Baltimore, Williams and Wilkins

37. Schaefer SD, Close LG (1990) Endoscopic management of frontal sinus disease. Laryngoscope 100:155–160

38. Schaeffer JP: Cited by Sier (1911) Rouillons. Arch Int Laryngol 31:709

39. Schoenborn: Cited by Wilkop A (1894) Ein Beitrag zur Kasuistik der Erkrankungen des Sinus frontalis. Wuerzburg, F. Frome.

40. Sewall EC (1935) The operative treatment of nasal sinus disease. Ann Otol 44:307

41. Stankiewicz JA, Wachter B (2003) The endoscopic modified Lothrop procedure for salvage of chronic frontal sinusitis after osteoplastic flap failure. Otolaryngol Head Neck Surg 129(6):678–83

42. Tato JM, Bergaglio OE (1949) Cirurgia del frontal injerto de grosa. Nueva tecnica (Surgery of frontal sinus. Fat grafts, new technique. Otolaringologica, Oct. 1949) cited according Tato, Sibbald and Bergaglio. Laryngoscope (1954) 64: 504–521

43. Walsh TE (1943) Experimental surgery of the frontal sinus. The role of the ostium and nasofrontal duct in postoperative healing. Laryngoscope 53:75–92

44. Wells R (1870) Abscess of the frontal sinus. Lancet 1:694

45. Wells WA (1901) On sounding and irrigating the frontal sinus through the natural opening. Laryngoscope 10:262

46. Wide K, Sipila J, Suonpaa J (1997) Report on results of frontal sinus obliterations in Turku University Central Hospital, 1977–1994. Acta Otolaryngol 529(suppl):184–186

Chapter 2

Radiologic Anatomy of the Frontal Sinus

2

Ramon E. Figueroa, Joseph Sullivan

Core Messages

- The frontal sinus and its drainage pathway comprise one of the most complex anatomic areas of the anterior skull base, amplified by significant variability

- Improvements in radiologic imaging clarity along with multiplanar demonstration of frontal sinus complex anatomy have paralleled and augmented advances in the surgical management of the frontal sinuses

Contents

Introduction

The frontal sinus and its drainage pathway comprise one of the most complex anatomic areas of the anterior skull base. Its complexity is magnified by the frequency of anatomic variations which impact the direction of drainage, efficiency of mucociliary clearance, and morphology of the frontal recess. Recent significant advances in computed tomography (CT), especially the introduction of multidetector helical scanning and the routine availability of computer workstations, have made demonstration of this complex anatomy easier and more useful to rhinologic surgical approach. This improvement in imaging clarity and multiplanar demonstration of frontal sinus complex anatomy is now of even more clinical relevance in view of the extensive developments in powered instruments, better endoscopic devices, and surgical navigation with CT cross-registration.

Embryologic and Functional Concepts

The sinonasal embryologic development during the first trimester is characterized by the emergence of more than six ethmoturbinals, which progressively coalesce and differentiate into the final anatomy of the lateral nasal wall [6].

The ethmoturbinals give rise to the following structures:

- The most superior remnant of the first ethmoturbinal becomes the agger nasi mound
- The remnant of the descending portion of the first ethmoturbinal becomes the uncinate process
- The basal lamella of the second ethmoturbinal pneumatizes and gives origin to the bulla ethmoidalis
- The basal lamella of the third ethmoturbinal becomes the basal lamella of the middle turbinate.

2

The nasal mucosa invaginates at specific points in the lateral nasal wall, forming nasal pits that develop into the anlages of maxillary, frontal sinuses, and ethmoid cells [2]. The mesenchyme resorbs around the invagination of the nasal pits, allowing progressive development of the sinus cavity. The embryologic point at which the initial invagination occurs becomes the future sinus ostium. Cilia develop and orient towards this ostium, allowing mucus to flow towards and through the ostium. The efficiency of the mucociliary drainage is then dictated and impacted by the patency, tortuosity, and/or frank narrowing of the resulting drainage pathways, which are progressively modified by the sequential ongoing pneumatization process occurring during the patient's life. Typically the ethmoid cells and the maxillary antra are pneumatized at birth, with the maxillary antra progressively expanding into mature sinuses as the maxilla matures and the teeth erupt. The frontal sinus develops and expands in late childhood to early adolescence, and continues to grow into adulthood. The rate of sinus growth is modified by the efficiency of ventilation and mucociliary drainage, dictated by the sinus ostium and corresponding drainage pathways. The frontal sinus drainage pathway is the most complex of all sinuses, impacted by its anatomic relationships with the agger nasi, anterior ethmoid cells, and pattern of vertical insertion of the uncinate process [3].

Frontal Sinus Evaluation

CT of the paranasal sinuses classically has been performed with continuous coronal and axial 3-mm slices to provide two planes of morphologic depiction of sinus anatomy for presurgical mapping and evaluation [5]. Recent advances in CT scanner designs with the introduction of multidetector helical designs and much larger and faster computing processing capacities now allow for single-plane thin-section high-resolution databases to be acquired and postprocessed to depict the sinus anatomy in any planar projection with high definition of the underlying anatomy. This multiplanar capability has impacted the evaluation of the frontal sinus drainage pathways the most, since depiction of this region in a sagittal plane has become routine.

Typical high-resolution multidetector scanning is performed in the axial plane (Fig. 2.1A) following the long axis of the hard palate, using a low MA tech-

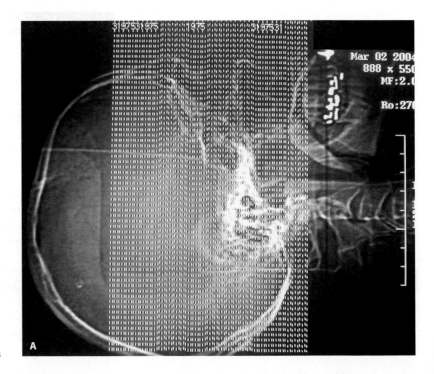

Fig. 2.1A,B.
High-resolution sinus navigation CT protocol. A Lateral scout view shows the typical prescription of axial thin section slices. B An axial image at the level of the nasal cavity helps prescribe the sagittal reformatted images

Fig. 2.1B.

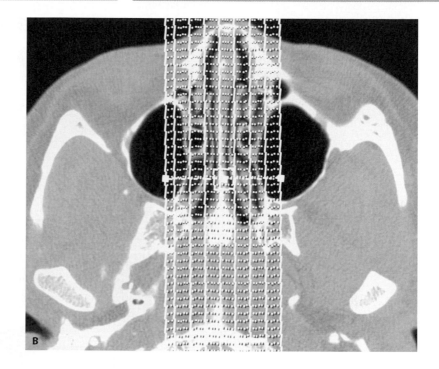

nique, a small field of view (18–20 cm), and 1.25 mm collimation, with data back-processed in 0.65-mm thickness in bone algorithm and displayed in mucosal (window of 2000, level of –200) and bone (3500/800) detail. Most centers use this pattern of data acquisition for 3D computer-assisted surgical navigation. Interactive evaluation of the data is then performed on the CT workstation to define a sagittal plane perpendicular to the hard palate, prescribing a set of sequential sagittal sections to encompass both frontal sinuses and their corresponding drainage pathways (Fig. 2.1B).

Frontal Sinus Drainage Pathway

The frontal sinus grows and expands within the diploic space of the frontal bone from the frontal sinus ostium medial and superior to the orbital plates, enclosed anteriorly by the cortical bone of the anterior frontal sinus wall and posteriorly by the cortical bone of the skull base and posterior frontal sinus wall (-which is also the anterior wall of the anterior cranial fossa). Each frontal sinus grows independently, with its rate of growth, final volume, and configuration

dictated by its ventilation, drainage, and the corresponding growth (or lack of it) of the competing surrounding sinuses and skull base.

The frontal sinus narrows down inferiorly and medially into a funnel-shaped transition point, which is defined as the frontal sinus ostium (Fig. 2.2A,B), extending between the anterior and posterior frontal sinus walls at the skull base level. This point is typically demarcated along its anterior wall by the variably shaped bone ridge of the nasofrontal buttress, frequently called the "nasal beak" (Fig. 2.2C). The frontal sinus ostium is oriented nearly perpendicular to the posterior wall of the sinus at the level of the anterior skull base [3].

The Anatomic Terminology Group defined the frontal recess as "the most anterior and superior part of the anterior ethmoid complex from where the frontal bone becomes pneumatized, resulting in a frontal sinus" [7]. In sagittal plane, the frontal recess frequently looks like an inverted funnel (Fig. 2.2C) that opens superiorly to the frontal sinus ostium. The anatomic walls of surrounding structures dictate its walls and floor. The lateral wall of the frontal recess is defined by the lamina papyracea of the orbit (Fig. 2.3). The medial wall is defined by the vertical attachment

2

Fig. 2.2A–C.
The frontal sinus ostium. Axial (A),
coronal (B), and sagittal (C) images at
the level of the frontal sinus illustrate
the frontal sinus ostium (arrows), the
frontal recess (*), the nasal beak
(NB), and the agger nasi (AN) cells

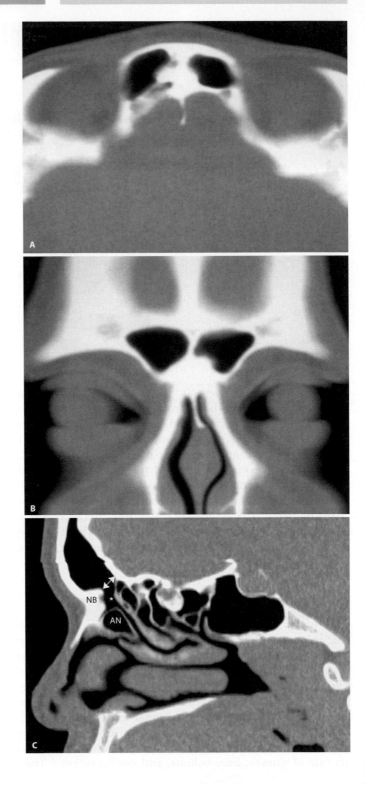

of the middle turbinate (its most anterior and superior part). Its posterior wall is variable, depending on the basal lamella of the bulla ethmoidalis reaching (or not) the skull base, if it is dehiscent allowing a communication with the suprabullar recess, or if it is hyper-pneumatized producing a secondary narrowing of the frontal recess from it posterior wall [2].

The agger nasi cells and the uncinate process dictate the floor and the pattern of drainage of the frontal recess. The frontal recess can be narrowed from the anterior-inferior direction by hyper-pneumatized agger nasi cells (Fig. 2.3). Its inferior drainage is dictated by the insertion of the vertical attachment of the uncinate process, a sagittally oriented hook-like bony leaflet (Fig. 2.4). Whenever the uncinate process attaches to the skull base or the superior-anterior portion of the middle turbinate, the frontal recess drains into the superior end of the ethmoidal infundibulum (Fig. 2.4A). If the uncinate process attaches laterally into the lamina papyracea of the orbit (Fig. 2.4B), the frontal recess opens directly into the superior aspect of the middle meatus, and the ethmoidal infundibulum ends blindly into a "terminal recess".

The ethmoidal infundibulum is a true three-dimensional space defined laterally by the lamina papyracea, anteromedially by the uncinate process, and posteriorly by the bulla ethmoidalis (Fig. 2.5A). It opens medially into the middle meatus across the hiatus semilunaris inferior, a cleft-like opening between the free posterior margin of the uncinate process and the corresponding anterior face of the bulla ethmoidalis (Fig. 2.5B). It is the functional common pathway of mucociliary drainage for the anterior ethmoid, agger nasi, and maxillary sinus mucus. The frontal sinus drainage can also drain through the ethmoidal infundibulum if the uncinate process does not attach to the lamina papyracea of the orbit.

Fig. 2.3A–C.
The frontal recess. A large right agger nasi cell (AN) is stenosing the right frontal recess (***), which is opacified by congested mucosa and can be followed on coronal and sequential axial images. The left frontal recess (*) is well aerated

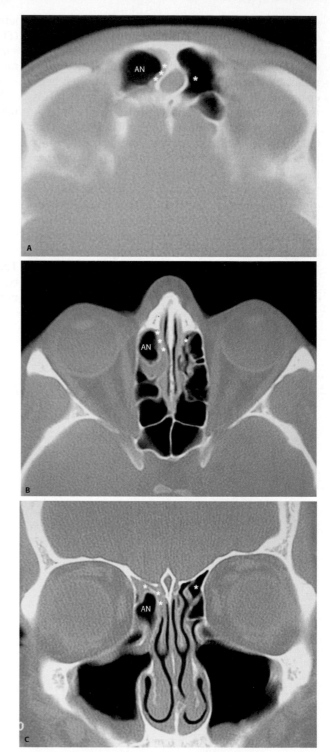

Fig. 2.4A,B.
The uncinate process. In coronal image (A) the uncinate process attaches to the skull base (black arrow), with the frontal recess (***) continuing downwards between the agger nasi cell (AN) and the uncinate process. In coronal image (B) the uncinate process attaches to the lamina papyracea (black arrow), with the frontal recess (***) opening directly to the middle meatus, and the ethmoidal infundibulum (EI) ending in a blind end or "terminal recess" (TR)

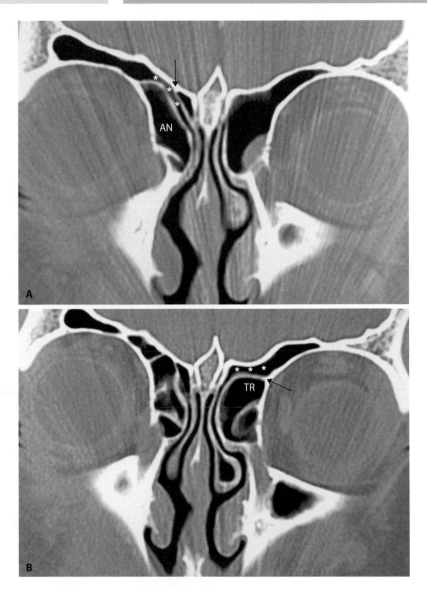

2

Fig. 2.5A,B.
The ostiomeatal complex. In coronal
image (A) the ethmoid infundibulum
(EI) lies between the uncinate process
(UP) and the bulla ethmoidalis (BE),
opening into the middle meatus
across the hiatus semilunaris inferior
(*). Notice the bilateral concha bullo-
sa and the deep olfactory fossae (Keros type III). In sagittal image (B) the
uncinate process (UP), bulla ethmoidalis (BE), and hiatus semilunaris
inferior (*) are shown better as sagittally oriented landmarks

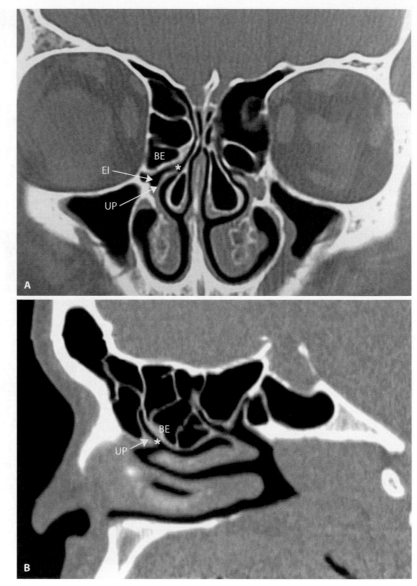

Anatomic Variants

Several important anatomic variants impact on the anatomy of the frontal sinus drainage pathways and the anterior skull base. Familiarity with these anatomic variants is required for safe anterior skull base and frontal recess surgical considerations.

Frontal Cells

The frontal cells are rare anatomic variants of anterior ethmoid pneumatization that impinge upon the frontal recess and typically extend within the lumen of the frontal ostium above the level of the agger nasi cells (Fig. 2.6). Bent and coworkers described four types of frontal cells [1]. All frontal cells can be clinically significant if they become primarily infected or if they obstruct the frontal sinus drainage, leading to secondary frontal rhinosinusitis.

The different types of frontal cells as described by Bent are [1]:

- Type I frontal cell, a single frontal recess cell above the agger nasi cell (Fig. 2.6A)
- Type II frontal cells, a tier of cells above the agger nasi cell, projecting within the frontal recess
- Type III frontal cell is defined as a single massive cell arising above the agger nasi, pneumatizing cephalad into the frontal sinus (Fig. 2.6B)
- Type IV frontal cell is a single isolated cell within the frontal sinus, frequently difficult to visualize due to its thin walls (Fig. 2.6C)

Supraorbital Ethmoid Cell

This is a pattern of pneumatization of the orbital plate of the frontal bone posterior to the frontal recess and lateral to the frontal sinus (Fig. 2.7), frequently developing from the suprabullar recess [2]. The degree of pneumatization of the supraorbital ethmoid cells can reach the anterior margin of the orbital plate and mimic a frontal sinus. Tracing back the borders of the air cell towards the anterior ethmoid behind the frontal recess allows us to recognize this variant better.

Depth of Olfactory Fossa

The orbital plate of the frontal bone slopes downwards medially to constitute the roof of the ethmoid labyrinth (foveola ethmoidalis), ending medially at the lateral border of the olfactory fossa (Fig. 2.8). This configuration makes the olfactory fossa the lowermost point in the floor of the anterior cranial fossa, frequently projecting between the pneumatized air cells of both ethmoid labyrinths [7]. The depth of the olfactory fossa into the nasal cavity is dictated by the height of the lateral lamella of the cribriform plate, a very thin sagittally oriented bone that defines the lateral wall of the olfactory fossa.

2

Fig. 2.6A–C.
Frontal cells. Frontal cells are rare air cells above agger nasi that impinge upon the frontal recess and frontal sinus. Type I is a single cell above agger nasi, while type II is a tier arrangement above agger nasi. Type III is a single large frontal cell projecting into the frontal sinus lumen. Type IV is a large cell completely contained in the frontal sinus ("sinus within a sinus)

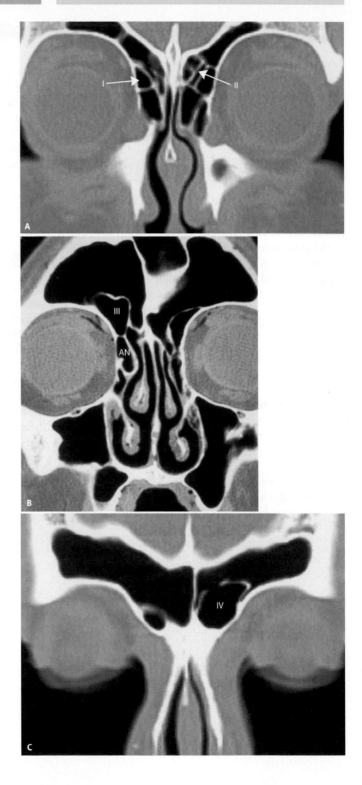

Fig. 2.7A–C.
Supraorbital Ethmoid Cells. In the
sequential axial images A–C the
supraorbital ethmoid cells (SOEs)
expand and pneumatize anteriorly
into the orbital plate of the frontal
bone, not to be confused with the
frontal sinus (FS)

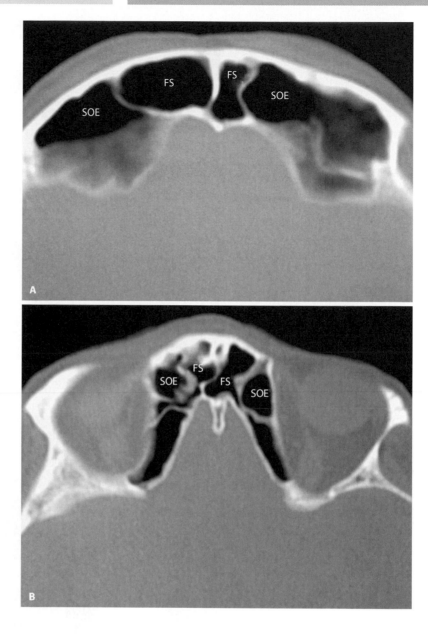

2

Fig. 2.7C.

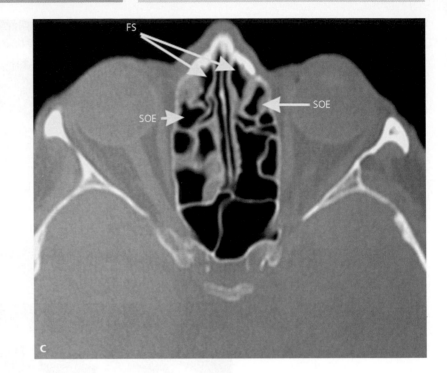

Fig. 2.8A–C.
Depth of olfactory fossa. The length
of the lateral lamella of the cribriform plate (white arrows) determines
the depth of the olfactory fossa,
categorized by Keros in Type I
(A, 1–3 mm deep), Type II
(B, 4–7 mm deep) and Type III
(C, 8–16 mm deep)

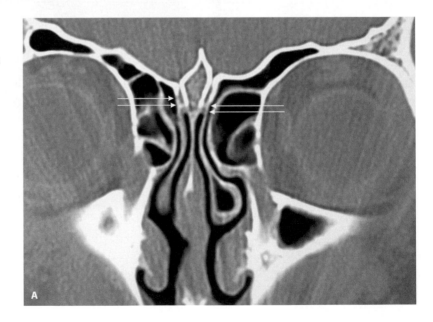

Fig. 2.8B,C.

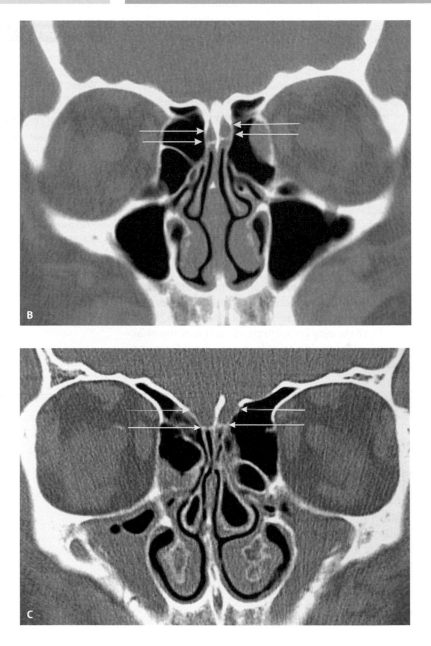

2

Keros described the anatomic variations of the ethmoid roof and the olfactory fossa, classifying it in three surgically important types [4]:

- Type I has a short lateral lamella, resulting in a shallow olfactory fossa of only 1–3 mm in depth in relation to the medial end of the ethmoid roof
- Type II has a longer lateral lamella, resulting in an olfactory fossa depth of 4–7 mm
- Type III olfactory fossa has a much longer lateral lamella (8–16 mm), with the cribriform plate projecting deep within the nasal cavity well below the roof of the ethmoid labyrinth.

The type III configuration represents a high-risk area for lateral lamella iatrogenic surgical perforation in ethmoid endoscopic surgical procedures. Occasionally there may be asymmetric depth of the olfactory fossa from side to side, which must be recognized and considered prior to surgery.

Conclusion

The frontal sinus drainage pathways and the surrounding anterior ethmoid sinus represent one of the most complex anatomic regions of the skull base. An intimate knowledge of its anatomy and a clear understanding of its physiology and anatomic variants are required for safe and effective surgical management of frontal sinus drainage pathway problems.

References

1. Bent JP, Cuilty-Siller C, Kuhn FH (1994) The frontal cell as a cause of frontal sinus obstruction. 4:185–191
2. Bolger WE, Mawn CB (2001) Analysis of the suprabullar and retrobullar recesses for endoscopic sinus surgery. Ann Oto Rhinol Laryngol 110:3–14
3. Daniels DL, Mafee MF, Smith MM, et al (2003) The frontal sinus drainage pathway and related structures. Am J Neuroradiol 24:1618–1626
4. Keros P (1965) Uber die praktische bedeutung der niveauunterschiede der lamina cribosa des ethmoids. Laryngol Rhinol Otol (Stuttgart) 41:808–813
5. Melhelm ER, Oliverio PJ, Benson ML, et al (1996) Optimal CT evaluation for functional endoscopic sinus surgery. Am J Neuroradiol 17:181–188
6. Stammberger HR (1991) Functional endoscopic sinus surgery. BC Decker, Philadelphia
7. Stammberger HR, Kennedy DW, Bolger WE, et al (1995) Paranasal sinuses: anatomic terminology and nomenclature. Ann Rhinol Otol Laryngol (suppl) 167:7–16

Chapter 3

Surgical Anatomy and Embryology of the Frontal Sinus

Carlos S. Duque, Roy R. Casiano

Core Messages

- **(Overview)** A thorough knowledge of frontal sinus anatomy is critical when performing even basic endoscopic sinus surgical procedures. Every endoscopic sinus surgeon must be aware of all the normal, as well as the abnormal, variants that may exist

- The number and size of the paranasal sinuses are determined early during embryologic development. Disease processes during childhood or early adulthood may modify this anatomy or its relationship to neighboring structures

- The close relationship between the frontal sinus and neighboring orbit or anterior skull base makes it particularly vulnerable to complications from disease or surgery

Contents

Introduction

As with any surgical procedure, a thorough knowledge of anatomy is the one most important factors in minimizing complications and maximizing one's chances of a good surgical outcome. This is particularly important for otolaryngologists performing endoscopic sinus surgery, as each and every one of the paranasal sinuses are in close proximity to critical orbital and skull base structures. A good knowledge of anatomy will enable the surgeon to operate with more confidence, by improving one's ability to correctly interpret normal variants from abnormal or pathological conditions, and determine an appropriate surgical treatment plan to reestablish mucociliary flow to the sinus. This is even more critical for distorted anatomy, due to previous surgery or neoplasms. Furthermore, CT imaging has become an integral part of the diagnostic armamentarium for sinus surgeons. Technological advancements such as intraoperative navigational devices depend on the surgeon's proper identification of normal or abnormal structures on CT or MRI scans. However, despite this technology's intent of reducing complications, failure to know the sinus anatomy or properly identify critical structures on the scan may still result in disastrous consequences.

The frontal sinus hides in the anterior cranial vault surrounded by two thick layers of cortical bone. Its naturally draining "ostium", or frontal infundibulum, remains immersed in an intricate complex area covered by ethmoid cells and other anatomical structures that may not be so easy to find. In order to better understand frontal sinus anatomy, one must begin with its embryological development.

3

Embryology of the Frontal Sinus

It is important to know that all of the development of the head and neck, along with the face, nose, and paranasal sinuses, takes place simultaneously in a very short period of time. Frontal sinus development begins around the fourth or fifth week of gestation, and continues not only during the intrauterine growth period, but also in the postnatal period through puberty and even early adulthood.

By the end of the fourth week of development, one begins to see the development of the branchial arches, along with the appearance of the branchial pouches and the primitive gut. This gives the embryo its first appearance of an identifiable head and face, with an orifice in its middle, called the stomodeum (Fig. 3.1). This structure is surrounded by the mandibular and maxillary arches or prominences, bilaterally. Both of these prominences are derivatives of the first branchial arch. This arch will ultimately give rise to all of the vascular and neural structures supplying this area. The newly developed stomodeum is

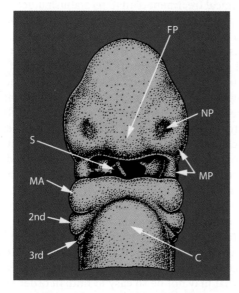

Fig. 3.1. Ventral view of a 5-week-old embryo, showing the stomodeum (S), mandibular arch (MA), 2nd branchial arch (2nd), 3rd branchial arch (3rd), frontonasal prominence (FP), nasal placode (NP), maxillary prominences (MP), and cardiac bulge (C)

limited superiorly by the frontonasal prominence and inferiorly by the mandibular arch [10, 15, 16].

The frontonasal prominence differentiates inferiorly with two nasal projections, or nasal placodes, that will be invaded by the growing ectoderm and mesenchyme. These structures later fuse and form the nasal cavity and primitive choana, separated from the stomodeum by the oronasal membrane. The primitive choana will be the point of development for the posterior pharyngeal wall as well as the different sinuses. The oronasal membrane will be fully formed by the end of the fifth week of development, to form the floor of the nose (palate). As the embryo grows, the maxillary processes and the nasal placodes come together in the midline, to form the maxillary bone and the beginning of the external nose. The frontonasal prominence will also develop a caudal mesodermic projection that will form the nasal septum, diving the nose into two chambers [15–17].

Simultaneously, while all these changes are starting to take place, the cranial and facial bones are forming as well. The skeletal system develops from the mesoderm, from which mesenchyme develops, forming the connective tissue (fibroblasts, chondroblasts, osteoblasts) that eventually differentiates into the various support structures of the nose and paranasal sinuses. The neural crest cells and mesenchyme migrate to the occipital area and the future site of the cranial cavity, and disperse in order to form the hyaline cartilage matrix that will later become ossified. Each cranial bone is formed by a series of bone spicules that grow from the center towards the periphery, to occupy its place. At birth, all cranial bones are separated by layers of connective tissue that later become fused and ossified in the postnatal period. Although all of these cranial structures are made out of cartilage and eventually will become ossified, they can still be invaded by neighboring epithelial cells (from the nasal cavity), eventually giving rise to the future paranasal sinuses [16, 17].

Around the 25th to 28th week of development, three medially directed projections arise from the lateral wall of the nose. This begins the process of defining the anatomical structures of the paranasal sinuses. Between these projections small lateral diverticula will invaginate into the lateral wall of the primitive choana to eventually form the nasal meati (Fig. 3.2) [15–17].

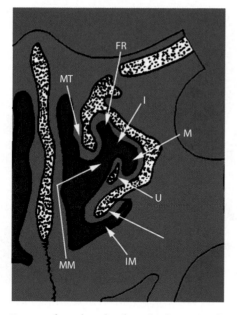

Fig. 3.2. Between the 25th and 28th week of gestation, lateral diverticula will invaginate into the lateral wall of the primitive choana to eventually form the nasal meati. Between these invaginations lie the prominences that later form the middle turbinate (MT), inferior turbinate (IT), and uncinate process (U). The infundibulum (I), maxillary sinus (M), and frontal recess (FR) are seen as small blind recesses or pockets within the middle meatus (MM). The inferior meatus (IM) is also noted

The medial projections of ectodermal tissue form the following structures:

- The anterior projection forms the agger nasi
- The inferior projection (the maxillo-turbinate) forms the inferior turbinate and maxillary sinus [16, 17]
- The superior projection, known as the ethmoido-turbinate, forms the middle and superior turbinate as well as the small ethmoidal cells, with their corresponding draining meati, between the septum and the lateral wall of the nose. Between the already formed inferior turbinate and the middle turbinate, the middle meatus will develop [14–16]

The middle meatus invaginates laterally giving shape to the embryonic infundibulum, along with the unci-

form process. During the 13th week of development the infundibulum continues expanding superiorly, giving rise to the frontonasal recess. It has been proposed that the frontal sinus might develop during the 16th week simply as a direct elongation of the infundibulum and frontonasal recess, or as an upwards epithelial migration of the anterior ethmoidal cells that penetrate the most inferior aspect of the frontal bone between its two tables. Primary pneumatization of the frontal bone occurs as a slow process up to the end of the first year of life. Up to this moment, the frontal sinus remains as a small, smooth, blind pocket, and will remain this way until the infant reaches approximately 2 years of life, when the process of secondary pneumatization begins. From 2 years of age until adolescence, the frontal sinus will progressively grow and become fully pneumatized (see Fig. 3.3) [14, 15, 17]. Between 1 and 4 years of age, the frontal sinus starts its secondary pneumatization, forming a cavity no bigger than 4–8 mm long, 6–12 mm high, and 11–19 mm wide. After 3 years of age, the frontal sinus may be seen in some CT scans. When a child reaches 8 years of age, the frontal sinus becomes more pneumatized, and will be seen by most radiological studies. Significant frontal pneumatization is generally not seen until early adolescence, and continues until the child reaches 18 years of age.

Frontal sinus development may be variable. On cadaveric and radiological (CT) studies, the frontal sinus is only identifiable in less than 1.5% of infants less than one year of age [6, 8, 9]. During this period, the frontal sinus remains as a potential pocket and has been referred to as a "cellulae ethmoidalis", since the findings point clearly to its close embryological and anatomical relationship with anterior ethmoid air cells [19, 20, 25].

The frontal sinuses develop within the frontal bones. Each bone remains separated by a vertical (sagittal) suture line that becomes ossified. This will eventually form the frontal sinus intersinus septum. It is not clear which factors trigger the formation of the frontal sinuses. Some authors have speculated that the adolescent growth phase may be stimulated by the different hormonal changes or even by the process of mastication itself [13, 19, 20, 25]. The right and left frontal sinuses develop independently. Each side undergoes separate reabsorption of bone, with the formation of one, two, or even multiple cells, di-

Fig. 3.3.
Sagittal and coronal views of the frontal sinus noting its progressive secondary pneumatization between the ages of 3 and 18 years of age. Between 1 and 4 years of age (1), the frontal sinus starts its secondary pneumatization. After 4 years of age, the frontal sinus may be seen as a small, but definable, cavity (2) . When a child reaches 8 years of age (3), the frontal sinus becomes more pneumatized. Significant frontal pneumatization is generally not seen until early adolescence (4), and continues until the child reaches 18 years of age (5). The agger nasi air cell (AN), type III frontal infundibular cell (III), ethmoid bulla (B), suprabullar cell (SB), middle turbinate (MT), and orbit (O) are marked

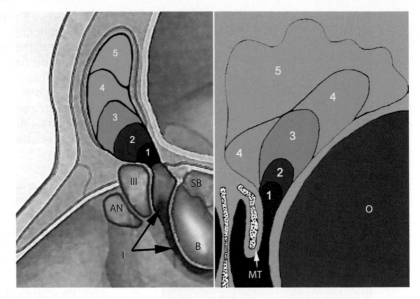

vided by various septae. Occasionally, frontal sinuses may develop asymmetrically, or even fail to develop at all. It is not uncommon to find one frontal sinus that is more "dominant" on one side, and a hypoplastic, or even aplastic frontal sinus, on the other side (Figs. 3.4 and 3.5). Aplasia of both frontal sinuses has been reported in 3%–5% of patients, depending on the study. The presence of only one well-developed frontal sinus (with a contralateral aplastic sinus) ranges from 1% to 7%. In some rare cases, pneumatization can be significant, extending out to remote areas like the sphenoid ala, orbital rim, and even the

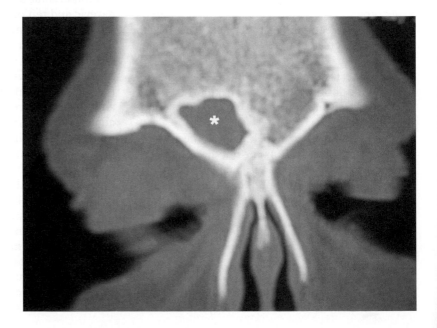

Fig. 3.4.
CT of a patient with chronic rhinosinusitis, a hypoplastic right frontal (asterisk), and aplastic left frontal

Fig. 3.5.
CT of bilaterally aplastic frontal
sinuses

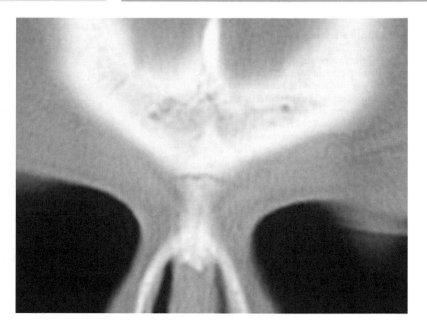

temporal bone. Race, geography, and climate are just
a few factors that have been implicated in the abnormal development of the frontal sinus [1, 5, 19, 21, 23].
For example, bilaterally aplastic frontal sinuses have
been seen in as many as 43% of Alaskan or Canadian
Eskimos. Additional normal variants of frontal sinus
development include the formation of as many as five
frontal sinus cells, each cell with its own independently draining outflow tract into the middle meatus
[5, 20].

Surgical Anatomy of the Frontal Sinuses

As seen in the previous section, the frontal sinus
shares a common embryological and anatomical relationship with the ethmoid sinus, to the point that
several authors and researchers have referred to this
sinus as a "large ethmoidal cell" or simply the termi-
nation or upper limit of the intricate ethmoidal labyrinth [14, 15, 17].

In an adult, two frontal sinuses are usually seen.
Each frontal sinus cavity takes on the shape of a pyramid, with a thick anterior table and a thinner posterior table.

The anterior wall of the frontal sinus begins at the
nasofrontal suture line and ends below the frontal
bone protuberance, along the vertical portion of the
frontal bone. The height of the cavity at its anterior
wall ranges from 1 to 6 cm, depending on the degree
of pneumatization [15, 16]. It is made up of thick cortical bone measuring an average of 4 to 12 mm in
thickness. This thick anterior table is covered by the
pericranium (thick external periosteal layer), followed more superficially by the frontalis muscle, subcutaneous fat, and skin. This very vascularized pericranium is frequently used for reconstruction of
large anterior skull base defects or for frontal sinus
obliteration [14, 24].

The posterior wall of the frontal sinus forms the
most anteroinferior boundary of the anterior cranial
fossa, and is in close contact with the frontal lobes,
separated only by the dura mater [8, 11, 14, 16, 18, 19,
24]. It has a superior vertical, and a smaller inferior
horizontal, portion. The horizontal portion will form
part of the orbital roof. Both posterior walls join inferiorly to form the internal frontal crest, to which
the falx cerebri inserts (Fig. 3.6). The posterior table
of the frontal sinus can also be inherently thin (less
than a millimeter in some areas), and prone to gradual erosion and subsequent mucocele formation

3

Fig. 3.6.
View of the anterior cranial fossa and orbital roof. The posterior table and extent of the frontal sinuses (F) are identified. The crista galli (CG) and superior saggital sinus (SS) demarcate the approximate level of the intersinus septum separating the right and left frontal sinuses. The crista galli is also continuous with the perpendicular plate of the ethmoid inferiorly. The cribriform plate (C) is seen on either side of the crista galli. Branches of the anterior ethmoid artery (EA) are seen reentering intracranially anterior to the cribriform plate. The optic nerve (ON) is seen entering the optic canal medial to the anterior clinoid process (AC)

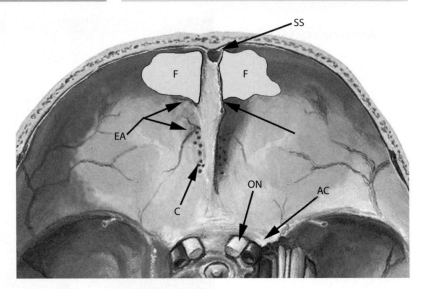

from chronic inflammatory conditions [5]. The absence of bony walls cannot be addressed through a physical or endoscopic exam. However, with today's imaging studies this type of abnormality should be easily detected preoperatively.

A triangular-shaped intersinus septum separates the frontal sinuses into separately draining sinus cavities. It is the continuation, anteriorly, of the fused and ossified embryologic sagittal suture line. Although the intersinus septum may vary in direction and thickness as it proceeds superiorly, the base of the intersinus septum will almost always be close to the midline at the level of the infundibulum. At this level, the intersinus septum is continuous with the crista galli posteriorly, the perpendicular plate of the ethmoid inferiorly, and the nasal spine of the frontal bone anteriorly (Fig. 3.7). The falx cerebri inserts into the posterior table of the frontal sinus, at a point corresponding to the posterior edge of the intersinus septum. Additional intersinus septum cells may exist within this intersinus septum. Pneumatization from these intersinus cells may occasionally extend all the way into the crista galli. These cells tend to drain into the nose through their own outflow tract, adjacent to the normal frontal sinus out flow tract, at the level of the infundibulum, on one or both sides of the nose.

Inferiorly, the frontal sinus cavity is limited by the supraorbital rim and wall (or roof), through which

the supraorbital neurovascular pedicle courses towards the forehead skin via the supraorbital foramen. At this level, the frontal sinus is funnel-shaped, forming the base of a pyramid. As it forms the roof of the orbit, it is also the point of insertion for the superior oblique muscle. Supraorbital pneumatization may extend as far as the lesser wing of the sphenoid. With the exception of the thin septations of the ethmoidal cells, this inferior wall of the frontal sinus makes up one of the thinnest walls of all the sinus cavities. Like the posterior table of the frontal sinus, this area is also prone to gradual erosion from chronic inflammatory conditions, giving rise to mucoceles with subsequent proptosis and orbital complications. Fortunately, the orbital periosteum (periorbita) acts as an effective barrier to serious consequences, in most of these cases.

Laterally the cavity extends itself as far as the angular prominence of the frontal bone. The superior border of the frontal sinus is the non-pneumatized cancellous bone of the frontal bone.

The frontal sinus outflow tract has been described in many ways and given all sort of names, depending on the surgical approach or perspective by which the frontal sinus is visualized [6, 9, 11]. However, today most authors agree that the frontal sinus outflow tract has an hourglass shape with its narrowest point at the level of the frontal sinus infundibulum (Fig.

Fig. 3.7.
CT of a normal well pneumatized frontal sinus in an adult. The intersinus septum (IS) of the frontal sinus (F) is continuous with the crista galli posteriorly, the perpendicular plate of the ethmoid (PP) inferiorly, and the nasal spine of the frontal bone anteriorly. In well-pneumatized frontal sinuses, the inferomedial portion of the frontal sinus may be accessible through the nose directly via transseptal (TS) or supraturbinal approach (ST). The asterisk demarcates the anterior attachment of the middle turbinate

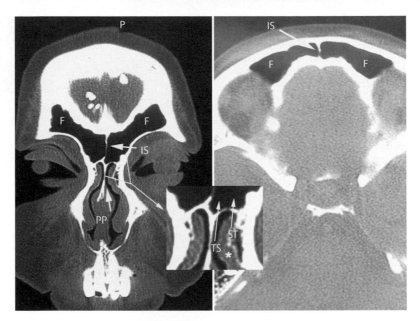

Fig. 3.8.
Sagittal section through the agger nasi (A), ethmoid bulla (B), suprabullar cells (SB), posterior ethmoid (PE), and lateral sphenoid (S). The frontal sinus (F) outflow tract is noted by the dotted arrow, coursing through the frontal infundibulum (the narrowest area in this hourglass-shaped tract), and into the ethmoid infundibulum, before exiting into the middle meatus. The uncinate process has been removed to expose the maxillary ostium (M). The tail of the middle turbinate (MT) is also noted

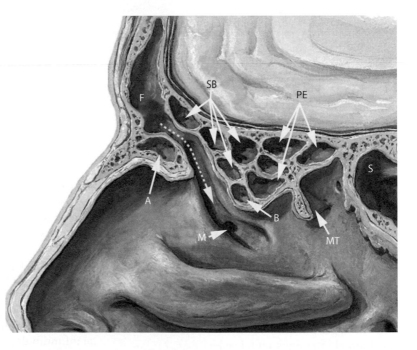

3.8). The frontal sinus infundibulum is formed by the most inferior aspect of the frontal sinus. It has the form of a funnel that points towards the ethmoid in a posteromedial direction. The angulation (postero-medially) and maximum diameter of this funnel may vary greatly between patients, or even between sides (Fig. 3.9) [2–4, 9, 12, 13, 16, 22].

3

Fig. 3.9.
The right frontal sinus infundibulum
is very narrowed and surrounded by
thick bone. Unlike the left frontal infundibulum (which is very wide and
accessible through a transnasal or
supraturbinal approach), this right
frontal infundibulum may be more
prone to easy obstruction due to persistent inflammatory disease or from
inadvertent surgical trauma with subsequent fibrosis or osteoneogenesis

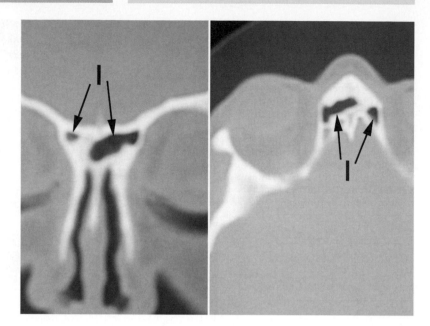

The frontal sinus infundibulum is bounded by the
following structures:

- The lamina papyracea laterally in its superior
  portion
- The middle turbinate anteriorly
- The vertical lamella medially
- The agger nasi anteroinferiorly
- The ethmoid suprabullar air cells posteriorly

A series of "accessory" ethmoidal cells may line the
frontal sinus outflow tract along the frontal recess
and infundibulum. These cells receive different
names according to the location where they impinge
on the frontal recess.

These cells include:

- The agger nasi cell
- Frontal intersinus septal cells
- Suprabullar cells (with or without supraorbi-
  tal pneumatization)
- The frontal or infundibular cells.

It is important to know that these cells might be
present in any given patient, not only because they
might alter the normal sinus drainage if inflammatory conditions are present, but also because an endoscopic surgeon not aware of these cells might confuse
them with the frontal sinus. This could result in a surgical failure due to inadequate reestablishment of
frontal sinus outflow drainage and continued frontal
sinus symptoms [2–4, 13].

The agger nasi cell is one of these cells. Located
anterior to the superior membranous attachment of
the uncinate process, the agger nasi cell is sometimes
difficult to differentiate on CT imaging and even during surgery. However, with experience, its presence
can be documented with CT scan in up to 98% of the
cases [2, 3, 9, 13]. It is intimately related to the anteri-
or head of the middle turbinate, along the ascending
intranasal portion of the maxillofrontal suture line,
and adjacent posteriorly to the lacrimal sac.

The frontal sinus can also be confused with "frontal infundibular cells". These represent a series of anterior ethmoidal cells directly superior to the agger
nasi cell, coursing along the anterior wall of the frontal outflow tract. Bent and Kuhn have divided frontal
infundibulum cells into four categories, based on

their relationship to the agger nasi cell and the orbital roof (Fig. 3.10) [2, 6, 9, 13].

The types frontal infundibulum cells are:

- Type I frontal cell represents a single air cell above the agger nasi.
- Type II frontal cells correspond to a series of small cells above the agger nasi, but below the orbital roof.
- Type III frontal cells extend into the frontal sinus, but remain contiguous with the agger nasi cell.
- Type IV cell corresponds to a completely isolated frontal cell (not contiguous with the agger nasi cell) within the frontal sinus cavity

Supraorbital cells may also disturb the normal frontal sinus outflow tract in diseased states. On CT these supraorbital cells are essentially suprabullar cells with significant pneumatization over the orbital roof [3, 4, 12].

The frontal sinus obtains its vascular supply from terminal vessels of the sphenopalatine artery and internal carotid artery (via the anterior and posterior ethmoid arteries). Terminal branches of the sphenopalatine artery make their way towards the frontal sinus by way of the nasofrontal recess and infundibulum. The anterior ethmoid artery (and more rarely the posterior ethmoid artery) also gives off some branches to supply the posterior aspect of the frontal sinus cavity. Most of the frontal sinus venous blood supply consists of a compact system of valveless diploic veins, which communicate intracranially, intraorbitally, and with the midfacial and forehead skin. The posterior wall drains into the superior sagittal sinus, intracranially [1, 17].

Microscopic channels provide lymphatic drainage to the frontal sinus through the upper nasal (midfacial) lymphatic plexus, for most of the anterior and inferior part of the sinus. The remaining portion of the frontal sinus drains into the subarachnoid space.

Branches of the ethmoidal, nasal, supraorbital, and supratrochlear nerves provide the frontal sinus cavity with an extensive array of sensory innervation. Autonomic innervation of mucosal glands accompanies the neurovascular bundle supplying the frontal sinus.

The frontal sinus mucosa resembles the rest of the upper respiratory mucosa with its ciliated columnar

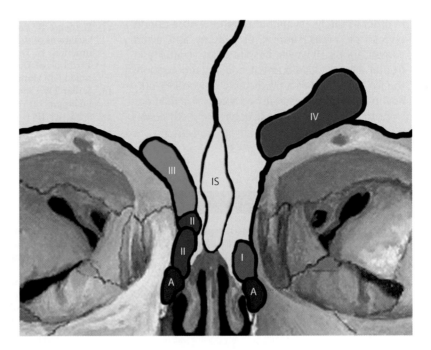

Fig. 3.10.
Bent and Kuhn's classification of frontal infundibular air cells based on its proximity to the agger nasi (A) and orbital roof. Types I, II, III, and IV are shown. In addition, one or more intersinus septal cell (IS) may also exist

3

respiratory epithelium, along with numerous glands and goblet cells that produce serous and mucinous secretions. The frontal sinus mucosa is constantly producing secretions in order to ensure that the cavity is at all times cleared of particulate matter, and that proper humidification is achieved. Although the final destination of the secretions is the frontal recess, the secretions might recirculate several times through the entire frontal sinus cavity, via its intersinus or intrasinus septae before they finally make their way out into the nose through the frontal infundibulum [8, 11, 13]. Failure to maintain the frontal sinus outflow tract patent (because of edema, fibrosis, polyps, and/or neoplasm) may trigger a vicious cycle of events that results in retained secretions, secondary bacterial colonization, hypoxia, pH changes, and ciliary dysfunction. Any or all of these physiological changes may culminate in chronic rhinosinusitis [13].

Conclusions

Frontal sinus anatomy can be challenging even for the most experience surgeon. A thorough knowledge of the most common normal variants is critical in order to safely navigate through the nose during endoscopic sinus surgical procedures and avoid complications. However, despite great variability in frontal air cell development and pneumatization, the frontal sinus has a predictable mucociliary outflow tract with well established anatomical relationships to neighboring vital structures and ethmoidal air cells.

References

1. Aydinhoglu A, , Kavakli A, Erdem S (2003) Absence of frontal sinus in Turkish individuals. Yonsei Medical Jnl 44(2): 215–18
2. Bent J, Kuhn FA, Cuilty C (1994) The frontal cell in frontal recess obstruction Am J Rhinol 8:185–191
3. Bolger WE, Butzin CA, Parsons DS et al (1991) Paranasal sinus bony anatomic variations and mucosal abnormalities: CT analysis for endoscopic sinus surgery. Laryngoscope 101(1pt 1):56–64
4. Bolger WE, Mawn (2001) CB analysis of the suprabullar recess for endoscopic sinus surgery. Ann Otol Rhinol Laryngol Suppl 186:3–14
5. Cryer MH (1907) Some variations in the frontal sinus. JAMA 26:284–289
6. Friedman M, Bliznikas D, Ramakrishnan V et al (2004) Frontal sinus surgery 2004: Update of clinical anatomy and surgical techniques. Oper Tech Otolaryngol Head Neck Surg 15(1):23–31
7. Hajek M (1926) Pathology and Treatment of the Inflammatory Diseases of the Nasal Accessory Sinuses. Fifth ed. CB Mosby, St. Louis pp 34–52
8. Kuhn FA (2001) Surgery of the frontal sinus in diseases of the sinuses diagnosis and management. In Kennedy DW et al "Diseases of the Sinuses", B.C. Decker, Hamilton. London pp 281–301
9. Lang J (1989) Clinical Anatomy of the Nose, Nasal Cavity and Paranasal Sinuses. Thieme Medical Publishers, New York pp 1–3
10. Lothrop HA (1898) The anatomy and surgery of the frontal sinus and anterior ethmoidal cells. Annals of Surg 28: 611–638
11. Loury MC (1993) Endoscopic frontal recess and frontal sinus ostium dissection. Laryngoscope 103(4 pt 1):455–458
12. McLaughlin RB Jr., Rehl RM, Lanza DC et al (2001) Clinically relevant frontal sinus anatomy and physiology. In Kennedy DW, Lanza DC, Current Concepts in The Surgical Management of Frontal Sinus Disease. Otolaryngol Clin North Am 34(1):1–21
13. Mosher HP (1904) The applied anatomy of the frontal sinus. Laryngoscope 14:830–855
14. Navarro JA (1997) Cavidade do Nariz e Seios Paranasales Anatomia Cirurgica 1, All Dent Brazil pp 3–24
15. Peynegre R, Rouvier P (1996) Anatomy and anatomical variations of the paranasal sinuses. Influence on sinus dysfunction. In Diseases of the Sinuses: A Comprehensive Textbook of Diagnosis and Treatment, Gershwin ME, Incaudo GA, Humana Press, New Jersey 1996: 3–32
16. Sadler TW (2004) Langman's Medical Embryology, Ninth Ed Lippincott Williams & Wilkins, Philadelphia pp 363–401
17. Schaeffer JP (1916) The genesis, development, and adult anatomy of the nasofrontal region in man. Am J Anatomy 20(1): 125–145
18. Shah R, Dhingra JK, Carter BL et al (2003) Paranasal Sinus development: A radiographic study. Laryngoscope 113(2): 205–209
19. Spaeth J, Krugelstein U, Schlondorff G et al (1997) The paranasal sinuses in CT-imaging: Development from birth to age 25. Int J Pediatr Otorhinolaryngol 39(1):25–40
20. Tilley H (1896) An investigation of the frontal sinus in 120 skulls from a surgical aspect, with case illustrating methods of treatment of disease in this situation. Lancet 2: 866–870
21. Van Alyea QE (1941) Frontal cells: An anatomic study of these cells in consideration of their clinical significance. Arch Otolaryngol 34:11–23
22. Vidic B (1969) Extreme development of the paranasal sinuses. Ann Otol Rhinol Laryngol 78(6):1291–1298

23. Williams PW (1910) Rhinology: A text book of diseases of the nose and nasal accessory sinuses. Longmans Green, New York pp 34–54

24. Wolf G, Anderhuber W, Kuhn F et al (1993) Development of the paranasal sinuses in children: Implications for parana-sal sinus surgery. Ann Otol Rhinol Laryngol 102(9): 705–711

25. Worldmald P (2003) The agger nasi cell: The key to under-standing the anatomy of the frontal recess. Otolaryngol Head Neck Surg 129(5): 497–507

Chapter 4

Acute Frontal Sinusitis

4

Douglas Reh, Peter H. Hwang

Core Messages

- Although uncomplicated acute frontal sinus-itis (AFS) is a self-limited disease, complica-tions associated with it can be catastrophic

- Uncomplicated AFS is most often associated with a viral upper respiratory tract infection. Bacterial infection is suspected if symptoms are persistent for at least 10 days

- The diagnosis of AFS is considered in patients who meet the general diagnostic criteria for acute sinusitis and have symp-toms localized to the forehead region

- The predominant organisms cultures from patients with uncomplicated AFS are *Hemophilus influenza*, *Streptococcus pneu-moniae*, and *Moraxella catarrhalis*

- When indicated, uncomplicated AFS should be treated with 10 to 14 days of antibiotics

- Complicated AFS is suspected when symp-toms are protracted and severe

- Work up of complicated AFS should include CT scans with IV contrast

- Intracerebral abscess is the most common intracranial complication of AFS

- Patients with complicated AFS should be admitted for intravenous antibiotic therapy, intravenous hydration, and serial neurologic examinations

- Treatment of complicated AFS often requires surgery in addition to antibiotic therapy

Contents

Introduction

Acute sinusitis is one of the leading diagnoses made in ambulatory medicine. The National Ambulatory Medical Care Survey (NAMCS) estimates that 20 mil-lion cases of acute bacterial rhinosinusitis (ABRS) occur each year [1]. The incidence of acute frontal si-nusitis (AFS) specifically is considerably lower, less common than maxillary sinusitis in adults and eth-moid sinusitis in children. Medical therapies for acute sinusitis result in expenditures of $3.5 billion per year in the United States. Of all antibiotics pre-scribed in 2002, 9% of pediatric prescriptions and 18% of adult prescriptions were written for a diagno-sis of acute sinusitis [1].

AFS occurs most commonly in adolescent males and young men. While the reasons for the male predilection are unknown, the age predilection appears likely due to the peak vascularity and peak development of the frontal sinuses between the ages of 7 and 20. Although AFS is largely a self-limited disease, complications of acute sinusitis can have catastrophic clinical consequences if not detected promptly.

Etiology and Pathophysiology of Acute Frontal Sinusitis

Acute frontal sinusitis is most commonly preceded by a viral upper respiratory tract infection. Human rhinovirus is implicated in 50% of cases, but other viruses may include coronavirus, influenza, parainfluenza, respiratory syncytial virus, adenovirus, and enterovirus. The peak prevalence of these viruses occurs in early fall and spring, which parallels the peak incidence of ABRS. Viruses upregulate pro-inflammatory cytokines such as interleukin-1, interleukin-6, interleukin-8, tumor necrosis factor-α, as well as other inflammatory mediators such as histamine and bradykinin. Viruses also suppress neutrophil, macrophage, and lymphocyte function and can thereby inhibit the immune response [2]. The viral induction of the inflammatory cascade results in acute mucosal edema, occlusion of sinus ostia, and impaired mucociliary clearance. Mucus stasis can then favor the proliferation of pathogenic micro-organisms, resulting in acute bacterial sinusitis. Other risk factors for acute sinusitis include a variety of host factors: septal deviation, nasal polyposis, and immunodeficiency/immunosuppression, among others.

While acute sinusitis typically affects the ethmoid and maxillary sinuses, progression of disease to involve the frontal sinus may be influenced by anatomic variations of the frontal sinus. The frontal sinus begins developing at age 3. Four frontal pits along the upper lateral wall of the embryological middle meatus differentiate into the anterior ethmoid cells. The second of these furrows evaginates from the anterior ethmoid region into the frontal bone, creating the frontal sinus [3]. Because the frontal sinus is embryologically derived from pneumatization of the ethmoid, frontal sinus outflow is thus influenced and defined by the degree of pneumatization of the ethmoid labyrinth. A variety of ethmoid-derived structures that comprise the frontal recess can thus narrow the outflow tract and predispose to acute frontal sinusitis. These structures may include agger nasi cells anteriorly, the bulla lamella posteriorly, supraorbital ethmoid cells laterally, and type I–IV frontal cells [3].

Uncomplicated Acute Frontal Sinusitis

Diagnosis

AFS is principally a clinical diagnosis based on type and duration of symptoms. CT scans, when ordered to diagnose acute bacterial sinusitis, may yield false positives. Gwaltney et al. showed that 87% of adults with acute onset of upper respiratory tract infection (URI) symptoms demonstrate CT evidence of nasal cavity mucosal thickening and sinus opacification [4]. They also showed that after 2 weeks without antibiotic therapy, repeat CT scans showed improvement in 79% of 14 patients with these findings. Sinus aspiration studies have shown that significant bacterial growth occurs in approximately 60% of patients with URI symptoms lasting for 10 days or more [5]. Therefore persistent or worsening symptoms after 10 days may indicate a bacterial infection [1].

In 1997 the American Academy of Otolaryngology-Head and Neck Surgery Foundation assembled the Rhinosinusitis Task Force (RSTF) to develop clinical definitions of rhinosinusitis. Rhinosinusitis as defined by the RSTF is "inflammation of the nasal cavity and paranasal sinus" [6]. The RSTF subclassified rhinosinusitis into three major clinical categories based on duration of symptoms: acute, with symptoms lasting less than 4 weeks; subacute, between 4 and 12 weeks; and chronic, greater than 12 weeks.

By RSTF guidelines, patients with rhinosinusitis must meet a variety of symptomatic major and minor criteria.

The major criteria defined by the RSTF include:

- Facial pain or pressure
- Nasal congestion
- Nasal obstruction
- Purulent rhinorrhea
- Hyposmia or anosmia
- Fever (for acute rhinosinusitis only)
- Purulence on nasal exam

The minor criteria defined by the RSTF include:

- Headache
- Nonacute fever
- Halitosis
- Fatigue
- Dental pain
- Cough
- Ear pain or pressure

A diagnosis of rhinosinusitis requires either two major factors, one major and two minor factors, or purulence in the nasal cavity on physical exam [6].

There are no site-specific criteria for the diagnosis of AFS. Generally frontal sinus symptoms are localized to the brow, temple, and frontal bone region. Frontal headache is the most prevalent symptom of AFS [7]. Thus, a diagnosis of AFS should be considered in patients who meet RSTF criteria for acute sinusitis, in whom symptoms localize to the forehead region. In some cases, the acute onset of frontal headache, even in the absence of more classic symptoms such as nasal congestion and rhinorrhea, should prompt the physician to consider a diagnosis of AFS. This is especially true in those patients without a history of chronic headache.

Although most cases of acute rhinosinusitis can be diagnosed by symptoms alone, the physical examination can provide helpful adjunctive diagnostic information. Transillumination and palpation, while classically described for physical exam of the sinuses, are relatively nonspecific tests. Anterior rhinoscopy and nasal endoscopy, however, can be useful adjunctive diagnostic tools. Examination of the nasal cavity may reveal mucosal edema, purulent discharge, or anatomic obstructions such as septal deviation or polyposis. Purulent secretions may be aspirated under endoscopic visualization and cultured to guide antimicrobial therapy. During aspiration and culture, the endoscope should be used to retract the nasal vestibule away to minimize contamination of the culture device by normal nasal vestibular flora.

Unless a complication of acute sinusitis is suspected, imaging studies such as CT and MRI are not necessary in making the diagnosis of AFS.

Bacteriology

While the bacteriology of acute maxillary sinusitis has been well documented by maxillary tap studies, the bacteriology of AFS has not been well studied. Data are limited principally because of the difficulty of accessing the frontal sinus for cultures. Brook obtained aspirates from the frontal sinuses of 15 patients with acute infection [8]. Twenty isolates were grown from 13 of the specimens. The predominant aerobic and facultative organisms were *Haemophilus influenzae* (6/13), *Streptococcus pneumoniae* (5), and *Moraxella catarrhalis* (3). B-lactamase producing organisms were isolated in 33% of the specimens. Limitations of this study were its small numbers and the lack of documentation of sampling technique.

Given that AFS typically occurs in conjunction with acute maxillary and ethmoid sinusitis, it seems reasonable to extrapolate data for acute maxillary sinusitis to that for AFS. Indeed, the organisms cultured in the Brook study did parallel those obtained from the maxillary sinuses in other studies; namely, *Streptococcus pneumoniae*, *Haemophilus influenzae* and *Moraxella catarrhalis* [1].

Treatment

The goals of treating uncomplicated AFS are:

- to control the infectious component of the disease process using antimicrobial therapy
- to reduce the edematous, obstructive component of the disease process and restore sinus patency using decongestant therapy
- Uncomplicated AFS is almost exclusively treated medically; surgical therapy is rarely indicated.

Antibiotic therapy should be selected for coverage of the primary organisms associated with acute rhinosinusitis: *S. pneumoniae*, *H. influenzae*, and *M. catarrhalis*. Drug resistance has become an increasing concern in the treatment of ABRS. Since the early 1990's, the rates of penicillin resistance in *S. pneumoniae* have increased dramatically, with 15% of iso-

4

Table 4.1. U.S. penicillin resistance rates of *S. Pneumoniae* by region, 1999–2000

Geographic Location	No. of isolates	Intermediate resistance (%)	High-level resistance (%)
West			
San Diego, CA	30	10.0	23.30
Los Angeles, CA	51	5.9	15.70
San Francisco, CA	52	9.6	23.10
Portland, OR	22	22.7	31.80
Seattle, WA	50	18.0	18.00
Denver, CO	51	21.6	13.70
Salt Lake City, UT	50	16.0	16.00
Phoenix, AZ	59	10.2	35.60
Midwest			
Iowa City, IA	54	11.1	16.70
Indianapolis, IN	56	10.7	19.60
Chicago, IL	41	14.6	12.20
Milwaukee, WI	53	11.3	32.10
Detroit, MI	58	8.6	5.20
Cleveland, OH	52	7.7	34.60
East			
Rochester, NY	50	18.0	22.00
Boston, MA	31	6.5	19.40
New York, NY	59	15.3	20.30
Philadelphia, PA	52	19.2	7.70
Washington DC	20	5.0	35.00
South			
Chapel Hill, NC	41	9.8	56.10
Mobile, AL	49	10.2	16.30
Houston, TX	55	20.0	38.20
Dallas, TX	44	11.4	15.90
Miami Beach, FL	21	19.1	28.60

From [10]

lates showing intermediate resistance and 25% showing high resistance. Macrolide- (18%) and trimethoprim/sulfamethoxazole (TMP/SMX) (20%)-resistant strains of *S. pneumoniae* are also significant in the United States [9]. Thirty percent of *H. influenzae* and greater than 95% of *M. catarrhalis* cultured are B-lactamase-producing isolates [1]. Resistance patterns and prevalence differ by geographic region. Table 4.1 shows differences in bacterial resistance by U.S. region [10].

The Sinus and Allergy Health Partnership recently published antibiotic recommendations for the treatment of mild to moderate ABRS. These recommendations are based on clinical efficacy and reflect drug resistance patterns. These recommendations are summarized in Table 4.2 [1]. AFS should be treated with a minimum of 10 to 14 days of antibiotics when possible. If the patient's symptoms fail to resolve, the antibiotic course should be extended by 2 weeks [11] and consideration should be given to endoscopic exam and culture.

Adjunctive medical treatment in AFS is aimed primarily at re-establishing the patency of the frontal recess and ostiomeatal complex through which the frontal sinus drains. Topical (oxymetazoline, phenylephrine) and oral (pseudoephedrine) decongestants and mucolytics (guaifenesin) may improve drainage of the affected sinuses. Selected patients with known inflammatory dysregulation, such as those with atopic disease, aspirin sensitivity, or nasal polyposis may benefit from oral steroids. When used in carefully selected patients, steroids can acutely reduce inflammation and facilitate drainage of affected sinuses [11].

Complicated Acute Frontal Sinusitis

Diagnosis

Occasionally, patients with AFS may present in acute distress with toxic clinical features. Clinical findings such as prostration, severe headache, or orbital complaints should raise suspicion for an infectious complication of AFS.

Complications from AFS principally involve:

- extension to intracranial structures
- the orbits may occasionally be affected

Although the true incidence of AFS-related complications is unknown, a study of 649 patients admitted to the hospital for sinusitis showed an intracranial complication rate of 3.7% [12].

The frontal sinus is susceptible to extrasinus spread of infection in part because its venous drainage occurs through diploic veins that traverse the posterior table and communicate with the venous supply of the meninges, cavernous sinus and dural sinuses. These venous channels may be more porous in the developing sinus, and thus adolescents and young

Table 4.2. Recommended antibiotic therapy for adults with mild or moderate ABRS

Initial therapy	Calculated clinical efficacy (%)	Calculated bacteriologic efficacy (%)	Switch therapy options (no improvement after 72 hours)
Mild disease with no recent antimicrobial use in past 4–6 weeks			
Amoxicillin/clavulanate (1.75–4 g/250 mg/d)	90–91	97–99	
Amoxicillin (1.5–4 g/d)	87–88	91–92	Gatifloxacin/levofloxacin/moxifloxacin
Cefpodoxime proxetil	87	91	Amoxicillin/clavulanate (4 g/250 mg)
Cefuroxime axetil	85	87	Ceftriaxone
Cefdinir	83	85	Combination therapy
B-Lactam Allergic			
TMP/SMX	83	84	
Doxycycline	81	80	Gatifloxacin/levofloxacin/moxifloxacin
Azithromycin/erythromycin/clarithromycin	77	73	Rifampin plus clindamycin
Mild disease with recent antimicrobial use in past 4–6 weeks or moderate disease			
Gatifloxacin/levofloxacin/moxifloxacin	92	100	
Amoxicillin/clavulanate (4 g/250 mg)	91	99	Reevaluate patient
Ceftriaxone	91	99	
B-Lactam Allergic			
Gatifloxacin/levofloxacin/moxifloxacin	92	100	Reevaluate patient
Clindamycin and rifampin			

From [1]

adults (especially male) are at increased risk for complications of AFS.

Suspicion for complicated AFS should be elevated when:

- Symptoms are protracted or more severe than would be expected for a typical case of acute sinusitis
- On physical examination, there is periorbital edema or discoloration, which can indicate a preseptal cellulitis, or painful or restricted eye movement, which may indicate an orbital cellulites or abscess
- Neurologic findings such as altered mental status, seizure, or cranial neuropathy are present, which may indicate intracerebral complications

As in uncomplicated AFS, nasal endoscopy may yield cultures of purulent material that can guide antimicrobial therapy. Lumbar puncture may also be indicated to obtain CSF cultures and to rule out meningitis. Consultations with an ophthalmologist, neurosurgeon, neurologist, or infectious disease specialist should be considered.

In contrast to uncomplicated AFS, radiologic studies play an important role in confirming and characterizing the extent of extrasinus infectious involvement. CT scan is the imaging modality of choice in evaluating intracranial or orbital complications of AFS. Studies should be performed with IV contrast in axial and coronal planes. With bone and soft tissue algorithms, CT scans can characterize bony erosions of the frontal sinus as well as phlegmons or fluid collections in adjacent orbital and intracranial soft tissue. Serial imaging studies should be considered in patients who appear clinically unresponsive to initial treatment.

4

Intracerebral abscess is the most common intracranial complication of AFS. The frontal lobe is most frequently involved, although hematogenous seeding of distant brain structures may be observed less commonly [12]. Headache is the most common early symptom, although subsequently there may be a quiescent asymptomatic phase during which an abscess has coalesced [13]. Overall mortality reported in the literature ranges widely from 0% to 53% [13,14].

Meningitis is another important neurologic complication of AFS [12].

Symptoms suggestive of meningitis include:

- High fever
- Photophobia
- Neck pain or stiffness
- Severe headache
- Mental status changes

Mortality is reported as high as 45% [15]. While meningitis is the second most common intracranial complication of acute sinusitis in general, the frontal sinus as a site of origin is less common than the sphenoid (most common) and the ethmoid sinuses. Advanced cases of frontal sinusitis with meningitis may also be associated with subdural or epidural abscesses. When these abscesses occur they typically develop immediately posterior to the frontal sinus along pathways of venous drainage [14].

Osteomyelitis of the frontal sinus may be caused by direct extension of infection or by thrombophlebitis of the diploic veins. Of all the paranasal sinuses, the frontal sinus is most commonly associated with osteomyelitis. When osteomyelitis involves the anterior table, a subperiosteal abscess may develop, presenting as a subcutaneous fluctuant protuberance over the brow or forehead. This abscess is known as Pott's Puffy Tumour, which was first described by Sir Percival Pott in 1775 [16]. Strictly an infectious complication and not neoplastic in any way, Pott's Puffy Tumour may present with severe headache, fever, and photophobia.

Cavernous sinus thrombosis and superior sagittal sinus thrombosis comprise another important class of complications associated with AFS.

Patients with cavernous sinus thrombosis develop:

- Ophthalmoplegia
- Proptosis
- Visual loss
- Trigeminal nerve (V2 and V3) deficits

Early clinical recognition is important, as symptoms can quickly progress, and mortality exceeds 30% [17–19]. Superior sagittal sinus thrombosis is associated with subdural abscess and has a high mortality rate, 80% [18].

Isolated AFS rarely causes orbital complications. However, AFS in the context of pansinusitis is associated with 60–80% of orbital complications [20,21]. Although direct spread to the orbits from the frontal sinus is possible, the ethmoid sinuses are more commonly implicated in the development of orbital complications.

Bacteriology

The organisms cultured from the sinuses of patients with intracranial abscesses include [12]:

- *Staphylococcus aureus*
- Anaerobic streptococci
- *Streptococcus epidermidis*
- *Streptococcus pneumoniae*
- *Staphylococcus intermedius*
- Beta-hemolytic streptococci
- Gram-positive aerobes and anaerobes are the predominant bacteria in complicated AFS

Table 4.3 summarizes the organisms cultured from paranasal sinuses in patients with intracranial complications [12]. Table 4.4 shows Goldberg et al.'s summarization of the common organisms associated with AFS complications and the recommended primary antibiotic therapy based on the Sanford Guide to Antimicrobial Treatment [14].

Treatment

Treatment of complicated AFS includes aggressive medical therapy and surgery to drain both the involved sinus and the abscess collection if present.

Because of the acuity and morbidity of complicated frontal sinusitis, patients should be admitted for

intravenous antibiotic therapy, serial neurologic examination, and intravenous hydration. Empiric antibiotic therapy should be initiated immediately, choosing broad-spectrum agents that have favorable penetration of the blood-brain barrier. If cultures can be obtained, antibiotic therapy may be tailored accordingly. It should be noted that a significant percentage of cultures from patients with intracranial complications are negative. This may perhaps occur because antibiotic therapy is often initiated emergently before cultures can be obtained. Antila et al. obtained 103 frontal sinus cultures in patients with AFS and simultaneous maxillary sinusitis [22]. Only 30% of these cultures were positive for bacteria. Twenty-one percent of the cultures in Clayman et al.'s study were negative [12]. In such cases, bacteriologic data from historical cohorts may be used to guide antibiotic selection.

Depending on the degree of morbidity, many patients will require continuation of intravenous antibiotic therapy as an outpatient after resolution of the acute phase of illness. Oral antibiotic therapy may be appropriate in selected patients. Duration of treatment varies with the nature and severity of the complication, as well as the response to initial therapy.

The use of intravenous corticosteroids in patients with AFS complications is controversial. Some stud-

Table 4.3. Organisms cultured from paranasal sinuses with associated intracranial complications

Organism	n (%)
Negative cultures	5 (21)
S. aureus	5 (21)
Anaerobic streptococci	3 (12)
S. epidermidis	2 (8)
S. pneumoniae	2 (8)
S. intermedius	2 (8)
b-Hemolytic streptococci	2 (8)
S. viridans	1 (4)
Actinomycoses sp.	1 (4)
Fusobacterium necrosporum	1 (4)
Bacteroides melaninogenicus	1 (4)

From [12]

Table 4.4. Common organisms associated with ABRS-related complications and recommended empiric antibiotic therapy

Disease	Most common organism	Primary drug choice	Alternative 1
Pott's tumor (acute osteomyelitis)	S. aureus, streptococci, anaerobes, polymicrobial	Pencillinase-resistant penicillin and metronidazole, consider vancomycin	Third-generation cephalosporin and vancomycin and metronidazole
Intracranial abscess	Streptococci, Bacteroides sp.	3rd generation cephalosporin and metronidazole	High-dose PCN G and metronidazole
Orbital complication	S. pneumococcus, H. influenzae, M. catarrhalis, S. aureus	2nd and 3rd generation cephalosporin or ampicillin/ sulbactam	Ticarcillin/ clavulanate or piperacillin and tazobactam
Meningitis	S. pneumococcus, H. influenzae	3rd generation cephalosporin and vancomycin	Meropenem and vancomycin
Dural sinus thrombophlebitis	S. aureus, group A streptococcus, H. influenzae, fungal organisms	Pencillinase-resistant penicillin and 3rd generation cephalosporin	Imipenem or meropenem and vancomycin

From [14]

ies have advocated their use in patients with cerebral edema and clinical deterioration [23], while others argue that they may interfere with antibiotic penetration and immune response [12]. No prospective studies or animal models have conclusively shown that steroids improve mortality or morbidity associated with cerebral edema; thus the use of corticosteroids should be considered on an individual basis.

Treatment of complicated AFS often involves surgery in addition to antibiotic therapy. Patients with intracranial abscesses may require neurosurgical drainage concurrently with surgical treatment of the frontal sinus.

Methods of draining the frontal sinus include:

- Trephination
- Endoscopic frontal sinusotomy
- External ethmoidectomy

Advantages and Disadvantages of Trephination

Advantages

- Technical simplicity
- Efficacy of draining the sinus
- Access to the sinus lumen for irrigation

Disadvantages

- Scar
- Potential injury to the supraorbital nerve
- The critical area of impaired outflow of the sinus is not addressed

In experienced hands, endoscopic frontal sinusotomy may be an alternative surgical technique in complicated AFS. The endoscopic approach provides a minimally invasive means of draining the sinus and anatomically improving frontal outflow. Disadvantages of the endoscopic approach include its techni-

cal complexity as well as the difficulty of adequate visualization in the acutely infected milieu. External frontoethmoidectomy is less commonly used in managing complicated AFS. This technique may be associated with frontal mucocele formation (20%–30% of cases) and frontal stenosis [24].

References

1. Sinus and Allied Health Partnership (2004) Antimicrobial treatment guidelines for acute bacterial rhinosinusitis. Otolaryngol Head Neck Surg 130(1):1–45
2. Patel J, Faden H, Sharma S, et al (1992) Effect of respiratory syncytial virus on adherence, colonization and immunity of non-typable Haemophilus influenzae: implications for otitis media. Int J Pediatr Otorhinolaryngol 23:15–23
3. Kuhn FA (2001) Surgery of the Frontal Sinus. In: Kennedy DW, Bolger WE, Zinreich SJ "Diseases of the Sinuses", B.C. Decker, Hamilton, Ontario, pp 281–301.
4. Gwaltney JM Jr, Scheld WM, Sande MA, et al (1992) The microbial etiology and antimicrobial therapy of adults with community-acquired sinusitis: A fifteen year experience at the University of Virginia and review of other selected studies. J Allergy Clin Immunol 90:457–461
5. Gwaltney JM Jr, Phillips CD, Miller RD, et al (1994) Computed tomographic study of the common cold. N Engl J Med 330:25–30
6. Report of the Rhinosinusitis Task Force Committee Meeting (1997) Alexandria, Virginia, August 17, 1996. Otolaryngol Head Neck Surg 117(3 Pt 2):S1–68
7. Seiden A, Martin V (2001) Headache and the frontal sinus. Otolaryngol Clinics North Am 34(1):227–241
8. Brook I (2002) Bacteriology of acute and chronic frontal sinsusitis. Arch Otolaryngol Head Neck Surg 128:583–555
9. Hoban DJ, Doern GV, Fluit AC, Roussel-Delvallez M, Jones RN (2001) Worldwide prevelance of antimicrobial resistance in *Streptococcus pneumoniae, haemophilus influenzae*, and *Moraxell catarrhalis* in the SENTY antimicrobial surveillance program, 1997–1999. Clinic Infectious Disease 32(Suppl 2):S81–93
10. Doern GV, Heilmann K, Brueggemann A, et al (2001) Antimicrobial resistance among clinic isolates of streptococcus pneumoniae in the United States during 1999–2000, including a comparison of resistance rates since 1994–1995. Antimicrob Agents Chemother 45(6):1721–1729
11. Maccabee M, Hwang P (2001) Medical therapy of acute and chronic frontal sinusitis. Otolaryngol Clinics North Am 34(1):41–7
12. Clayman GL, Adams GL, Paugh DR, Koopmann CF (1991) Intracranial complications of paranasal sinusitis: A combined institutional review. Laryngoscope 101:234–239
13. Giannoni CM, Stewart MG, Alford EL (1997) Intracranial complications of sinusitis. Laryngoscope 107(7):863–867

14. Goldberg AN, Oroszlan G, Anderson TD (2001) Complications of frontal sinusitis and their management. Otolaryngol Clinics North Am 34(1):211–225
15. Singh B, Dellen VJ, Ranjettan S, et al (1995) Sinogenic intracranial complications. J Laryngol Otol 1109:945
16. Pott P (1775) The Chirurgical Works of Percival Pott. London, Hayes W. Clarke and B. Collins
17. Morgan PR, Morrison WV (1980) Complications of frontal and ethmoid sinusitis. Laryngoscope 90:661
18. Southwick FS, Richardson EP, Swartz M (1986) Septic thrombosis of the dural venous sinuses. Medicine 65:82
19. Stankiewitz JS, Newell DJ, Park AH (1993) Complications of inflammatory diseases of the sinuses. Otolaryngol Clin North Am 26:63
20. Jackson K, Baker SR (1986) Clinical implications of orbital cellulitis. Laryngoscope 96:568
21. Schramm VL, Curtin HD, Kennerdell JS (1982) Evaluation of orbital cellulitis and results of treatment. Laryngoscope 92:732
22. Antila J, Suonpaa J, Lehtonen O (1997) Bacteriological evaluation of 194 adult patients with acute frontal sinusitis and findings of simultaneous maxillary sinusitis. Acta Otolaryngol Suppl (Stockh) 529:162
23. Gallagher RM, Gross CW, Phillips D (1998) Suppurative intracranial complications of sinusitis. Laryngoscope 108:1635
24. Lang EE, Curran AJ, Walsh MA, et al (2001) Intracranial complications of acute frontal sinusitis. Clin Otolaryngol 26:452–457

Chapter 5

Chronic Frontal Rhinosinusitis: Diagnosis and Management

Michael Sillers

Core Messages

- Despite significant advances in surgical techniques, technology, and knowledge of pathophysiology, management of chronic frontal rhinosinusitis remains one of the most challenging problems for otolaryngologists

- Medical therapy for chronic frontal rhinosinusitis is analogous to the therapy for chronic ethmoid rhinosinusitis

- Long-term management success is best achieved in a setting of an integrated medical and surgical approach

Chronic frontal rhinosinusitis represents perhaps one of the most difficult areas within the paranasal sinuses to manage. A current search of the literature will result in numerous publications describing medical therapy, imaging techniques, and surgical procedures specifically for the treatment of symptomatic chronic frontal rhinosinusitis.

This chapter will attempt to discuss a workable rationale for the appropriate diagnosis and treatment of patients with this troublesome disease by presenting the following:

- Anatomic review of the frontal sinus outflow tract
- Current diagnostic criteria
- Endoscopic evaluation techniques
- Advanced CT imaging
- Strategies for medical therapy
- An integrated surgical approach

Contents

Anatomy of the Frontal Sinus Outflow Tract

There has been much confusion regarding the anatomy of and drainage from the frontal sinus. The term "nasofrontal duct" has been entrenched in our literature for many years when, in fact, there is no "duct" leading from the frontal sinus into the nasal cavity [12]. Understanding this complicated anatomic region does not come easily but only after extensive study. The frontal sinus outflow tract (FSOT) can be envisioned as an hourglass with three basic components [16]. The frontal sinus infundibulum is the inferior aspect of the frontal sinus into which "pours" the mucus generated by the respiratory epithelium which lines the frontal sinus. The frontal sinus os-

5

tium is the inferiormost aspect of the frontal sinus proper, beyond which lays the frontal recess. The frontal recess is a space dependent on the pneumatization of several distinct ethmoid air cells, described by Bent et al., and tends to be the most varied component of the FSOT [2]. The degree to which these cells develop determines the complexity of the frontal recess and in many instances will dictate a specific surgical approach when medical therapy fails.

The frontal recess is bound by:

- The posterior wall of the agger nasi region anteriorly
- The anterior wall of the ethmoid bulla posteriorly
- The lamina papyracea laterally
- The anterior vertical portion of the middle turbinate medially
- The ethmoid roof superiorly

The agger nasi region ("agger nasi" means "mound in the nose") will pneumatize in almost all circumstances [4]. The degree to which it pneumatizes varies and has a great influence on the dimensions of the frontal recess and the frontal sinus (Figs. 5.1, 5.2). Ethmoid cells located above the agger nasi cell are designated as frontal cells and are further classified based on their size and number. Suprabullar, supraorbital ethmoid, and intersinus septal cells can all influence the frontal recess. Each of these cells can be confused with the frontal sinus itself during an attempted endoscopic intranasal frontal sinusotomy, and need to be distinguished on the patient's preoperative CT images and anticipated at the time of surgery. Sagittal reconstructed images are indispensable in the accurate diagnosis of pathology in this region.

Current Diagnostic Criteria

Patients with chronic frontal rhinosinusitis frequently have associated disease in the remaining paranasal sinuses. Isolated frontal sinus disease occurs rarely. Patients present with a history of symptoms of 3 months or more duration as defined by the most recent report of the rhinosinusitis task force [1] (Table 5.1). Symptoms are not generally sensitive or specific for uncomplicated frontal sinus disease. Notable exceptions are frontal sinus osteomas, frontal sinus and supraorbital ethmoid mucoceles, and frontal sinus neoplasm, in which cases patients may have localized pain.

Table 5.1. Diagnostic criteria for chronic rhinosinusitis

1. Continuous symptoms and/or physical finding ≥ 12 weeks
2. One inflammatory sign associated with symptoms
a. Discolored mucus, nasal polyp, or polypoid swelling
b. Edema or erythema of the middle meatus
c. Generalized edema, erythema, or granulation tissue. If not involving the middle meatus or ethmoid bulla, must have radiographic confirmation of inflammation.
d. Imaging modalities:
i.   CT showing diffuse signs of inflammation
ii. Plain radiograph with > 5 mm mucosal thickening or opacification
iii. MRI not recommended

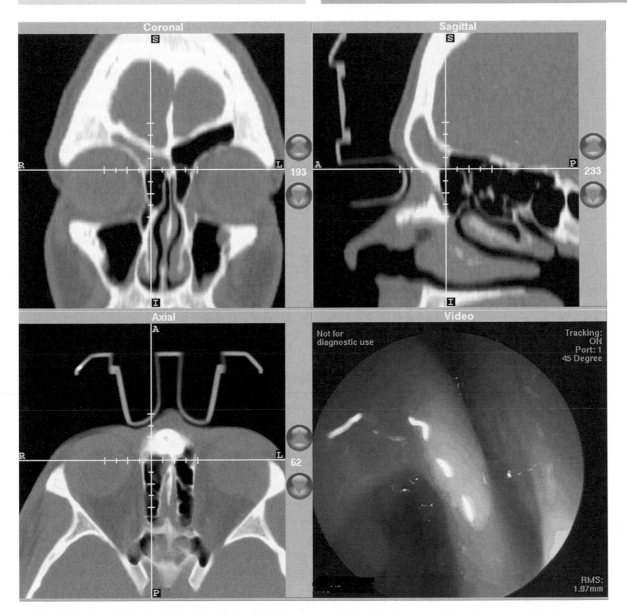

Fig. 5.1. Intraoperative computer-assisted surgery view of large agger nasi cell and associated frontal sinus opacification

Endoscopic Evaluation

Diagnostic nasal endoscopy is the most comprehensive physical examination for the rhinologic patient. The nose should be examined in the natural and de-congested state. Careful note is made of differences between sides and in different areas; i.e., middle meatus vs. superior meatus vs. sphenoethmoidal recess. The presence and degree of edema as well as the character and color of secretions should be documented. Abnormal secretions should be collected

5

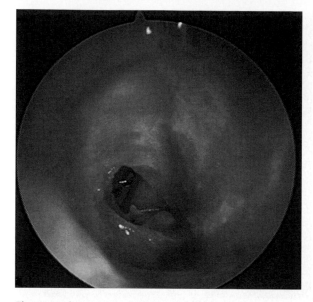

Fig. 5.2. Endoscopic view following removal of the roof of the agger nasi cell

with careful endoscopic technique and sent for appropriate staining and culture. Tantilipikorn et al. found no significant difference between endoscopically acquired cultures obtained through aspiration versus those obtained with a calcium-alginate tipped swab [13]. Often the volume of secretions is small and may be more amenable to a swab technique than an aspirate.

In patients who have undergone previous surgery, frontal sinus disease is suspected when the following are seen:

- Lateralized or amputated middle turbinate
- Synechia
- Polypoid edema in the anterior ethmoid cavity

An angled telescope (30° or more) is almost always required to adequately assess the frontal recess and frontal sinus (Fig. 5.3A–D.)

Advanced Imaging Techniques

Noncontrast CT imaging is the imaging modality of choice for the radiographic evaluation of patients with chronic uncomplicated rhinosinusitis. Standard axial and coronal images are necessary as a preoperative data set but may not be adequate to comprehensively depict the complexity of the FSOT anatomy. Specifically for patients with difficult frontal recess anatomy, sagittal reconstruction is vital. From sagittal images, the anterior to posterior dimensions of the frontal recess can be assessed, and the extent to which frontal recess cells impact the FSOT can be determined [8]. In general, sagittal reconstruction is performed from reformatted axial images. The thinner the axial image slice the better the resolution of the reconstructed sagittal image. These images can be acquired from the workstation in the radiology suite or on a surgical navigation workstation if available.

Computer-assisted sinus surgery has gained wide acceptance and has proven useful in functional endoscopic sinus surgery (FESS) in general. Perhaps one of its greatest areas of utility is in the FSOT. Patients with complex anatomy and/or scarring from prior surgery present a significant challenge to the endoscopic sinus surgeon. The ability to accurately track surgical instruments within a defined surgical volume to which multiplanar CT images are registered has enabled surgeons to safely and successfully treat patients who previously would have required more aggressive open procedures (Fig. 5.4).

Medical Management

There is no medical therapy designed specifically for the frontal sinus. In general there is currently no medical therapy that is FDA-approved for the treatment of *chronic* rhinosinusitis. The choice of therapeutic agents should be made thoughtfully and on an individualized basis. The microbiologic environment of acute rhinosinusitis is different from that in chronic rhinosinusitis and includes primarily *Staphylococcus aureus*, coagulase-negative *Staph* and *Pseudomonas* species. Schlosser et al. specifically cultured

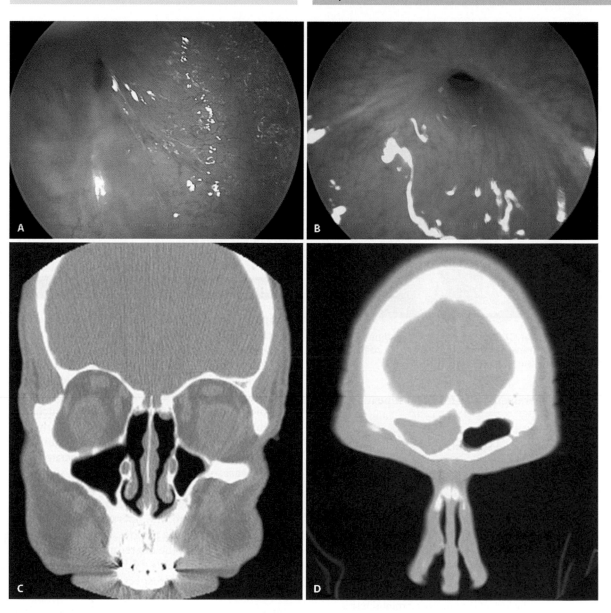

Fig. 5.3. Thirty-degree endoscopic views of left and right frontal recess and accompanying coronal CT in a patient with multiple prior surgeries. A Obstructed right frontal recess. B Patent left frontal recess. C Coronal CT depicting middle turbinate resection and osteoneogenesis along the ethmoid roof. D Coronal CT depicting patent left and opacified right frontal sinuses

patients with chronic frontal rhinosinusitis via a mini-trephination approach (Table 5.3). Patients undergoing primary surgery were more likely to have *H. influenza* while coagulase-negative *Staph* was more common in revision cases [11]. Because of these microbiologic differences, culture-directed therapy is likely to result in the most appropriate choice of antimicrobials in each individual patient. Adjuvant therapy focusing on the reduction of inflammation is also frequently recommended.

5

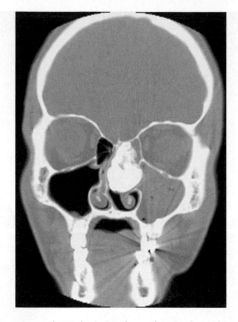

Fig. 5.4. Coronal CT depicting large frontoethmoid osteoma removed via transnasal endoscopic approach utilizing computer-assisted surgery

Adjuvant therapy in chronic frontal sinusitis may include:

- Intranasal and systemic steroids
- Topical and systemic decongestants
- Antihistamines
- Leukotriene modifiers
- Mucolytics
- Nasal saline nasal spray/irrigations

The recommendation for these medications should consider potential side effects, underlying comorbid-

Table 5.3. Microbiology of chronic frontal rhinosinusitis

Aerobic	
Staphylococcus aureus	– 21%
Coagulase negative Staph	– 21%
Haemophilus influenza	– 9%
Other	– 26%
Anaerobic	– 3%
No growth	– 38%
Fungus	– 4%

ities and their relative contraindications, drug interactions, and cost. There remains quite a debate as to what constitutes "maximal medical therapy" in both the degree as well as the duration. Adding to the confusion is the difference between patients such as one with aspirin-sensitive asthma and nasal polyposis versus one with limited maxillary and ethmoid infundibular disease. All chronic rhinosinusitis is not the same. In general, patients should have the benefit of therapy for 3–4 weeks followed by a posttreatment CT, at which time an assessment of their clinical response can be made. Symptomatic patients with evidence of chronic inflammatory changes on CT can be considered "medical failures" and appropriate surgery can be recommended.

An Integrated Surgical Approach

Multiple surgical procedures have been described for the treatment of chronic frontal rhinosinusitis. Montgomery popularized the osteoplastic frontal sinus fat obliteration that was the workhorse procedure for many years [7]. With the advent, widespread acceptance, and technical advances of functional endoscopic sinus surgery, this procedure is much less frequently utilized. As with medical therapy, the choice of approach to the frontal sinus should be made thoughtfully. Factors such as associated ethmoid disease, pneumatization patterns, suspected pathology, need for exposure, and operator experience should all influence the choice an appropriate surgical procedure; no one operation will work for every patient. A stepwise progression should be considered depending on the degree and type of pathology in individual patients (Table 5.4). Weber et al. published combined retrospective results of frontal sinus surgery in 1286 patients: 85% of patients underwent an endonasal approach while only 15% required an external procedure. They achieved success ranging from 79%–97.8% in patients with chronic frontal rhinosinusitis, neoplasm, and trauma [14].

It is important to recognize that mucosal disease in the frontal sinus is usually the result of outflow obstruction in the inferior portion of the frontal sinus outflow tract, i.e. the frontal recess. Notable exceptions include frontal sinus osteoma, inverting papilloma, and de novo mucocele. As a consequence, in many patients with limited mucosal thickening in the frontal sinus, the most appropriate procedure is a careful anterior ethmoidectomy, taking care not to violate the mucosa in the frontal recess. An intranasal frontal sinusotomy which entails the removal of all ethmoid air cell partitions in the frontal recess, pre-serving boundary mucosa, and visually identifying the frontal sinus is appropriate in patients with more severe frontal sinus disease, patients with severe polypoid disease in the frontal recess, and those who have failed prior anterior ethmoidectomy (Fig. 5.5). More advanced/aggressive intranasal endoscopic ap-

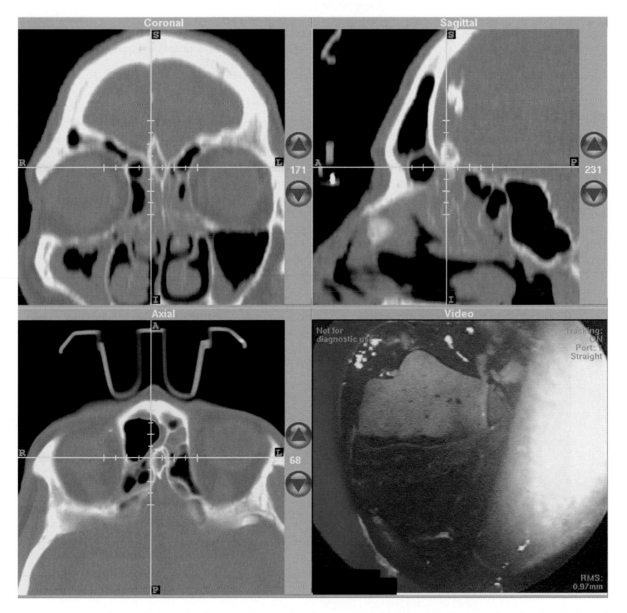

Fig. 5.5. Intraoperative computer-assisted surgery image of an obstructing Type III frontal cell removed to visualize the frontal sinus

Table 5.4. Integrated surgical approach

Procedure	Indication
Endoscopic anterior ethmoidectomy	Limited frontal sinus mucosal thickening
Intranasal frontal sinusotomy	Extensive frontal sinus mucosal thickening/opacification, nasal polyps, and/or failed ethmoidectomy
Frontal sinus rescue procedure	Failed intranasal frontal sinusotomy
Draf II/III, endoscopic modified Lothrop, trans-septal frontal sinusotomy	Extensive frontal sinus disease, neoplasm, osteoneogenesis, and failed intranasal frontal sinusotomy
Frontal sinus trephination	Frontal sinus pathology inaccessible via intranasal approach alone
External frontal sinusotomy	Neoplasm, trauma, or CSF leak requiring wide exposure

proaches (Draf II/III, frontal sinus rescue procedure, endoscopic modified Lothrop procedure, and trans-septal frontal sinusotomy) are chosen based on the patient's unique anatomy and usually the failure of prior endoscopic techniques [5, 6, 9, 10, 15].

External procedures are much less frequently required with advanced endoscopic techniques and computer-assisted surgery. A frontal sinus trephination can be performed in conjunction with endoscopic techniques when the disease process in the frontal sinus cannot be adequately reached from an intranasal approach alone. Laterally based frontal sinus mucoceles, small osteomas, and Type III/IV frontal cells are examples of pathology that may be successfully addressed by this "combined" approach [3] (Figs. 5.6, 5.7). External frontal sinusotomy via Lynch incision or through an osteoplastic flap approach is generally considered when wide exposure and visualization are needed such as with frontal sinus neoplasm, trauma, and frontal sinus CSF leak.

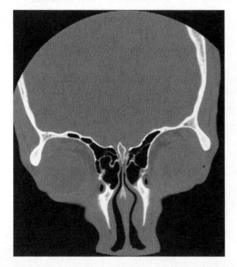

Fig. 5.6. Coronal view of Type III frontal cell

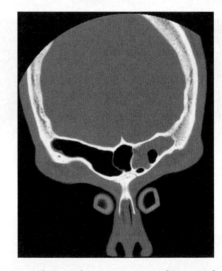

Fig. 5.7. Coronal view of superior extent of Type III frontal cell and associated frontal sinus opacification

Conclusion

Despite the tremendous advancements that have been made in the medical and surgical treatment of chronic rhinosinusitis, it remains one of the most challenging disease processes managed by otolaryngologists today. In 1946 Harris Mosher stated "frontal sinus surgery in my hands has been bitterly disappointing. Temporary favorable results have been common. Permanently favorable results I could never guarantee." His sentiment is true today, and only with long-term follow-up can we determine if our current treatment methods will result in consistent "permanently favorable results."

References

1. Benninger MS, Ferguson BJ, et al (2003) Adult chronic rhinosinusitis: Definitions, diagnosis, epidemiology and pathophysiology. Otolaryngol H N Surg 129(3 suppl): S1–S32
2. Bent JP, Cuilty-Siller C, Kuhn FA (1994) The frontal cell as a cause of frontal sinus obstruction. Am J Rhinol 8:185–191
3. Bent JP, Spears RA, Kuhn FA, et al (1997) Combined endoscopic intranasal and external frontal sinusotomy. Am J Rhinol 11:349–354
4. Bolger WE, Butzin CA, Parsons DS (1991) Paranasal sinus bony anatomic variations and mucosal abnormalities: CT analysis for endoscopic sinus surgery. Laryngoscope 101: 56–64
5. Draf W (1991) Endonasal micro-endoscopic frontal sinus surgery: The Fulda concept. Operative Techniques in Otolaryngology 2:234–240
6. Gross W, Gross C, Becker D et al (1995) Modified transnasal endoscopic Lothrop procedure as alternative to frontal sinus obliteration. Otolaryngol Head Neck Surg 113: 427–434
7. Hardy JM, Montgomery WW (1976) Osteoplastic frontal sinusotomy: An analysis of 250 operations. Ann Otol 85: 523
8. Jacobs JB, Lebowitz RA, Sorin A, Hariri S, Holliday R (2000) Preoperative sagittal CT evaluation of the frontal recess. Am J Rhinol 14(1):33–37
9. Kuhn FA, Javer AR, Nagpal K, Citardi MJ (2000) The frontal sinus rescue procedure: Early experience and three-year follow-up. Am J Rhinol 14(4):211–16
10. McLaughlin RB, Hwang PH, Lanza DC (1999) Endoscopic trans-septal frontal sinusotomy: The rationale and results of an alternative technique. Am J Rhinol 13:279–287
11. Schlosser RJ, London SD, Gwaltney JM Jr, Gross CW (2001) Microbiology of chronic frontal sinusitis. Laryngoscope 111(8):1330–32
12. Stammberger H, Kennedy DW, et al (1995) Paranasal sinuses: Anatomic terminology and nomenclature. The anatomic terminology group. Ann Otol Rhinol Laryngol 167 (-suppl):7–16
13. Tantilipikorn P, Fritz M, Tanabodee J, Lanza DC, Kennedy DW (2002) A comparison of endoscopic culture techniques for chronic rhinosinusitis. Am J Rhinol 16(5): 255–260
14. Weber R, Draf W, Kratzsch B, Hosemann W, Schaefer SD. Modern concepts of frontal sinus surgery. Laryngoscope 111(1):137–46
15. Wormald PJ, Xun-Chan SZ (2003) Surgical techniques for the removal of frontal recess cells obstructing the frontal ostium. Am J Rhinol 17(4): 221–226
16. Zeifer B (1998) Update on sinonasal imaging anatomy and inflammatory disease. Neuroimaging Clin North Am 8: 607–614

Microbiology of Chronic Frontal Sinusitis

6

Birgit Winther, Jack Gwaltney

Core Messages

- Because of limitations in sampling techniques, microbiology of chronic frontal rhinosinusitis remains poorly understood

- Obstruction of the frontal sinus outflow in the presence of pathogenic bacteria may yield frontal infection

- Surgical manipulation of the sinuses appears to impact subsequent microbiology of the disease process

Contents

Introduction

The microbiology of chronic rhinosinusitis is poorly understood. A major problem has been the sampling method used for collecting specimens for cultures. Most studies have employed surgical or swab specimens obtained during endoscopic surgery. It is not possible to know whether these specimens are contaminated with bacteria from the nasal passages as the result of surgical manipulation during the procedure. Only a few studies have employed the technique of aseptic sinus aspiration prior to beginning the surgical procedure. Another problem is that the bacteriological findings from pre- and postsurgery patients have often not been distinguished, although the two conditions are obviously different.

Chronic frontal sinusitis is less common than chronic maxillary sinusitis. A limited number of published studies have reported the microbiologic findings in patients with chronic frontal sinusitis. This chapter will discuss the pathology of frontal sinusitis and review current knowledge on its bacteriology.

Definitions

The clinical definition of acute infectious sinusitis has been based on a combination of various signs and symptoms and demonstration of a high titer ($\geq 10^4$ cfu/ml of sinus secretion) of bacteria in the sinus aspirate.

Histopathologic findings include [4]:

- Edema
- Massive infiltration with neutrophils
- Increased lymphocytes and plasma cells

- Microabcesses
- In severe cases thrombosed blood vessels and necrotic foci

The epithelial surface remains intact. Neutrophil infiltration has also been reported in viral rhinosinusitis [18]. The clinical definition of chronic sinusitis also depends on selected signs and symptoms, but a bacteriologic criterion is not well established. In fact the role of bacteria in the initial etiology of chronic sinusitis is not well established.

6

Pathologic findings in chronic sinusitis include [13]:

- Swelling of the ciliary membrane
- Formation of compound cilia
- Dropping of epithelial cells
- Metaplasia

The number of inflammatory cells correlates with the thickened antral mucosa and with amount of purulent secretion [7].

Frontal Sinus Outflow Anatomy and Patency by CT Scanning

The normal frontal sinus is fully aerated and believed to be sterile except during periods of transient bacterial contamination. CT study utilizing application of intranasal contrast medium has suggested that there is an open and easy communication from the nasal cavity to the frontal sinus cavity. Nasal fluid containing contrast medium can be detected in the frontal sinus after noseblowing in normal adult volunteers (Fig. 6.1). In this study, noseblowing generated an intranasal pressure of 60–70 mmHg, which is sufficient to propel nasal fluid through the frontal duct into the sinus [8]. At times polypoid tissue from the frontal sinus mucosa and viscous mucopus may occlude the frontal duct. CT scanning cannot accurately distinguish between mucosal swelling or the presence of viscous exudate when obstruction is present in the frontal duct and opacification observed in the frontal sinus.

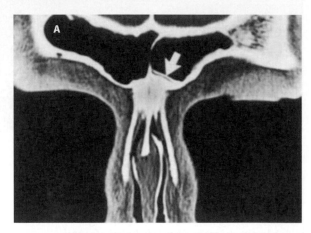

Fig. 6.1. Radiopaque contrast material (*arrow*) in the frontal sinus following noseblowing in healthy adult

Mucociliary Clearance in the Frontal Sinus

In the early 1930's Hilding [1] described the pattern of mucociliary clearance of the frontal sinus. Using fresh cadavers, ink was sprayed in a thin film over the mucosal surface of the sinus and was observed to be carried to the frontal ostium. Movements proceeded in a spiral pattern, and the velocity of flow increased as fluid approached the ostium.

Experimental Bacterial Infection of Canine Frontal Sinuses

In early work Arnold and coworkers [3] failed to produce experimental bacterial rhinitis by spraying bacteria into the nasal cavity in 42 healthy adults. They noted that 90%–95% of viable bacteria had disappeared within 5 to 10 min. Hilding [1] injected a bacterial suspension directly into the frontal sinus and also failed to produce infection; however, infection of the sinus was achieved by inoculation with a suspension of bacteria in warm milk. The milk coagulated after injection into the sinus and served to keep the bacteria in the sinus. No bacterial invasion of the frontal sinus mucosa was noted. During viral respiratory infection fibrin clots may be formed on the epithelial lining of the sinus [19], and similar to coagulated milk may provide substrate material to keep bacteria in the sinus.

Viral Rhino/Frontal Sinusitis

Viral respiratory tract infection produces a viscous exudate in the sinuses [9] and decreases the mucociliary clearance in the nose for several weeks [14]. Frontal sinus abnormalities with acute viral rhinosinusitis were demonstrated by CT scanning in 32% of 31 patients with acute viral rhinosinusitis [9]. It is unclear whether the frontal ostium also was occluded in those instances. The nasopharynx is believed to be the primary site of acute viral infection of the upper respiratory tract [20], but the nasal passage, paranasal sinuses, laryngeal and bronchial mucosa are also frequently involved. It is not clear how frequently respiratory viruses replicate in those secondary sites, but respiratory viruses have been recovered in cultures and identified by RT-PCR from sinus aspirates in patients with acute sinusitis [12, 15].

Chronic Bacterial Frontal Sinusitis

Specimens for bacterial cultures cannot be obtained from the frontal sinus cavity by way of the nasal passages. Frontal sinus mini-trephination is a technique that provides uncontaminated specimens from the sinus cavity for culture. Antila and co-workers recovered *H. influenza* and/or *S. pneumoniae* from 30% of 103 samples obtained by trephination of the frontal sinus in patients with acute frontal and maxillary sinusitis. Specimens were collected 24 h after initiation of antibiotic treatment [2]. In a study by Schlosser and co-workers [17] of 30 patients undergoing endoscopic surgery for chronic frontal sinus disease, 46 samples were obtained by trephination from the frontal sinus. Approximately one-third of the samples were negative for aerobic and anaerobic bacteria and fungi. There was a trend towards a different pattern of bacteria in patients with prior functional endoscopic sinus surgery (FESS) without frontal surgery versus patients with prior FESS with frontal "drill out" surgery, and compared to patients without any prior sinus surgery (Table 6.1). *H. influenzae* was isolated in two of eight samples from patients without prior FESS, but none of 21 samples from FESS patients without prior frontal sinus surgery (intact frontal sinus). *Staphylococcus aureus* and coagulase-negative Staphylococcus were isolated more frequently from patients with prior FESS with and with-

Table 6.1. Culture results of frontal sinus aspirates (46 trephines)

	No prior sinonasal surgery	Prior FESS[a] without frontal surgery	Prior surgery of frontal recess/sinus
No aerobic growth	37% (3/8)	38% (8/21)	33% (2/6)
Staphylococcus aureus	12% (1/8)	24% (5/21)	17% (1/6)
Coagulase-negative *Staphylococcus*	12% (1/8)	19% (4/21)	33% (2/6)
Haemophilus influenzae	25% (2/8)	0% (0/21)	17% (1/6)
Mixed oropharyngeal flora	12% (1/8)	5% (1/21)	17% (1/6)
Escherichia coli	0% (0/8)	5% (1/21)	0% (0/6)
Xanthamona	0% (0/8)	5% (1/21)	0% (0/6)
Group A *Streptococcus*	0% (0/8)	0% (0/21)	17% (1/6)
Serratia sp	0% (0/8)	0% (0/21)	17% (1/6)
Gram-negative rods-not specified	12% (1/8)	0% (0/21)	0% (0/6)
S. pneumonia	0% (0/8)	5% (1/21)	0% (0/6)
Anaerobic bacteria (Gram-Positive cocci)	0% (0/7)	0% (0/21)	25% (1/4)
Fungi (*Penicillium*)	0% (0/6)	7% (1/14)	0% (0/5)

[a] FESS, functional endoscopic sinus surgery.

With permission from The Laryngoscope [17].

6

out frontal surgery [43% (9/21) and 50% (3/6), respectively] compared to patients without FESS (25%; 2/8). One of six samples from patients with prior FESS with frontal sinus surgery had *H. influenzae* recovered. An array of other bacteria were also cultured, including mixed oropharyngeal flora, Group A Streptococcus, *S. pneumoniae, Escherichia coli, Serratia spp.*, and *Xanthomonas* (Table 6.1). Only one sample was positive for anaerobic bacteria, from a patient with prior FESS including frontal sinus surgery. This is in contrast to the studies by Brook, who reported frequent recovery of anaerobic bacteria when cultures were obtained through osteoplastic flaps from 13 patients with chronic frontal sinusitis [6]. The discrepancy between the studies is unexplained but may relate to the different sampling methods used.

Chronic Fungal Frontal Sinusitis

The frequency of isolation of fungi from the paranasal sinus of patients with chronic sinus disease has varied hugely. Ponikau and co-workers found at least one fungus in 96% of 210 patients with chronic sinusitis and from 100% of 14 healthy controls [16]. The fungal species recovered were similar in both groups. Fungal cultures from specimens obtained by mini trephination of the frontal sinus have recently been reported by Schlosser and co-workers [17]. They found penicillium in 4% of 24 samples from patients who had had prior FESS without frontal sinus surgery.

Chronic Inflammatory Sinus Disease in Postsurgery Patients

Bacteria are present in the nasopharynx at all times, while the mucosa of the intact sinus with normal mucociliary clearance is thought to be sterile [5].

Chronic sinus disease in patients with previous sinus surgery is characterized by:

- Decreased clearance of mucus from the paranasal sinuses
- Prolonged presence of gram-positive and/or gram-negative bacteria in the sinuses

Very little is known about the pathogenesis of chronic sinus disease in either the pre- or postsurgical state. The bacteria present in postsurgical patients do not appear to be the original cause of the disease. It is not clear to what extent the bacteria are responsible for the ongoing disease in patients who remain symptomatic after surgery, but they are believed to play a major role in the exudates and crusting which characterize the process. New information suggests their role may depend on the PAMP (pathogen-associated molecular pattern) of a given flora [10]. Toll-like receptors (TLRs) of the innate immune system are essential for shaping the adaptive immune response. The TLRs provide a signal that increases the antigenic function of immature dendritic cells, which influence the differentiation into Th1 or Th2 cytokine-producing T-lymphocytes [11]. A concurrent viral upper respiratory tract infection or allergen exposure may temporally change the existing balance of PAMP and the immune response in patients with chronic sinus disease. The degree of activation of pro-inflammatory signal cascades in response to bacterial flora in chronic sinus disease needs further investigation.

Conclusion

Microbiology of chronic frontal rhinosinusitis remains a controversial topic. Difficulty in specimen acquisition and occurrence of previous surgery are but two variables that may impact data. While the frontal sinuses are usually presumably sterile, in the setting of frontal outflow obstruction accompanied by bacterial inoculation of the sinus, infection may arise. However, the exact mechanism resulting in the development of chronic inflammation remains elusive.

References

1. Anderson Hilding (1934) Studies of common cold and nasal physiology. Trans Am Laryngol Assoc 56 : 253–271
2. Antila J, Suonpaa J, Lehtonen O (1997) Bacteriological evaluation of 194 adult patients with acute frontal sinusitis and finding of simultaneous maxillary sinusitis. Acta Otolaryngol (Stock) Suppl 529 : 162–164

3. Arnold L, Ostrom ML, Singer C (1928) Autosterilizing power of the nasal mucous membrane. Proc Soc Exp Biol and Med 25:624

4. Berger G, Kattan A, Bernheim J, Ophir D, Finkelsein Y (2000) Acute sinusitis: A histopathological and immunohistochemical study. Laryngoscope 110:2089–2094

5. Bjorkwall T (1950) Bacteriological examination in maxillary sinusitis: bacterial flora of the maxillary antrum. Acta Otolaryngol Suppl (Stockh) 83:1–58

6. Brook I (2002) Bacteriology of acute and chronic frontal sinusitis. Arch Otolaryngol Head and Neck Surg 128:583–585

7. Forsgren K, Fukami M, Penttila M, Kumlien J, Stierna P (1996) Endoscopic and Caldwell-Luc approaches in chronic maxillary sinusitis: A comparative histopathologic study on preoperative and postoperative mucosal morphology. Ann Otol Rhinol Laryngol 104:350–357

8. Gwaltney JM Jr, Hendley JO, Phillips CD, Bass CR, Mygind N, Winther B (2000) Nose blowing propels nasal fluid into the paranasal sinuses. Clin Inf Dis 30:387–391

9. Gwaltney JM Jr, Phillips CD, Miller DR, Riker DK (1994) Computed tomographic study of the common cold. New Eng J Med 330:25–30

10. Medzhitov R (2001) Toll-like receptors and innate immunity. Nature reviews. Immunology 1:135–45

11. Medzhitov R, Janeway C Jr (2000) Innate immunity. New Eng J Med 343:338–344

12. Hamory BH, Sande MA, Sydnor A Jr., Seale DL, Gwaltney JM (1979) Etiology and antimicrobial therapy of acute maxillary sinusitis. J Infect Dis 139:197–202

13. Ohashi Y, Nakai Y (1983) Functional and morphologic pathology of chronic sinusitis mucous membrane. Acta Otolaryngol (Suppl 397) 11–48

14. Pedersen M, Sakakura Y, Winther B, Brofeldt S, Mygind N (1983) Nasal mucociliary transport, number of ciliated cells, and beating pattern in naturally acquired common colds. Eur J Resp Dis 64(supp 128):355–364

15. Pitkaranta A, Arruda E, Malmberg H, Hayden FG (1997) Detection of rhinovirus in sinus brushing of patients with acute community-acquired sinusitis by reverse transcription-PCR. J Clin Microbiol 35:1791–1793

16. Ponikau JU, Sherris DA, Kern EB, Holmburger HA, Frigas E, Gaffey TA, Roberts GD (1999) The diagnosis and incidence of allergic fungal sinusitis. Mayo Clin Proc 74:877–884

17. Schlosser RJ, London SD, Gwaltney JM Jr., Gross CW (2001) Microbiology of chronic frontal sinusitis. Laryngoscope 111;1330–1332

18. Winther B (1994) Effects on the nasal mucosa of upper respiratory viruses (common cold). Danish Med Bull 41:193–204

19. Winther B, Gwaltney JM, Humphries, Hendley JO (2002) Cross-linked fibrin in nasal fluid of patients with the common cold. CID 34;708–710

20. Winther B, Gwaltney JM Jr., Mygind N, Turner RB, Hendley JO (1986) Intranasal spread of rhinovirus during point-inoculation of the nasal mucosa. J Am Med Assoc 256:1763–1767

Chapter 7

Orbital Complications of Frontal Sinusitis

Robert T. Adelson, Bradley F. Marple

Core Messages

- The most common cause of orbital infections is sinusitis, most often seen in the second to third decades of life

- The propagation of orbital infection is facilitated by the valveless veins of the orbit that allow free communication between facial, sinus, and surrounding venous networks

- Orbital complications most often arise from the ethmoid sinuses; however, frontal sinusitis complications may progress rapidly and result in worse outcomes

- The orbital septum is the key feature in the classification of orbital infections

- Ophthalmological consultation is critical when physical exam findings suggest postseptal spread of orbital infection

- The bacteriology of orbital complications of sinusitis is similar to that of the sinusitis itself

- Contrast CT scans can distinguish cellulitis or abscess and assist in the planning of surgery when it is indicated

- The most common orbital complication of sinusitis is orbital cellulitis, which most often responds rapidly to intravenous antibiotics. Progression of symptoms or failure to respond to antibiotic treatment is an indication for surgical therapy

- Surgical intervention in postseptal orbital complications of sinusitis is frequently required (12%–66%)

Contents

Introduction

Sinusitis, in the antibiotic era, is a disease process for which infectious complications have become increasingly uncommon. It is estimated that a maximum of 1%–3% of all sinus infections result in intraorbital or intracranial complications [22]. The preantibiotic era was witness to a 17% incidence of death and 20% incidence of blindness in postseptal infections, declining in the modern era to 1%–2% and 1%–8%, respectively [6, 22]. The persistence of such morbidities demands further study of the complications of sinusitis.

Frontal sinusitis and orbital complications thereof is a narrow clinical window that demands both a high level of diagnostic acumen and technical ability to engender a successful outcome. A thorough understanding of the pathogenesis, diagnosis, and current treatment recommendations for orbital complications of frontal sinusitis will allow physicians to decrease the morbidity and mortality associated with this condition.

Demographics

The overwhelming majority of orbital infections are a result of sinusitis, representing greater than 70% of cases in most series [8, 10, 11].

The most common complications of sinusitis in order of frequency are [1, 19, 20, 28]:

- Orbital involvement
- Intracranial complications
- Frontal bone osteomyelitis
- Soft tissue abscesses

Several case series have characterized further the population of patients affected by orbital complications of sinusitis, particularly in those patients with frontal sinusitis. Eighty-five percent of patients with orbital complications of paranasal sinusitis are within the pediatric age group, and within this group 68% are less than 15 years old [15, 24]. As the frontal sinus does not begin to pneumatize significantly until six - years of age, the population experiencing complications related to the frontal sinus is correspondingly narrowed [1, 11]. Orbital complications of frontal sinusitis are most common in patients in the second to third decades of life (average age of 25 years), in males more so than in females (ratio of 2.6:1 to 3.3:1), and involve the left eye more frequently than the right [19, 20, 24, 28]. The discrepant age, sex, and laterality trends have been noted by multiple authors, yet convincing explanations are lacking.

Relevant Orbital and Sinus Anatomy

The intimate relationship between the paranasal sinuses and the vital surrounding organs is foremost in the mind of surgeons whose routine operative approaches demand expert navigation of this compact, complex anatomy. In the context of acute sinusitis with orbital complications, anatomic landmarks are further obscured and surgery made cumbersome by the bleeding tendencies of inflamed sinonasal mucosa.

The orbit is separated from the ethmoid sinuses medially by a thin and often dehiscent lamina papyracea, from the maxillary sinus by a similarly thin orbital floor, and from the frontal sinus by a portion of the orbital roof. The bony orbit is vulnerable to spread of infection, directly or by thrombophlebitic spread, via the numerous fissures and foramina that transmit vessels and nerves through the sinuses, orbit, and intracranial space [15]. The periosteal lining of the orbital bones, the periorbita, is an additional layer of separation between the orbital contents and the sinuses. This fibrous tissue is firmly adherent to underlying bone at the orbital rims, suture lines, orbital fissures, and lacrimal crest but loosely adherent elsewhere, allowing infection to dissect into these potential subperiosteal spaces [3]. The orbital septum, a key feature of the classification of orbital infections, arises from the union of the periorbita with the periosteum of the forehead and cheekbones at the orbital rim (the *arcus marginalis*) [3, 21]. The orbital septa of the upper and lower eyelids form an anatomic barrier to infection and define the preseptal and postseptal spaces [4].

The valveless veins of the orbit play a key role in propagation of orbital infections, as they allow free communication between the facial, sinus, orbital, and intracranial venous network [25]. The superior ophthalmic vein is a well-defined vessel formed by the union of the angular and supraorbital veins, which receives multiple tributaries as it travels posterolaterally through the orbit to exit via the superior orbital fissure to enter the cavernous sinus [3, 13]. The inferior ophthalmic vein is a less well-defined structure, originating near the anterior orbital floor and terminating by sending one branch to the pterygoid plexus via the inferior orbital fissure and a second, larger contribution to the superior ophthalmic vein; both will ultimately drain into the cavernous sinus [3].

Although previously it had been widely accepted that lymphatics are absent within the orbit, orbital lymphangiomas have been reported and recent histochemical studies have confirmed the presence of lymphatics within the lacrimal gland and in the dura mater of the optic nerve [3, 6, 21, 22, 26]. The anatomy of the orbital lymphatic system is still under active investigation, and while its role in orbital complications of sinusitis is not likely to be of any real clinical significance, a definitive answer is not yet available. In contradistinction, the upper and lower eyelids have well-described lymphatic networks, and these preseptal tissues drain into preauricular and submandibular nodes [21].

The anatomy of the frontal sinus foreshadows its potential for development of orbital and intracranial complications of sinusitis. The horizontal orbital plate of the frontal bone, the thinnest wall of the frontal sinus, forms the roof of the orbit and articulates with the ethmoid bone to contribute to both the roof of the nasal cavity and the floor of the anterior cranial fossa [16]. Venous drainage from the frontal sinus begins in diploic veins which pass through the multiple anterior and posterior table foramina (Breschet's canals), coalescing in sequentially larger diploic veins, developing into the frontal diploic vein that joins at the supraorbital notch with the supraorbital vein to create the superior ophthalmic vein described above [16]. Although not specifically addressed in this chapter, the diploic veins of Breschet contribute significantly to frontal bone osteomyelitis and intracranial complications of sinusitis via their communications with dural sinuses and the marrow cavity of the frontal bone [6, 15, 16].

Pathogenesis of Orbital Complications of Sinusitis

Orbital complications of sinusitis are most often attributable to the ethmoid sinuses, though 84% of cases have radiographic evidence of disease involving two or more sinuses, and some series establish a minimum pattern of concomitant maxillary, ethmoid, and frontal sinusitis in 79% of those cases with orbital complications [6, 22, 10, 19, 29].

It is generally accepted that orbital infections arising from a sinonasal source can arise by two mechanisms [5, 6, 10, 15, 18, 23, 27, 28, 29]:

- Direct extension
- Retrograde thrombophlebitis

The bony limits of the orbit are not perfect barriers to direct extension of infection into the orbit. Congenital or acquired bony dehiscences, neurovascular foramina, and open suture lines all constitute mechanisms by which direct extension can occur [5, 6, 23, 11, 18, 28]. The valveless veins of the sinonasal cavity and orbit provide a more circuitous route by which a septic thrombophlebitis can extend to involve the orbit [5, 6, 11, 18, 23, 28].

Classification of Orbital Complications of Sinusitis

An understanding of the relevant sinonasal and orbital anatomy as well as the mechanisms by which orbital complications develop is required to classify the disease state so that treatment recommendations can be made and outcomes studied. Hubert proposed the earliest well-documented classification scheme based on his experience with 114 patients in the preantibiotic era [14]. The classification of patients into five groups based on the anatomy involved, perceived progression of infection, responsiveness to treatment, and general prognosis is a convention that is still in use today, though as the widely accepted schema proposed by Chandler [5]. Chandler's work solidified the utility of this classification system, and his therapeutic principles characterize the modern approach to managing orbital complications of sinusitis (Table 7.1) [5, 13, 25].

Table 7.1. Chandler classification systems for orbital complications of sinusitis

Group 1	Inflammatory edema (preseptal cellulitis)
Group 2	Orbital cellulitis
Group 3	Subperiosteal abscess
Group 4	Orbital abscess
Group 5	Cavernous sinus thrombosis

From [5]

- Group I – Inflammatory edema (preseptal cellulitis) represents swelling of the eyelids anterior to the orbital septum thought to be secondary to restricted venous drainage. The eyelids are usually not tender and, as inflammation does not involve the postseptal structures, chemosis, extraocular muscle movement limitations, and vision impairment should be absent [5, 6, 11, 18]. Authors disagree regarding the absence [5, 10, 27] or presence of mild proptosis at this stage [6, 22]. The degree of preseptal inflammation may hamper accurate assessment of proptosis, especially when examining pediatric patients.

- Group II – Orbital cellulitis results in a pronounced edema and inflammation of the orbital soft tissue without frank abscess formation [5, 6, 22]. It is vital to detect the signs of proptosis and decreased extraocular motility, as these are considered reliable signs of orbital soft tissue involvement [10, 19, 23]. Chemosis is almost always present to varying degrees, yet vision loss is very unusual in this stage, but should be monitored carefully [6, 18, 22].

- Group III – Subperiosteal abscess develops in the potential space between periorbita and bone [5]. The orbital contents are displaced by the mass effect of a collection of subperiosteal pus, frequently in an inferolateral direction. Chemosis and proptosis are reliably present, although decreased ocular mobility and vision loss may take some time to develop and are not always present early in the course of this stage [10, 15, 22, 24, 25, 27].

- Group IV – Orbital abscess, a collection of purulent, necrotic material within the orbital tissue, can develop as a result of a progressive orbital cellulitis or from the rupture of a subperiosteal abscess [5, 6, 15]. Severe proptosis and near complete ophthalmoplegia are noted, and visual loss is increasingly common within this group [10, 22, 27, 29].

- Group V – Cavernous sinus thrombosis may include such nonspecific signs and symptoms as fever, headache, periorbital edema, and photophobia in addition to more specific findings of proptosis, chemosis, ophthalmoplegia, and decreased visual acuity; however, the development of *bilateral* ocular symptoms is the classic finding in this condition [6, 15, 10, 23]. A more expeditious diagnosis is possible when patients demonstrate palsies of those cranial nerves transmitted through the cavernous sinus (III, IV, V1, V2, VI) or develop meningitic symptoms in the presence of a unilateral orbital infection [15, 24, 25].

Despite the clarity and near-ubiquitous application of Chandler's classification system, several other authors have modified his work, and their contributions are useful in highlighting focal changes in our concepts of orbital infections as well as advances in diagnostic technology over the last 34 years.

Schramm's large series of orbital cellulitis allowed him to identify periorbital (preseptal) cellulitis with chemosis as a distinct grouping intermediate in prognosis between Chandler's group I and group III (Table 7.2) [24]. Those patients with periorbital cellulitis with chemosis did not always respond to parenteral antibiotic therapy alone, and therefore frequent serial examinations and a lower threshold for surgical intervention are warranted [11, 24].

Moloney modified Chandler's classification to assign lower priority to orbital infections anterior to the septum, and then delineated the progression of postseptal, intraorbital infections (Table 7.3) [17]. Mortimore and Wormald applied advanced computed tomography (CT) imaging to Moloney's concept of dividing preseptal and postseptal infections, relying upon further radiologic differentiation to be made between cellulitis and an abscess [19, 20]. It is not clear that further, more stringent classifications of orbital infections have altered therapeutic strategies.

Table 7.2. Orbital cellulitis

Periorbital cellulitis
Periorbital cellulitis with chemosis
Orbital cellulitis
Subperiosteal abscess
Orbital abscess
Cavernous sinus thrombosis

From [24]

Table 7.3. Comparison of Moloney classification and the Groote Shuur modification of Moloney

Moloney	Groote Schuur modification
Pre-septal cellulitis	Pre-septal a. Cellulitis b Abscess
Subperiosteal abscess	Post-septal (subperiosteal) a. Phlegmon/cellulitis b. Abscess
Orbital cellulitis	Post-septal (intraconal) a. Cellulitis b. Abscess
Orbital abscess	I. Localized II. Diffuse
Cavernous sinus thrombosis	Considered intracranial

From [19]

Bacteriology

Orbital complications do not have a bacterial profile different from that of acute rhinosinusitis [6, 10, 11, 15, 22].

The most commonly cultured organisms in orbital infections are [1, 6, 10, 15]:

- *Streptococcus pneumoniae*
- *Haemophilus influenzae*
- *Moraxella catarrhalis*
- *Staphylococcus aureus*
- *Streptococcus pyogenes*

A study of patients with simultaneous frontal and maxillary sinusitis found *H. influenzae* and *S. pneumoniae* to be the most commonly isolated organisms [2].

The existing literature does not support a substantial difference in the bacterial populations implicated in frontal sinusitis from that of ethmoid sinusitis. The frontal sinus is the most frequent culprit for intracranial complications of sinusitis, and in these instances, *S. aureus* and polymicrobial infections are found at a slightly increased frequency [11]. The incidence of bacteremia in patients with orbital complications is greatest in children and declines steadily with age [6]. Schramm et al. reported bacteremia in 33% of children under 4 years old, yet demonstrated positive blood cultures in only 5% of the adult patients in a large case series [24].

Diagnostic Evaluation

The various systems for classifying orbital infections emphasize the importance of accurately differentiating between preseptal and postseptal involvement.

Patients typically present with:

- A history of recent upper respiratory infection or symptoms of acute bacterial rhinosinusitis
- And demonstrate:
- Fever
- Edematous eyelids
- Conjunctival injection
- Varying degrees of discomfort

Preseptal cellulitis is the most commonly encountered orbital complication of sinusitis, with multiple large studies documenting a frequency of 48% of such complications seen at tertiary referral centers and nearly 80% of the orbital complications seen overall [6, 10, 24, 28, 29]. Preseptal infections do not require imaging studies [6, 7, 10, 22, 23, 29].

Physical exam findings can be suggestive of a postseptal process, particularly the development of gaze restriction and proptosis [5, 15, 18, 27].

Signs of postseptal involvement include:

- Proptosis
- Gaze restriction
- Decreased visual acuity
- Color vision changes
- Afferent pupillary defect

Ophthalmologic examination is critical in measuring proptosis, evaluating extraocular motility, and, if

7

necessary, determining intraocular pressure. Traditionally, imaging studies are obtained when the history and physical exam are consistent with postseptal disease [7, 15, 19, 28, 29]. To further clarify those signs of postseptal infection, Younis suggested that the indications for obtaining a CT scan are identical to the indications for surgery, as addressed below [9, 29].

Contrast-enhanced CT scans of the sinuses in axial and coronal planes are essential to surgical planning, as the modality accurately distinguishes between cellulitis and abscesses and identifies which sinuses will need surgical drainage [6, 15, 20, 23, 25]. Magnetic resonance imaging (MRI) offers superior soft-tissue resolution and is most appropriate in the context of intracranial complications, while CT remains the standard initial, and often definitive, modality in the diagnosis of sinusitis and its orbital extension [29]. In one well-controlled study, clinical examination correctly diagnosed 81% of the cases of orbital complications of sinusitis, while 91% accuracy was achieved on the basis of CT findings alone [29]. Despite the advances in technology, CT findings are not absolute. Patt and Manning attribute four cases of blindness in a series of 159 patients with complicated acute sinusitis to negative or equivocal CT findings that delayed surgical therapy [23]. Radiographic imaging is integral to the diagnosis, staging, and surgical therapy for postseptal infections, but does not substitute for therapeutic decision-making.

Frontal sinus disease can be well-delineated only on CT imaging. Preoperative recognition of a frontal sinus etiology or an abscess in proximity to the frontal sinus is essential to proper surgical planning [7, 9]. There is some indication that frontal sinusitis complications may progress rapidly and result in worse outcomes than those infections arising from other paranasal sinuses [1]. Owing to the proximity and intimate connections of the frontal sinus to both the intracranial and orbital anatomy, response to therapy and progression of symptoms are especially important in patients with complicated frontal sinusitis.

Treatment of Orbital Complications of Sinusitis

Therapeutic options for the orbital complications of sinusitis generally correlate with the classification of

infections. In general, treatment options will be based on the presence or absence of orbital signs (gaze restriction and proptosis), location of infection with regard to the orbital septum, progression of symptoms, responsiveness to medical therapy, and additional patient characteristics such as immune status and status of the contralateral eye [22, 23, 28].

Medical Therapy for Orbital Complications

Preseptal cellulitis, the most common orbital complication, is treated empirically with broad-spectrum intravenous antibiotics that cover the organisms listed above, have meaningful cerebrospinal fluid (CSF) penetration, and possesses activity against β-lactamase producing strains [6, 22]. Adjunctive topical and parenteral decongestants are often added, though steroids are not thought to be helpful [19, 24]. Patients who lack signs of postseptal involvement, such as proptosis, gaze restriction, decreased visual acuity, color vision changes, or afferent pupillary defect may be observed with serial ophthalmologic exams while receiving intravenous antibiotic therapy, deferring a CT scan for 24–48 h [6, 8, 10, 15, 19, 22, 28]. Progression of symptoms or failure to respond to antibiotics within 48 h of treatment necessitates a CT scan and is, in itself, an indication for surgical therapy.

Surgical Therapy for Orbital Infections

True preseptal cellulitis responds rapidly to intravenous antibiotics, and only in the rare case will surgery be required; typically the incision and drainage of a coalescing lid abscess [22]. In contrast, surgical intervention in postseptal disease is required in 12% to 66% of orbital complications of acute sinusitis [12, 24]. The indications for surgical therapy in postseptal infections comprise an evolving consensus of opinions from a number of large case series.

Surgery is recommended if any one of the following four indications is met [6, 23, 24, 28]:

■ CT evidence of abscess formation
■ Decreased visual acuity on presentation (20/60 or worse)

- Severe orbital complications on initial presentation with ipsilateral sinusitis (blindness, afferent papillary reflex, ophthalmoplegia)
- Progression of symptoms or failure to improve during the first 48 h of appropriate medical treatment

Immunocompromised patients (diabetes, chemotherapy, HIV) should be approached with a lower threshold for surgical intervention [23].

Though the above recommendations are widely accepted, dissenting opinions do exist. Souliere reported successful treatment with decongestants and intravenous antibiotics in five pediatric patients with subperiosteal abscesses and anterior ethmoiditis (Chandler Group III) [26]. In contrasting the risks of death or blindness resulting from progression of postseptal infection with the risks of endoscopic surgical techniques, our practice has been to favor operative exploration with regard to the indications listed above.

A number of different surgical techniques are applicable to the treatment of orbital complications of orbital sinusitis, though it is universally agreed that operative intervention should address the orbit and the paranasal sinuses simultaneously [6]. The advent of endoscopic surgical techniques has greatly reduced the morbidity of operative treatment. Chandler groups II (orbital cellulitis) and III (subperiosteal abscess) are routinely treated endoscopically; however, when inflammation precludes adequate drainage of the orbital infection, or ventilation of the involved sinuses, external techniques may be employed [20, 22, 25]. Chandler group IV usually requires an external ethmoidectomy and orbitotomy, though endoscopic techniques are gaining favor [6]. Cavernous sinus thrombosis, Chandler group V, is increasingly considered an intracranial complication of sinusitis, and as such its management should include neurosurgical consultation. Intravenous antibiotics are the primary therapeutic measure, though endoscopic surgery directed toward the involved sinuses (usually the ethmoid and sphenoid) is always recommended [6, 15, 19, 20, 22, 28]. Less clear is the utility of adjunctive steroids and heparin. Recent literature supports the use of steroids for cases of pituitary insufficiency; however, systemic anticoagulation remains controversial, balancing the bleeding risks with a potential decrease in thrombus propagation [6, 22].

Treatment of Orbital Complications of Frontal Sinusitis

The role of surgery in treating the orbital complications of frontal sinusitis is highlighted by the technical difficulties of operating on the acutely inflamed frontal sinus. Though the frontal sinus is only the third most frequently involved sinus in orbital infections, Hawkins' series found surgery to be required in every case of complicated frontal sinusitis [12]. Again, authors intimate that although frontal sinusitis is a less common source of orbital complications, those that take their origin from this sinus tend to be more aggressive in nature and portend more difficult clinical courses.

External frontoethmoidectomy had been an effective, commonly performed technique in the acute setting; however, complications including stenosis of the frontal sinus drainage tract (30%), CSF leak (5%), and diplopia (2%) have allowed endoscopic techniques to supplant this approach [20]. Frontal sinus trephine is an older technique that still has clinical value in the era of endoscopic sinus surgery. This simple and safe procedure can be employed acutely to treat complicated frontal sinusitis, allowing the surgeon to defer an endoscopic frontal sinusotomy until a time at which the operative field surrounding the frontal recess is less obscured by inflammation [20].

Conclusion

Orbital complications of sinusitis, though less frequent in the antibiotic era, are a source of morbidity and mortality that can be reduced further by attentive physical examination, prompt medical therapy, and strict adherence to the recommendations for surgical intervention. Orbital infections resulting from frontal sinusitis may be associated with a more

7

aggressive course, require surgery at a higher rate, and require external procedures if the challenging frontal recess anatomy is sufficiently obscured by inflammation. The role of intraoperative CT guidance in specifically treating orbital complications of sinusitis may have particular utility in allowing a wholly endoscopic approach to treating infections arising from acute frontal sinusitis.

References

1. Altman KW, Austin MB, Tom LWC et al (1997) Complications of frontal sinusitis in adolescents: Case presentations and treatment options. Int J Pediatr Otorhinolaryngol 41: 9–20
2. Antila J, Suonpaa J, Lehtonen O (1997) Bacteriological evaluation of 194 patients with acute frontal sinusitis and findings of simultaneous maxillary sinusitis. Acta Otolaryngol Suppl 529: 162–169
3. Bedrossian EH (2002) Surgical anatomy of the orbit. In: Della Rocca RC, Bedrossian EH, Arthurs BP (eds) Ophthalmic plastic surgery: Decision making and techniques. McGraw-Hill, New York, pp 207–227
4. Bedrossian EH (2002) Surgical anatomy of the eyelids. In: Della Rocca RC, Bedrossian EH, Arthurs BP (eds) Ophthalmic plastic surgery: Decision making and techniques. McGraw-Hill, New York, pp 25–41
5. Chandler JR, Langenbrunner DJ, Stevens ER (1970) The pathogenesis of orbital complications in acute sinusitis. Laryngoscope 80: 1414–1428
6. Choi SS, Grundfast KM (2001) Complications in sinus disease. In: Kennedy DW, Bolger WE, Zinreich SJ (eds) Diseases of the sinuses: Diagnosis and management. B.C. Decker, Ontario, Canada, pp 169–177
7. Clary RA, Cunningham MJ, Eavey RD (1992) Orbital complications of acute sinusitis: Comparison of computed tomography scan and surgical findings. Ann Otol Rhinol Laryngol 101: 598–600
8. Davis JP, Stearns MP (1994) Orbital complications of sinusitis: Avoid delays in diagnosis. Postgrad Med J 70: 108–110
9. Garcia CE, Cunningham MJ, Clary RA et al (1993) The etiologic role of frontal sinusitis in pediatric orbital abscesses. Am J Otolaryngol 14: 449–452
10. Goodwin WJ (1995) Orbital complications of ethmoiditis. Otolaryngol Clin North Amer 18: 139–147
11. Goldberg AN, Oroszlan G, Anderson TD (2001) Complications of frontal sinusitis and their management. Otolaryngol Clin North Amer 34: 211–225
12. Hawkins DB, Clark RW (1977) Orbital involvement in acute sinusitis. Clin Pediatr 16: 464–471
13. Healy GB (1997) The pathogenesis of orbital complications in acute sinusitis. Laryngoscope 107: 441–446
14. Hubert L (1937) Orbital infections due to nasal sinusitis. NY Med J 37: 1559–1564
15. Kendall KA, Senders CW (1996) Orbital and intracranial complications of sinusitis in children and adults. In: Gershwin ME, Incaudo GA (eds) Diseases of the sinuses: A comprehensive textbook of diagnosis and treatment. Humana Press, Totowa, New Jersey, pp. 247–272
16. McLaughlin RB, Rehl RM, Lanza DC (2001) Clinically relevant frontal sinus anatomy and physiology. Otolaryngol Clin North Amer 34: 1–22
17. Moloney JR, Badham NJ, McRae A (1987) The acute orbit, preseptal (periorbital) cellulitis, subperiosteal abscess and orbital cellulitis due to sinusitis. J Laryngol Otol 101 (12supp): 1–18
18. Morgan PR, Morrison WV (1980) Complications of frontal and ethmoid sinusitis. Laryngoscope 90: 661–666
19. Mortimore S, Wormald PJ (1997) The Groote-Schuur hospital classification of the orbital complications of sinusitis. J Laryngol Otol 111: 719–723
20. Mortimore S, Wormald PJ (1999) Management of acute complicated sinusitis: A five year review. Otolaryngol Head Neck 121: 639–642
21. Nerad JA (2001) Clinical anatomy. In: Nerad JA, Krachmer, JH (eds) Occuloplastic surgery: The requisites in ophthalmology. Mosby, St. Louis, Missouri, pp. 25–70
22. Osguthorpe JD, Hochman M (1993) Inflammatory sinus diseases affecting the orbit. Otolaryngol Clin North Am 26: 657–671
23. Patt BS, Manning SC (1991) Blindness resulting from orbital complications of sinusitis. Otolaryngol Head Neck Surg 104: 789–795
24. Schramm VL, Curtin HD, Kennerdell JS (1982) Evaluation of orbital cellulites and results of treatment. Laryngoscope 92: 732–738
25. Shahin J, Gullane PJ, Dayal VS (1987) Orbital complications of acute sinusitis. 16: 23–27
26. Souliere CR, Antoine GA, Martin MP et al (1990) Selective non-surgical management of subperiosteal abscess of the orbit: Computerized tomography and clinical course as indication for surgical drainage. Int J Pediatr Otorhinolaryngol 19: 109–119
27. Wagenmann M, Naclerio RM (1992) Complications of sinusitis. J Allergy Clin Immunol 90: 552–554
28. Younis RT, Lazar RH, Bustillo A et al (2001) Orbital infection as a complication of sinusitis: Are diagnostic and treatment trends changing? Ear Nose Throat J 81: 771–775
29. Younis RT, Anand VK, Davidson B (2002) The role of computed tomography and magnetic resonance imaging in patients with sinusitis with complications. Laryngoscope 112: 224–229

Chapter 8

CNS Complications of Frontal Sinus Disease

Andrew P. Lane

Core Messages

- **(Overview)** Although less common since the advent of antibiotics, CNS complications of frontal sinusitis still occur and warrant a high index of suspicion to permit timely diagnosis and management

- CNS complications of frontal sinusitis include meningitis, epidural abscess, subdural empyema, intracerebral abscess, and thrombosis of the cavernous sinus or superior sagittal sinus

- The frontal sinus is the most common sinus source of CNS complications

- Infection spreads to the CNS through vascular communications between the frontal sinus diploic veins and the dural venous plexus

- Progressive headache and fever are the most common presenting signs of CNS complications, although some may present silently

- The single most important study to obtain in the diagnosis of CNS complications of frontal sinusitis is a CT scan with and without contrast

- CNS complications of frontal sinusitis have a high incidence of long-term morbidity and mortality even with antibiotic therapy

- Treatment of CNS complications generally includes medical management with intravenous antibiotics, as well as surgical drainage of the frontal sinus and intracranial collections as indicated

Contents

Introduction

In the antibiotic era, intracranial complications of sinusitis have become less commonplace, but nevertheless continue to occur and be associated with significant morbidity and mortality. The frontal sinus is the most common source of intracranial complications of sinusitis, followed by the ethmoid, sphenoid, and maxillary sinuses [1]. Spread of infection from the frontal sinus to the intracranial space typically occurs by hematogenous spread through a communicating venous system. The small, valveless diploic veins (veins of Breschet) that extend through the posterior table of the sinus directly contribute to the venous plexi of the dura and periosteum [26]. Bacterial thrombi can travel throughout this network and seed intracranial sites remote from the frontal sinus, leading to meningitis, epidural or intracerebral abscesses, or subdural empyema. In some instances, a retrograde thrombophlebitis can develop and cause the further complications of cavernous or superior sagittal sinus thrombosis. Such life-threatening conditions must be recognized promptly and treated aggressively.

Epidemiology

Frontal sinusitis occurs most commonly in adolescent and young men, correlating with the time of peak development of the vascularity and pneumatization of the frontal sinus [19, 20, 32, 33]. The true incidence of frontal sinusitis complications today is unknown. Although the incidence of frontal sinusitis has not changed, it is clear that complications of sinusitis have become much less common, as antibiotic use has increased. More than a decade ago, a study of patients hospitalized for sinusitis showed an incidence of intracranial complications of 3.7% in that group [8]. Another study from the 1960's reported a 10% incidence of intracranial complications among patients admitted to the hospital for frontal sinusitis [2]. Regardless of how often it occurs, there continues to be a significant degree of morbidity and mortality associated with intracranial complications of acute frontal sinusitis, particularly if intervention is delayed.

Signs and Symptoms

The typical presentation of CNS complications of frontal sinusitis is characterized by:

■ Acute or progressive headache
■ Fever

The process may be silent until serious neurological symptoms and signs develop such as:

■ Focal neurological deficits
■ Change in mental status
■ Lethargy
■ Seizure
■ Coma

The presentation depends in part on the location of the infection; for example, with frontal lobe involvement, the only manifestation may be a subtle change in personality. Superior sagittal sinus thrombosis is frequently associated with nausea and vomiting, in addition to severe headache. Patients do not necessarily complain of rhinosinusitis symptoms such as nasal congestion and rhinorrhea at the time of presentation, but may give a history of sinusitis symptoms and localizing frontal pressure or discomfort. In a small number of cases, there may be osteomyelitis of the anterior frontal sinus table, causing overlying edema of the forehead or even a pericranial abscess (Pott's Puffy Tumor).

Clinical Features and Diagnostic Evaluation

Patients with suspected intracranial complications of frontal sinusitis should undergo high-resolution computed tomography (CT) with and without contrast as the primary diagnostic test [8]. Input from otolaryngology, neurosurgery, ophthalmology, and infectious diseases services are important in creating a multidisciplinary approach to the care of the patient [21]. The need for lumbar puncture to rule out meningitis must be weighed against the risk of precipitating brain herniation, as determined by the imaging studies and signs of increased intracranial pressure. If elevated intracranial pressure has been excluded, lumbar puncture should be performed, with cytological, microbiological, and laboratory analysis of the cerebrospinal fluid [15].

Patients with sinusitis and the following signs should be presumed to have meningitis until proven otherwise:

■ Persistent high fever
■ Severe headache
■ Meningismus
■ Photophobia
■ Irritability
■ Altered mental status

However, meningitis is seldom caused by isolated frontal sinusitis, and it is more likely to result from ethmoid or sphenoid sinusitis or intracranial abscesses, which may occur in the epidural space, the subdural space, or intraparenchymally [9].

Epidural abscesses most commonly occur directly behind an intact posterior table of the frontal sinus. The dura is loosely attached in this region, allowing pus to collect and expand [1]. Symptoms may be very mild until the collection becomes large enough to increase intracranial pressure. Because of the proximity to the orbit, orbital swelling is common, together with forehead edema and tenderness. Other than the increased pressure, lumbar punctures are usually normal with epidural abscesses [25, 26].

Infections in the subdural space also do not yield diagnostic lumbar punctures, but may be associated with increased pressure, elevated protein, and pleocytosis, with normal glucose and lack of organisms [1, 20]. The subdural space is a potential space between the arachnoid matter and the dura. The arachnoid prevents extension of the infection to the leptomeninges, but allows transmission of local inflammation through to the underlying cortex [6]. Pus in the subdural space also precipitates vasculitis and septic venous thrombosis. The inflammatory edema and venous obstruction tends to lead to a cycle of increasing edema and infarction, creating a far greater degree of intracranial hypertension than the mass effect of the empyema itself [27]. The infection may spread freely in the subdural space, posteriorly over the cerebral hemisphere and inferiorly into the interhemispheric fissure. The infection may then spread to the contralateral side of the brain under or through the falx cerebri [26].

Subdural empyema usually presents with:

- Increasing headache
- Fever
- Elevated white blood cell count
- Meningeal signs

As the process progresses, cortical signs and symptoms develop such as:

- Hemiparesis
- Hemiplegia
- Cranial neuropathies
- Seizure

Ultimately, the increase in intracranial pressure causes [1, 26]:

- Nausea
- Vomiting
- Slowed heart rate
- Hypertension
- Decreased level of consciousness

Death may occur from transtentorial herniation, which may be precipitated by lumbar puncture in the setting of markedly elevated intracranial pressures [20].

Dural sinus thrombosis can result directly from septic emboli from the frontal sinus, or secondary to epidural, subdural, or brain abscesses. Patients with thrombosis of the superior sagittal sinus or the cavernous sinus are generally very ill appearing [15]. Meningeal signs and/or focal neurologic deficits are almost always evident at presentation.

In cavernous sinus thrombosis, the key findings are:

- Proptosis
- Chemosis
- Ophthalmoplegia
- Cranial nerves II and III palsies
- Visual loss develops as the disease process worsens
- Contralateral involvement is pathognomic

In addition to the physical exam findings, dural sinus thrombosis is usually evident on contrast CT, MRI, and MR venogram [11]. Venous engorgement, particularly of the superior ophthalmic vein in cavernous sinus thrombosis, is an important diagnostic finding. Lumbar puncture is not diagnostic.

Brain abscesses due to frontal sinusitis most commonly derive from septic emboli that travel to the frontal lobe via retrograde venous communications. Typically, there will be liquefaction necrosis of the brain surrounding the infected vein, with surrounding edema [32]. Because the blood supply is less robust, abscesses tend to form in the white matter rather than the gray matter, and they become encapsulated over weeks [24]. The initial symptoms of brain abscess may be very mild or nonexistent. Only with significant edema can focal neurologic signs or signs of increased intracranial pressure be seen. Unfortunately, brain abscesses may not be apparent until they rupture into the ventricular system, causing rapid death. In other cases, rapid growth of the abscess and reactive edema may cause uncal herniation through mass effect (Figs. 1–3).

Treatment

The organisms most commonly cultured either from the frontal sinus or from intracranial collections are staphylococcus and streptococcus species [18, 19]. Other gram-positive bacteria may be found, as well as anaerobes, and gram negatives such as *H. influenzae* [4]. Patients with intracranial complications of frontal sinusitis should be admitted to the hospital for aggressive intravenous antibiotic therapy with broad-spectrum agents that penetrate the blood-brain barrier. Culture results will ultimately direct the choice of antibiotic, but agents such as penicillinase-resistant penicillins, vancomycin, and third-generation cephalosporins provide appropriate initial coverage [15]. The roles of mannitol and corticosteroids for brain edema, and anticoagulants for dural sinus thrombosis, are controversial, but may be indicated in certain situations [29, 30]. Currently, anticoagulation is favored in superior sagittal sinus thrombosis (SSST) but not cavernous sinus thrombosis, as long as there is no gross blood on CT or lumbar puncture [31]. After neurological consultation, anticonvulsants may also be administered because of the significant association of seizures with intracranial complications.

Management principles of frontal sinus-related intracranial complications:

- In most cases, management of intracranial complications requires surgery in addition to medical therapy
- Ideally, when indicated, both the intracranial process and the sinus infection should be addressed at the same surgical procedure [8, 18,

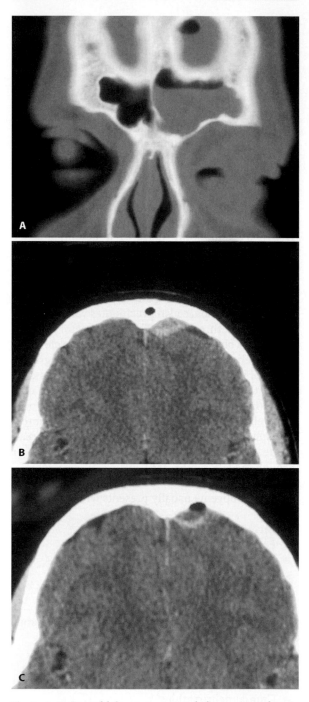

Fig. 8.1A–C. Frontal lobe pneumococcal abscess secondary to frontal sinusitis. A Coronal CT showing opacification of left frontal sinus. B Axial CT demonstrating abscess of frontal lobe

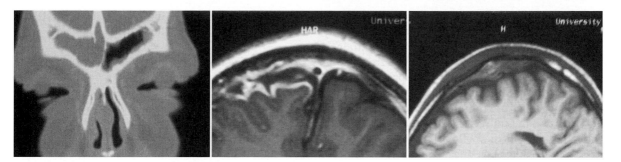

Fig. 8.2. Frontal sinusitis causing meningitis and frontal lobe abscess. Cultures of CSF and the abscess revealed staphylococcus A

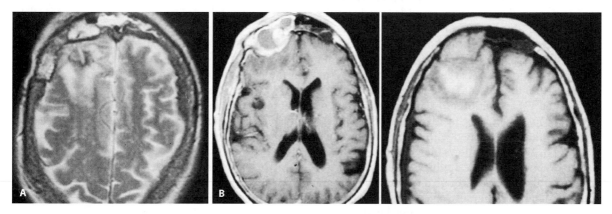

Fig. 8.3A,B. Frontal sinusitis causing septic thrombophlebitis and hemorrhagic brain infarction. A T2-weighted MRI demonstrating abscess. B T1-weighted image with higher signal intensity in the area of brain infarction

21, 26]. This theoretically prevents further seeding of the intracranial space from the infected sinus and has been shown to decrease the incidence of neurosurgical and sinus re-exploration.

■ In the acute setting, drainage of the frontal sinus takes precedence over establishing improved intranasal outflow. Typically, the surgical intervention of choice is a frontal sinus trephination with drainage of the infected material and irrigation of the sinus [12, 21].

The trephination may be combined with an endoscopic frontal sinusotomy if the conditions are favorable [13], or a catheter may be brought out through the brow incision to allow for postoperative irrigation and to prevent re-accumulation of purulence. If the frontal table of the sinus is necrotic or eroded by osteomyelitis, wide surgical debridement of the bone is necessary, along with prolonged intravenous antibiotic therapy. Reconstruction of the defect is delayed until the infection is resolved, as demonstrated by gallium-67 citrate scan [12].

Surgical treatment of uncomplicated epidural abscess involves creation of burr holes without opening the dura [35]. In the pediatric age group, there is evidence that this type of neurosurgery may not always be necessary, provided that adequate sinus drainage is achieved, there is minimal mass effect from the abscess, and the patient is given appropriate antibiotic therapy [16]. Subdural empyema may be managed by either burr holes or craniotomy, with opening of the dura to drain the collection [8]. Craniotomy provides wider access and may allow recognition of extensions of the empyema that would be missed with burr holes alone. On the other hand, with improved radiologic studies to localize the abscess, burr holes are sufficient in most cases [3]. When there is a brain abscess, the need for surgery depends largely on the extent of the abscess. Small or multiple abscesses, particularly in a stable patient or when located in an inaccessible area, are often managed medically with close observation [34]. Larger abscesses need to be drained to relieve the mass effect, which can be accomplished via aspiration or excision. Aspiration, or repeated aspiration, has the advantage of being less traumatic and is associated with fewer long-term sequelae [23]. Aspiration allows identification of the infecting organism to guide antibiotic therapy. Surgical excision of the abscess through a craniotomy is more definitive and may be desirable in a stable patient when the abscess is large, well-encapsulated, and not involving primary cortical areas. Excision may also be necessary when aspirations are unsuccessful [1].

The role of surgery in the management of dural sinus thrombosis is not completely defined, other than drainage of the frontal sinus source. Exploration of the cavernous sinus is generally not recommended, although it has been reported. Similarly, superior sagittal sinus thromboses are usually not explored, except in rare instances when thrombectomy is performed for very extensive thrombi [10]. Another interventional approach in this situation is the local infusion of thrombolytic agent into the dural sinus system [7, 14].

Prognosis

With the availability of antibiotic therapy, the incidence of intracranial complications of frontal sinusitis has decreased considerably. However, the mor-

bidity and mortality of intracranial complications, once they occur, remains high.

A large series from 1991 reported a 33% incidence of long-term morbidity following intracranial complications of sinusitis, with the following sequelae being the most common [8]:

- Hemiparesis
- Hypesthesia
- Seizure disorder

Delay in surgical intervention was shown to correlate with increased long-term morbidity. In general, neurologic morbidities from meningitis are common, and systemic postinfection sequelae may also occur in the pediatric population [17]. Subdural empyema and brain abscess have greater mortality rates than meningitis, and survivors frequently suffer from the morbidities mentioned above, as well as variable cognitive deficits or focal cranial neuropathies [23]. Of all the CNS complications, the mortality from dural sinus thrombosis is the greatest, perhaps as high as 50%–80% [30]. Prior to antibiotics, these complications were virtually uniformly fatal.

Conclusion

Potent antibiotics and modern advancements in radiology have made intracranial complications of acute frontal sinusitis far less common than they once were. Nevertheless, such complications continue to occur and can result in long-term morbidities, particularly if diagnosis is delayed. It is therefore essential for the otolaryngologist to be cognizant of the potential for CNS complications, in order to initiate prompt, aggressive medical and surgical therapy. With early recognition and a multidisciplinary approach to management, improved outcomes may be possible for these serious disease processes.

CNS Complications of Frontal Sinusitis

- Meningitis
- Epidural abscess
- Subdural empyema
- Brain abscess
- Cavernous sinus thrombosis
- Superior sagittal sinus thrombosis
- Frontal bone osteomyelitis

Management of Suspected CNS Complications of Frontal Sinusitis

- Admit to hospital
- High-resolution CT scan with contrast of the head and paranasal sinuses
- Consider head MRI or MR venogram for dural sinus thrombosis
- Lumbar puncture if no evidence of increased intracranial pressure
- Neurosurgery, ophthalmology, infectious diseases consultations
- Broad-spectrum antibiotics that cross blood-brain barrier
- Drainage of affected frontal sinus via trephination
- Consider intranasal frontal sinusotomy if conditions favorable
- Coordinate with neurosurgery if drainage of intracranial abscess indicated
- Focus antibiotic coverage once cultures available
- Monitor for clinical and radiographic improvement

References

1. Blitzer A, Carmel P (1985) Intracranial complications of the disease of the paranasal sinuses. In: Blitzer A, Lawson W, Friedman WH, eds. Surgery of the paranasal sinuses. Philadelphia, PA: WB Saunders Co 328–337
2. Bluestone CD, Steiner RE (1965) Intracranial complications of acute frontal sinusitis. South Med J 58:1–10
3. Bok AP, Peter JC (1993) Subdural empyema: Burr holes or craniotomy? A retrospective computerized tomography-era analysis of treatment in 90 cases. J Neurosurg 78(4): 574–578
4. Brook I (2002) Bacteriology of acute and chronic frontal sinusitis. Arch Otolaryngol Head Neck Surg 128(5): 583–585
5. Brook I (1981) Bacteriology of intracranial abscess in children. J Neurosurg 54(4):484–488
6. Choi SS, Grundfast KM (2001) Complications in sinus disease. In: Kennedy DW, Bolger WE, Zinreich SJ, eds. Diseases of the sinuses: Diagnosis and management. Hamilton, Ontario: BC Decker Inc 172–177
7. Cipri S, Gangemi A, Campolo C, Cafarelli F, Gambardella G (1998) High-dose heparin plus warfarin administration in non-traumatic dural sinuses thrombosis. A clinical and neuroradiological study. J Neurosurg Sci 42(1):23–32
8. Clayman GL, Adams GL, Paugh DR, Koopmann CF, Jr (1991) Intracranial complications of paranasal sinusitis: a combined institutional review. Laryngoscope 101(3): 234–239
9. Courville CB (1943) Subdural empyema secondary to purulent frontal sinusitis. Arch Otolaryngol 39:211–230
10. Ekseth K, Bostrom S, Vegfors M (1998) Reversibility of severe sagittal sinus thrombosis with open surgical thrombectomy combined with local infusion of tissue plasminogen activator: Technical case report. Neurosurgery 43(4): 960–965
11. Eustis HS, Mafee MF, Walton C, Mondonca J (1988) MR imaging and CT of orbital infections and complications in acute rhinosinusitis. Radiol Clin North Am 36(6): 1165–1183, xi
12. Gardiner LJ (1986) Complicated frontal sinusitis: Evaluation and management. Otolaryngol Head Neck Surg 95(3 Pt 1):333–343
13. Gerber ME, Myer CM, 3rd, Prenger EC (1983) Transcutaneous frontal sinus trephination with endoscopic visualization of the nasofrontal communication. Am J Otolaryngol 14(1):55–59
14. Gerszten PC, Welch WC, Spearman MP, Jungreis CA, Redner RL (1997) Isolated deep cerebral venous thrombosis treated by direct endovascular thrombolysis. Surg Neurol 48(3):261–266
15. Goldberg AN, Oroszlan G, Anderson TD (2001) Complications of frontal sinusitis and their management. Otolaryngol Clin North Am 34(1):211–225
16. Heran NS, Steinbok P, Cochrane DD (2003) Conservative neurosurgical management of intracranial epidural abscesses in children. Neurosurgery 53(4):893–897; discussion 897–898
17. Idriss ZH, Gutman LT, Kronfol NM (1978) Brain abscesses in infants and children: current status of clinical findings, management and prognosis. Clin Pediatr (Phila) 7(10): 738–740, 745–736
18. Kaufman DM, Litman N, Miller MH (1983) Sinusitis: Induced subdural empyema. Neurology 33(2):123–132

8

19. Kaplan RJ (1976) Neurological complications of infections of head and neck. Otolaryngol Clin North Am 9(3): 729–749

20. Kaufman DM, Miller MH, Steigbigel NH (1975) Subdural empyema: Analysis of 17 recent cases and review of the literature. Medicine (Baltimore) 54(6): 485–498

21. Lang EE, Curran AJ, Patil N, Walsh RM, Rawluk D, Walsh MA (2001) Intracranial complications of acute frontal sinusitis. Clin Otolaryngol 26(6): 452–457

22. Mamelak AN, Mampalam TJ, Obana WG, Rosenblum ML (1995) Improved management of multiple brain abscesses: A combined surgical and medical approach. Neurosurgery 36(1): 76–85; discussion 85–76

23. Maniglia AJ, Goodwin WJ, Arnold JE, Ganz E (1989) Intracranial abscesses secondary to nasal, sinus, and orbital infections in adults and children. Arch Otolaryngol Head Neck Surg 115(12): 1424–1429

24. Mohr RM, Nelson LR (1982) Frontal sinus ablation for frontal osteomyelitis. Laryngoscope 92(9 Pt 1): 1006–1015

25. Morgan PR, Morrison WV (1980) Complications of frontal and ethmoid sinusitis. Laryngoscope 90(4): 661–666

26. Remmler D, Boles R (1980) Intracranial complications of frontal sinusitis. Laryngoscope 90(11 Pt 1): 1814–1824

27. Renaudin JW, Frazee J (1980) Subdural empyema–Importance of early diagnosis. Neurosurgery 7(5): 477–479

28. Schlosser RJ, London SD, Gwaltney JM, Jr., Gross CW (2001) Microbiology of chronic frontal sinusitis. Laryngoscope 111(8): 1330–1332

29. Soleau SW, Schmidt R, Stevens S, Osborn A, MacDonald JD (2003) Extensive experience with dural sinus thrombosis. Neurosurgery 52(3): 534–544; discussion 542–534

30. Southwick FS, Richardson EP, Jr, (1986) Swartz MN. Septic thrombosis of the dural venous sinuses. Medicine (Baltimore) 65(2): 82–106

31. Stroke (1989) Recommendations on stroke prevention, diagnosis, and therapy. Report of the WHO Task Force on Stroke and other Cerebrovascular Disorders. Stroke 20(10): 1407–1431

32. Wald ER, Pang D, Milmoe GJ, Schramm VL, Jr (1981) Sinusitis and its complications in the pediatric patient. Pediatr Clin North Am 28(4): 777–796

33. Wenig BL, Goldstein MN, Abramson AL (1983) Frontal sinusitis and its intracranial complications. Int J Pediatr Otorhinolaryngol 5(3): 285–302

34. Yang SY, Zhao CS (1993) Review of 140 patients with brain abscess. Surg Neurol 39(4): 290–296

35. Younis RT, Lazar RH, Anand VK (2002) Intracranial complications of sinusitis: A 15-year review of 39 cases. Ear Nose Throat J 81(9): 636–638, 640–632, 644

Chapter 9

Frontal-Orbital-Ethmoid Mucoceles 9

James Palmer, Ioana Schipor

Contents

Introduction

Mucoceles are slow-growing, benign expansile lesions found in the paranasal sinuses. On histopathology, they are cyst-like structures lined with respiratory epithelium and filled with mucus. Infected mucoceles are known as mucopyoceles. Mucoceles are locally destructive lesions causing bony resorption and displacement of adjacent structures, most notably the orbital contents. Treatment is surgical, and originally involved removal/resection of the entire lesion. As surgical instrumentation has improved and the pathophysiology is better understood, surgical treatment of mucoceles has evolved into procedures that are less invasive and emphasize surgical drainage over ablation.

Epidemiology

Mucoceles are uncommon in adults [16, 25, 28, 32]. These lesions can form in any of the paranasal sinuses. The first series of 14 patients [15] reported the frontal sinus as their most common location. Subsequent series have shown that approximately 60%–89% occur in the frontal sinus, followed by 8%–30% in the ethmoid sinuses, and less than 5% in the maxillary sinus. Sphenoid sinus mucoceles are rare [1, 21]. There are several case reports of mucoceles occurring in unusual locations, such as the pterygomaxillary space, orbital floor, and middle turbinate.

Mucoceles can form at any age, but the majority are diagnosed in patients 40 to 60 years old [1]. Males and females are equally affected. The incidence of skull base bony destruction and intracranial extension has been reported to be between 10% and 55% [10, 19].

Paransal sinus mucoceles are extremely rare in children, although several case reports [13, 18] and a small series of pediatric mucoceles [13] have been published. Some authors have noted an association between mucoceles and cystic fibrosis patients [8]; however, this is not always the case, and most pediatric frontal sinus mucoceles appear to be idiopathic.

Pathophysiology

Mucoceles develop after obstruction of the sinus ostium. They enlarge slowly and fill the affected sinus cavity, expanding and eroding the adjacent bony structures. Secondary infection can lead to a period of rapid expansion with a resultant increased risk of complications, especially in the periorbital area [30].

One proposed mechanism for mucocele formation is cystic degeneration of a seromucinous gland, resulting in a retention cyst [3]. However, detailed histopathologic studies have shown little evidence for this mechanism and instead have pointed to the dynamic interface between bone and mucocele lining as being responsible for mucocele expansion. It is generally thought that following obstruction of the frontal recess and subsequent infection within the frontal sinus cavity, continued stimulation of lymphocytes and monocytes leads to the production of cytokines by the lining fibroblasts. These cytokines, in turn, promote bone resorption and remodeling and result in expansion of the mucocele [25]. Bone erosion results from mass effect as well as from the presence of cytokines such as IL-1 and IL-6 [24]. Cultured fibroblasts derived from frontoethmoidal mucoceles have been shown to produce significantly elevated levels of prostaglandin E2 and collagenase, compared with normal frontal sinus mucosa fibroblasts. This suggests that the lining fibroblasts represent a major source of bone-resorbing factors [23].

Common etiologic factors related to frontoethmoid mucocele formations include: a known history of sinusitis, previous sinus surgery, allergy, and trauma (Table 9.1). Surgery can lead to mucocele formation either by directly blocking the sinus ostium with scar tissue or by entrapping sinus mucosa. Postsurgical sinus mucoceles can occur up to several years after the initial operation. Frontal sinus mucoceles were reported in 9.3% of cases after osteoplastic flaps

Table 9.1. Paranasal sinus mucoceles: common etiologies

| Chronic rhinosinusitis |
| Previous sinus surgery |
| Previous maxillofacial trauma |
| Allergies |
| Tumors |
| Idiopathic |

[9]. Mucoceles have been described after both external and endoscopic sinus surgery [5, 12, 26, 28].

Uncommonly, mucoceles form as result of an ostial occlusion caused by a benign neoplasm (osteoma, fibrous dysplasia), or a malignant tumor [14, 30]. In as many as one-third of cases, however, the history is noncontributory and no demonstrable cause can be found [21].

Culture of the aspirated mucocele contents can sometimes confirm the presence of infection. A study demonstrated that the most common isolates were *Staphylococcus aureus*, alpha-hemolytic streptococci, *Haemophilus* species, and gram-negative bacilli. The predominant anaerobic isolates were *Propionibacterium acnes*, *Peptostreptococcus*, *Prevotella*, and *Fusobacterium* species [4].

Presentation

The expanding mucocele often compresses the orbit and, not surprisingly, many patients present initially to the ophthalmologist with orbital symptoms, such as pain, proptosis, diplopia, exophthalmos, globe dis-

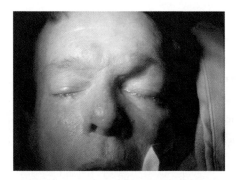

Fig. 9.1. Frontal sinus mucocele: left orbital proptosis

Table 9.2. Paranasal sinus mucoceles: common clinical presentations

Orbital symptoms: proptosis, globe displacement, diplopia, blurred vision, epiphora
Nasal symptoms: obstruction, mucopurulent rhinorrhea
Headaches
Facial or frontal swelling

placement, decreased visual acuity, or epiphora [2] (Fig. 9.1). Orbital expansion of the mucocele can lead to globe displacement, leading to exposure keratitis and central retinal block in more severe cases [7]. Other common presentations include headaches, facial pressure or swelling, nasal drainage, and obstruction (Table 9.2).

Intracranial extension through erosion of the posterior wall of the frontal sinus can lead to meningitis or CSF fistula [27, 31]. The posterior sinus wall is particularly prone to erosion because it is inherently thin. The tendency for bony erosion and intracranial extension is seen more often in the presence of infection.

Diagnosis

The diagnosis of a mucocele is based on the history, physical examination, and radiologic findings. Apart from the presenting features described above, often a palpable mass in the frontal region or in the area of the medial canthus accompany the proptosis and globe displacement. Office nasal endoscopy should assess other possible intranasal findings, such as polyposis, nasal septal deviation, etc., that may be addressed at the time of surgery.

Imaging plays a key role in the diagnosis of most mucoceles. Frontal sinus mucoceles can be seen on plain X-rays; however, lesions in the anterior ethmoids, sphenoid, and maxillary sinuses are difficult to diagnose using this modality.

The imaging of choice is CT scanning in both axial and direct coronal planes [21]. It clearly delineates the mucocele as a well-delineated, cyst-like, homogeneous lesion originating in a paranasal sinus and compressing surrounding structures. The bony changes surrounding the lesion can easily be seen (Fig. 9.2). The mucocele content demonstrates homogeneous mucoid attenuation (10–18 HU). Longstand-

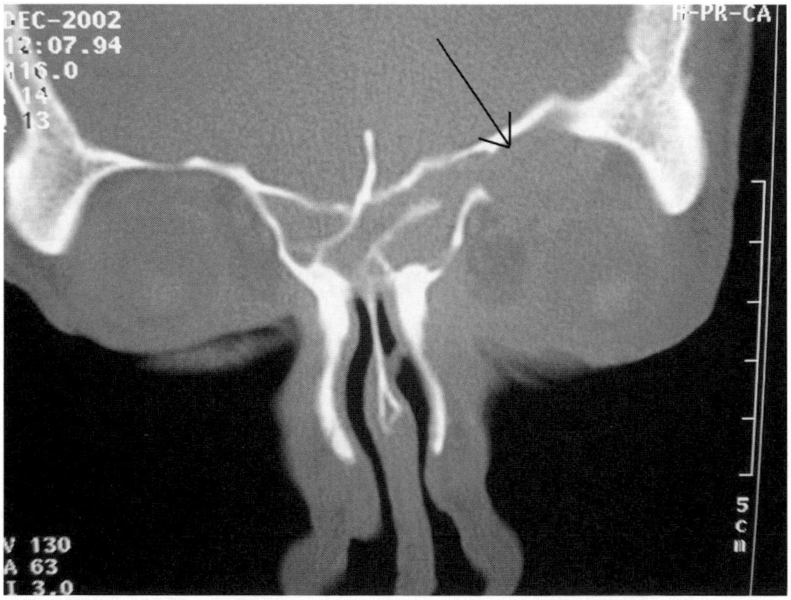

Fig. 9.2.
Coronal CT (bone windows) demonstrating opacification of the left frontal sinus with erosion of the orbital roof (*arrow*)

ing lesions have higher protein content and attenuate more (20–40 HU). Contrast enhancement is rarely necessary; however, after intravenous contrast medium injection the lesion shows rim enhancement.

Magnetic resonance imaging is useful when the diagnosis is uncertain and it is necessary to differentiate between different types of soft tissues within the sinonasal cavities, especially if the mucocele formed secondary to a neoplasm. Additionally, when the mucocele extends intracranially, MRI offers superior imaging of the surrounding brain. The usual signal characteristics for a mucocele are low T1 and high T2, but variations commonly occur depending on the presence of blood and the water content of the mucocele. Post-gadolinium images confirm the presence of fluid within the mucocele by showing absent signal [21]. Contrast-enhanced MRI is especially useful for delineating secondary mucocele formation: the nonenhancing mucocele is differentiated from the causative lesion (e.g. an obstructing tumor). It should be remembered that MRI does not provide the surgeon with the same bony detail that is available from CT.

9

Classification

Frontal sinus mucoceles can have various sizes and configurations. The degree of intraorbital involvement is not used to differentiate between the different types of lesions.

The following classification system was devised in order to standardize frontal sinus mucocele evaluation and management [11]:

- ■ Type 1. Limited to frontal sinus (with or without orbital extension)
- ■ Type 2. Frontoethmoid mucocele (with or without orbital extension)
- ■ Type 3. Erosion of the posterior sinus wall
  - – A. Minimal or no intracranial extension
  - – B. Major intracranial extension
- ■ Type 4. Erosion of the anterior wall
- ■ Type 5. Erosion of both anterior and posterior wall
  - – A. Minimal or no intracranial extension
  - – B. Major intracranial extension

Treatment

The treatment of mucoceles is surgical. The goals of surgery are eradication of the mucocele with minimal morbidity and prevention of recurrences. Surgical approaches are based on the size, location, and extent of the mucocele. In the presence of infection, adjuvant antibiotic treatment is indicated. Since many of these lesions have an intracranial or intraorbital component, ideally the surgery should not be performed in the setting of an infection. The exception is an acute symptomatic mucopyocele.

Traditional teaching in the United States emphasized that the entire lining of a sinus mucocele must be completely removed. Historically, surgical therapy involved an external approach (Lynch-Howarth frontoethmoidectomy) or osteoplastic flaps with sinus cavity obliteration. These procedures carried significant morbidity and cosmetic deformity, as well as a significant rate of recurrence [29]. Additionally, postoperative radiographic follow-up became difficult after obliteration.

- ■ More recent reports have shown that complete removal of the sinus lining is not necessary, and marsupialization is sufficient as long as ventilation of the sinus cavity is maintained [11]

Endoscopic drainage has been advocated in the belief that preservation of the frontal sinus mucosa and maintenance of a patent frontal recess result in a better clinical outcome [20].

In 1989 Kennedy et al. published the first series of 18 mucoceles treated by endoscopic marsupialization. Their study reported zero percent recurrence rate after follow-up averaging 18 months [18]. Another study, with longer follow-up, examined the recurrence rate in two groups of patients with sinus mucoceles: the first group was treated endoscopically (20 patients) and the second treated using a combined external and endoscopic approach (28 patients) [22]. The combined approach was used in the more severe cases where the anatomy, extent of disease, or previous surgery restricted endoscopic visualization and access to the frontal sinus, as well as in cases where a fistulous tract was present. There were no recurrences in the group managed exclusively via a transnasal endoscopic approach after a mean follow-up of 34 months. There were three recurrences (11%) in the combined endoscopic/external drainage group after a mean follow-up of 44 months. Although it is difficult to directly compare these recurrence rates given the difference in severity of disease in the two patient groups, the endoscopic approach was clearly shown to be safe and efficacious, with minimum associated morbidity (Figs. 9.3 and 9.4).

Har-El has published the largest series of patients with mucoceles in the English literature [10]. One hundred and three patients with 108 paranasal sinus mucoceles were treated by wide endoscopic marsupialization. Postoperative stents were used in frontal mucoceles. His recurrence rate was 0.9% (one patient) after a mean follow-up of 4.6 years. The rate of major complications was also very low, with only one patient experiencing an intraoperative CSF leak, which resolved after immediate repair and postoperative bedrest. The author concluded that the endo-scopic drainage should be considered the procedure of choice for management of paranasal sinus mucoceles.

The endoscopic approach is particularly useful when an extensive frontal mucocele has eroded the posterior frontal sinus wall. In these cases sinus obliteration is problematic given the difficulty of completely removing the lining mucosa from exposed dura [11].

No complications were reported in the small pediatric series reported by Hartley and Lund [13]. Seven children underwent endoscopic drainage of ethmoid and sphenoid mucoceles, and there were no recurrences after one-year follow-up.

Complex cases with extensive intracranial extension have been managed in a number of different ways. Neurosurgeons tend to use an open approach (craniotomy) and to remove the entire cyst lining [6]. Other authors have advocated wide marsupialization via an endoscopic transnasal approach [17]. Alternatively, mucoceles with intracranial extension are approached with a combined craniofacial and endoscopic approach [22].

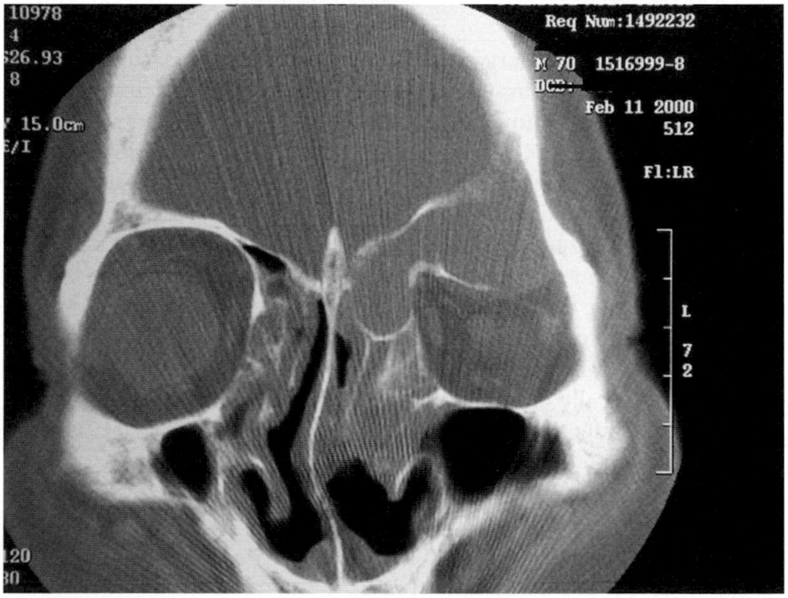

Fig. 9.3.
Preoperative CT of left frontal orbit mucocele eroding into the orbit

Fig. 9.4.
Postoperative CT after endoscopic
drainage of mucocele

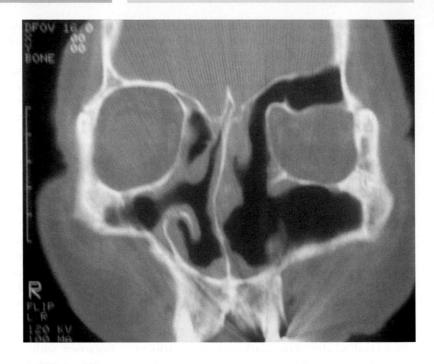

9

Surgical Technique

All patients should undergo preoperative CT scanning. The benefits of computer-aided, CT-based stereotactic navigation techniques have not yet been fully evaluated. In theory, however, stereotactic guidance may offer some advantages and may reduce the risk of surgical complications by being able to localize small mucoceles and by improving surgical orientation, especially in revision cases where anatomical landmarks may be distorted or missing.

The procedure can be performed either under local or, more commonly, under general anesthesia. The nose is topically decongested. Once the surgical landmarks are identified endoscopically, the mucocele is opened into the nasal cavity. The bone overlying the mucocele is usually thin and may be dehiscent [13]. Specimens should be sent for microbiology analysis. After entering the sac, the mucocele is then widely marsupialized in order to prevent reaccumulation. Occasionally the mucocele is filled with thin, clear fluid, raising suspicion of a CSF leak intraoperatively [22]. The medial orbital wall is often eroded in

the case of ethmoid mucoceles, and the globe is obviously at risk in these cases during the drainage procedure. Postoperative packing is not routinely used. Attention to postoperative nasal hygiene, including nasal irrigation and topical steroids is critical. If the contents of the mucocele are purulent or if the microbiological cultures are positive, oral antibiotics are used. Close endoscopic follow-up postoperatively should be continued until the cavity heals and mucociliary clearance re-establishes.

Postoperatively, temporary diplopia after globe repositioning can occur. Recurrences are possible, although not common.

Conclusion

Mucoceles are the most common benign lesions of the paranasal sinuses. Ninety percent occur in the frontal and ethmoid sinuses and frequently cause destruction of the surrounding bone, including the orbit. Diagnosis is made by CT scan. Over the past fifteen years the increasing use of endoscopic sinus surgery has resulted in safe and successful drainage of a large proportion of anatomically suitable lesions with minimal rates of recurrence and morbidity. Complex or revision cases may necessitate a combined endoscopic and external drainage procedure in order to prevent recurrence.

References

1. Arrue P, Thorn Kany M, Serrano E, et al (1998) Mucoceles of the paranasal sinuses: Uncommon location. J Laryngol Otol 112:840–844
2. Avery G, Tang RA, Close LG (1983) Ophthalmic manifestations of mucoceles. Ann Ophthalmol 15:734–737
3. Batsakis JG (1980) Tumours of the head and neck. Williams and Wilkins, Baltimore
4. Brook I, Frazier EH (2001) The microbiology of mucopyocele. Laryngoscope 111:1771–1773
5. Busaba NY, Salman SD (2003) Ethmoid mucocele as a late complication of endoscopic ethmoidectomy. Otolaryngol Head Neck Surg 128:517–522
6. Delfini R, Missori P, Iannetti G, et al (1993) Mucoceles of the paranasal sinuses with intracranial and intraorbital extension: Report of 28 cases. Neurosurgery 32:901–906
7. Garston JB (1968) Frontal sinus mucocele. Proc R Soc Med 61:549–551
8. Guttenplan MD, Wetmore, RF (1989) Paranasal sinus mucoceles in cystic fibrosis. Clin Pediatr 28:429–430
9. Hardy JM, Montgomery WW (1976) Osteoplastic frontal sinusotomy: An analysis of 250 operations. Ann Otol Rhinol Laryngol 85:523–532
10. Har-El G (2000) Endoscopic management of 108 sinus mucoceles. Laryngoscope 111:2131–2134
11. Har-El G (2001) Transnasal endoscopic management of frontal mucoceles. Otolaryngol Clin North Am 34:243–251
12. Har-El G, Balwally AN, Lucente FE (1997) Sinus mucoceles: Is marsupialization enough? Otolaryngol Head Neck Surg 117:633–640
13. Hartley BEJ, Lund VJ (1999) Endoscopic drainage of pediatric paranasal sinus mucoceles. Int J Pediatr Otorhinolaryngol 50:109–111
14. Hesselink JR, Weber AL, New PF, et al (1979) Evaluation of mucoceles of the paranasal sinuses with computed tomography. Radiology 133:397–400
15. Howarth, WG (1921) Mucocele and pyocele of the nasal accessory sinuses. Lancet 2:744–746
16. Hu XH, Lin DZ (1982) Mucocele des sinus. Rev de Laryngologie Otologie Rhinologie 103:199–201
17. Ikeda K, Takahashi C, Oshima T, et al (2000) Endonasal endoscopic marsupialization of paranasal sinus mucoceles. Am J Rhinol 14:107–111
18. Kennedy DW, Josephson JS, Zinreich SJ, et al (1989) Endoscopic sinus surgery for mucoceles: A viable alternative. Laryngoscope 99:885–895
19. Koike Y, Tokoro K, Chiba Y, et al (1996) Intracranial extension of paranasal sinus mucoceles: Two case reports. Surg Neurol 45:44–8
20. Kuhn FA, Javer AR (2001) Primary endoscopic management of the frontal sinus. Otolaryngol Clin North Am 34:59–75
21. Lloyd G, Lund VJ, Savy L, Howard D (2000) Optimum imaging for mucoceles. J Laryngol Otol 114:233–236
22. Lund VJ (1998) Endoscopic management of paranasal sinus mucoceles. J Laryngol Otol 112:36–40
23. Lund VJ, Harvey W, Meghji S, Harris M (1988) Prostaglandin synthesis in the pathogenesis of fronto-ethmoidal mucoceles. Acta Otolaryngol 106:145–151
24. Lund VJ, Henderson B, Song Y (1993) Involvement of cytokines and vascular adhesion receptors in the pathology of fronto-ethmoidal mucoceles. Acta Otolaryngol 113:540–546
25. Lund VJ, Milroy CM (1991) Fronto-ethmoidal mucoceles: A histopathological analysis. J Laryngol Otol 105:921–923
26. Moriyama H, Nakajima T, Honda Y (1979) Studies on mucoceles of the ethmoid and sphenoid sinuses. J Laryngol Otol 106:23–27
27. Nakayama T, Mori K, Maeda M (1998) Giant pyocele in the anterior intracranial fossa – Case report. Neurol Med Chir (Tokyo) 38:499–502
28. Natvig K, Larsen TE (1978) Mucocoele of the paranasal sinuses: A retrospective clinical and histological study. J Laryngol Otol 92:1075–1082
29. Rubin JS, Lund VJ, Salmon B (1986) Frontoethmoidectomy in the treatment of mucoceles. A neglected operation. Arch Otolaryngol Head Neck Surg 112:434–436
30. Stiernberg CM, Bailey BJ, Calhoun KH, et al (1986) Management of invasive frontoethmoidal sinus mucoceles. Arch Otolaryngol Head Neck Surg 112:1060–1063
31. Voegels RL, Balbani AP, Santos Junior RC, et al (1998) Frontoethmoidal mucocele with intracranial extension: A case report. Ear Nose Throat J 77:117–120
32. Zizmor J, Noyek AM (1968) Cysts and benign tumours of the paranasal sinuses. Semin Roentgenol 3:172–185

Pott's Puffy Tumor

10

Richard R. Orlandi

Contents

Introduction

Sir Percival Pott (1714–1788) was a surgeon of St. Bartholomew's Hospital in London who wrote a large number of treatises on subjects as varied as orthopedics, urology, and neurosurgery [6]. In 1760, he produced his *Observations on the Nature and Consequences of Wounds and Contusions of the Head, Fractures of the Skull, Concussions of the Brain, etc.* In this work he described "a puffy, circumscribed, indolent tumor of the scalp, and a spontaneous separation of the pericranium from the scull (sic.) under such a tumor" [3]. Hence was born the alliterative appellation, Pott's Puffy Tumor.

While originally described as a consequence of head trauma, this entity has become more commonly associated with complications of frontal sinusitis. The classic use of the Greek term "tumor" for swelling is rarely used today, instead having a modern connotation of a neoplasm. As defined by Pott, this "tumor" or swelling of the forehead is formed by a subperiosteal abscess. Pott termed this infectious collection as "matter" and went on to observe that it often appeared with "inflammation of the dura mater and the formation of matter between it and the skull" [2]. Patients with subperiosteal abscesses of the frontal bone typically demonstrate focal necrosis of the frontal bone as well. Thus intracranial and osteomyelitic complications of frontal sinusitis are often associated with what Pott originally described as a "puffy tumor."

Anatomy and Pathogenesis

The frontal sinuses form as pneumatic extensions of the anterior ethmoid complex that project into the diploic space of the frontal bone. This process begins in infancy but progresses slowly, only becoming radiologically evident at 6 years of age [5, 9]. For this reason, complications of frontal sinusitis, including Pott's puffy tumor, are relatively rare in younger children.

Infection from the frontal sinus may progress beyond the confines of the sinus by direct extension from either [1, 8]:

- Focal osteitis or osteomyelitis or
- Through infectious thrombophlebitis

The posterior table of the frontal sinus is almost completely composed of compact bone, whereas the anterior table contains both compact and cancellous bone. Aggressive infection of the frontal sinus mucosa can invade directly into the underlying bone. Progressive infection leads to the development and expansion of poorly vascularized or necrotic sequestra of bone. Osteitis can continue through the full thickness of the posterior table to the dura and epidural space, whereas transmural osteomyelitis of the anterior table can directly extend to the pericranium.

Progressive thrombophlebitis without overt bone infection is another potential source of Pott's puffy tumor and its frequently associated intracranial complications. Venous drainage of the frontal sinus mucosa passes through valveless diploic veins that extend posteriorly to the dura and anteriorly to the pericranium. Infectious thrombophlebitis can therefore extend posteriorly, causing epidural abscess or meningitis. More rarely, septic thromboemboli can lead to frontal lobe abscess. Thrombophlebitis of the anterior table can similarly lead to infection of the frontal pericranium and development of Pott's puffy tumor. As the pericranium is elevated off of the underlying frontal bone by expansion of the abscess, the vascular supply to the bone is further compromised, promoting necrosis and osteomyelitis.

Clinical Presentation

Pott's 18th century description of frontal subpericranial abscess still remains pertinent over 200 years later [2]:

- Patients typically do not have a history of chronic or recurrent acute frontal sinusitis
- Pott's puffy tumor can rarely complicate chronic frontal disease
- Symptoms of frontal sinusitis can be present for a variable amount of time prior to development of forehead swelling, ranging from just a few days to months
- Previous treatment with antibiotics is common

Focal doughy or pitting forehead swelling heralds the presence of a subpericranial abscess. Often significant tissue edema surrounds and overlies the abscess and may extend into the preseptal orbital tissues.

Associated symptoms include:

- Headache
- Fever
- Nasal drainage
- Frontal sinus tenderness

Males appear to be more commonly affected than females [1, 8].

As Pott noted in his 1760 description, intracranial complications are frequently associated with Pott's puffy tumor.

Pott's described an epidural abscess ("matter"), but conditions that can also complicate this disease include:

10

- Meningitis
- Venous sinus thrombosis
- Subdural abscess
- Brain abscess

Despite the presence of such serious intracranial sequelae, headache and doughy edema of the forehead may be the only presenting symptoms. For this reason, any patient presenting with Pott's puffy tumor should be evaluated radiographically for intracranial infection (Fig. 10.1) [2].

In addition to imaging the brain itself, imaging can also be helpful in delineating areas of chronic osteomyelitis and in defining the size of the subpericranial abscess. Imaging of the orbit is also indicated in the presence of preseptal cellulitis or when vision or extraocular muscle movements are compromised. A contrast-enhanced computed tomographic (CT) study is the most effective imaging modality. as it allows for soft tissue and bone evaluation [3]. In order to further delineate the degree of bone infection and

necrosis, nuclear medicine imaging may be useful. Merging nuclear medicine and CT imaging can yield precise localization of osteomyelitis [10].

Treatment

Once the extent of disease is defined, effective treatment can be initiated. The source of the infection, the frontal sinus, must be addressed as well as the subpericranial abscess and any bone or intracranial infection. Appropriate antibiotics must also be initiated.

Treatment of the frontal sinus is most easily accomplished through a trephine, although endoscopic treatment of the frontal sinusitis may also be effective [4]. Similarly, a limited subpericranial abscess can be drained through a small incision. The drawback of this minimally invasive approach is the inability to directly inspect the frontal bone for any necrotic areas.

When intracranial complications are present, simple drainage of the frontal sinus and the extracranial abscess will likely be insufficient. Because patients may deteriorate quickly from expansion of intracranial abscesses, prompt neurosurgical intervention is mandatory. Intracranial complications are typically treated with a bifrontal craniotomy, with thorough inspection of the frontal bone for necrotic areas and debridement of these areas when discovered [2]. This may necessitate a complete removal of posterior table of the frontal bone with cranialization of the frontal sinus or removal of the anterior table and collapse of the forehead skin onto the posterior table, known as a Riedel procedure (Fig. 10.2). The Riedel procedure carries with it significant aesthetic consequences which can be corrected with alloplastic or autogenous materials after sufficient time has passed to eradicate the original infectious process.

Materials used to reconstruct forehead contour after the Reidel procedure include:

- Split calvarial bone grafts
- Polymethyl-methacrylate
- Hydroxyapatite
- Titanium mesh

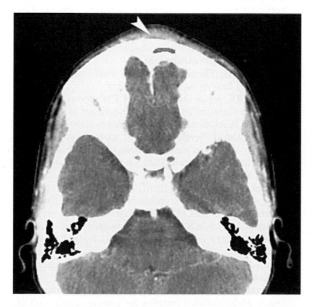

Fig. 10.1. Axial CT image demonstrating a small subperiosteal collection anterior to the frontal bone (*arrowhead*) with an associated intracranial abscess. Image courtesy of Albert Park, MD

10

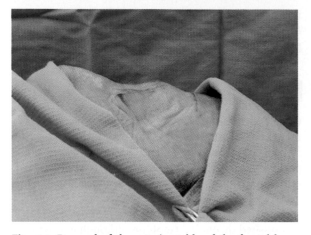

Fig. 10.2. Removal of the anterior table of the frontal bone (Riedel procedure) leaves a significant aesthetic defect

All these materials have been used successfully, and each has its inherent advantages and disadvantages [7].

In addition to prompt surgical intervention, intravenous antibiotics must be initiated early and continued for sufficient time, usually six weeks.

Organisms cultured from Pott's puffy tumor tend to be:

- Microaerophilic streptococci, including alphahemolytic streptococcus and peptostreptococcus
- Anaerobic bacteria

Obstruction of the frontal sinus by inflammatory edema likely leads to lower oxygen tension within the sinus, favoring the growth of microaerophilic and anaerobic bacteria. Empiric antimicrobial coverage started upon the diagnosis of Pott's puffy tumor must therefore include these organisms.

Conclusion

Pott's puffy tumor, described nearly 250 years ago, remains a rare complication of frontal sinusitis. Defined as a subpericranial abscess with surrounding edema, this entity is commonly accompanied by intracranial infectious complications. While rare in the post-antibiotic era, it may nevertheless develop despite previous antibiotics. Its associated intracranial complications and frontal bone infection and necrosis mandate quick diagnosis and treatment. Despite the presence of such complications, patients treated with drainage of abscesses, debridement of bone sequestra, and long-term intravenous antibiotics will most likely experience a favorable outcome.

References

1. Altman S, Austin MB, Tom LTC, Knox GW (1997) Complications of frontal sinusitis in adolescents: Case presentations and treatment options. Int J Ped Otorhinolaryngol 41:9–20
2. Bambidakis NC, Cohen AR (2001) Intracranial complications of frontal sinusitis in children: Pott's puffy tumor revisited. Ped Neurosurg 35:82–89
3. Blackshaw G, Thomson N (1990) Pott's puffy tumour reviewed. J Laryngol Otol 104:574–577
4. Chandra RK, Schlosser R, Kennedy DW (2004) Use of the 70-degree diamond burr in the management of complicated frontal sinus disease. Laryngoscope 114:188–192
5. Davis W (1914) Development and anatomy of the nasal accessory sinuses in man. Saunders, Philadelphia
6. Flamm ES (1992) Percival Pott: An 18th century neurosurgeon. J Neurosurg 76:319–326
7. Kuttenberger JJ, Hardt N (2001) Long-term results following reconstruction of craniofacial defects with titanium micro-mesh systems. J Cranio-Maxillofacial Surg 29:75–81
8. Marshall AH, Jones NS (2000) Osteomyelitis of the frontal bone secondary to frontal sinusitis. J Laryngol Otol 114:944–946
9. Onodi A (1911) Accessory sinuses of the nose in children. William Wood, New York
10. Strumas N, Antonyshyn O, Caldwell CB, Mainprize J (2003) Multimodality imaging for precise localization of craniofacial osteomyelitis. J Craniofacial Surg 14:215–219

Chapter 11

The Frontal Sinus and Nasal Polyps   11

James A. Stankiewicz, James M. Chow

Core Messages

■ **(Overview)** All patients with significant nasal polyposis generally have frontal sinus disease

■ Most patients prior to medical therapy or sinus surgery have minimal or no symptoms related to the frontal sinus

■ In most cases, surgical opening of the frontal ostia/sinuses is not necessary

■ Only patients with symptoms or signs referable to the frontal sinus refractory to medical therapy require frontal sinus surgery
  – Patients with pain, headaches, pressure
  – Patients with purulent drainage from the frontal sinus

■ Postoperatively, polyps will most likely return in the upper ethmoid/frontal recess and are not problematic in most cases

■ Medical therapy can control symptomatic recurrent frontal recess/sinus polyps in most cases

■ The choice of surgical procedure to control frontal sinusitis/polyps is dependent upon extent and location of disease and anatomy

Contents

Introduction

Nasal polyposis is a genetic disorder where upon reactive nasal/sinus mucosa fueled by chronic inflammation/infection from immunologic stimulation cause marked mucosal edema with development of nasal polyps. Several studies have discussed the etiology and pathogenesis of nasal polyps [10–12]. This chapter discusses how to clinically approach nasal polyps affecting the frontal recess and sinus from the viewpoint of observation versus that of medical therapy versus that of surgery in primary and revision case scenarios.

Nasal Polyps in the Primary Scenario

Nasal polyps, in most cases, even in obstructive polyposis, do not cause major symptoms ascribed to the frontal sinus. It is rare for these patients to complain of headache, pressure, or pain.

Most patients with nasal polyps complain of:

- Nasal obstruction
- Drainage
- Loss of smell related to nasal obstruction and/or infection

Rarely, polyposis can be so severe as to cause bone thinning and dehiscence in the frontal recess or frontal sinuses. More commonly, the CT scans show opacification or mucosal thickening of the frontal sinuses in these patients. No author has done a study to show what comprises frontal sinus opacification – polyps, fluid, or mucosal thickening.

- It is fair to say that diffuse polyposis, which exists in the lower sinuses, especially the ethmoid, does not occur to the same extent in the frontal.

The recent study by Larsen and Tos showed that most polyps originated from mucosa of the ostia, clefts or recesses which do not exist inside the frontal sinuses [10]. Of 69 autopsies reviewed, polyps existed in 32% but were symptomatically "silent". This would suggest that when considering surgical intervention in patients with medically refractory polyposis, conservatism in dealing with the frontal sinus should be the rule. In this chapter, we outline a protocol or care plan on how to deal with the frontal sinus in an operable nasal polyposis patient.

In patients in whom the symptoms are not related to the frontal sinus, the frontal sinus should be generally left untouched at the initial surgery. Del Gaudio reported that of 207 patients with frontal recess or frontal disease, only 32% of polyp patients had headaches [5]. Of patients with frontal sinus opacification, only 26% had pain or headache. Endoscopic removal of frontal recess polyps and agger nasi cells is all that is generally necessary. It is important in patients with asymptomatic frontal sinus disease that polyp disease in the frontal recess be removed without ostioplasty, taking care not to injure mucosa posteriorly, laterally, or medially. Irrigation of the frontal sinus can be performed to remove mucus or debris. Another study by Del Gaudio et al. nicely showed how

nasal polyposis can expand sinus walls [4]. It is not uncommon to see frontal recess/ostia expansion due to polyposis, which allows the frontal sinus better drainage and less chance of postoperative stenosis. If on CT scan the frontal ostium is dilated or widened, a curved microdebrider can remove polyps obstructing the recess/ostium up into the sinus without danger of stenosis. A narrow ostium on CT scan should not be instrumented except for irrigation. Also given the reason that the frontal/upper ethmoid area is the first area to develop recurrent polyps, rarely is aggressive frontal ostioplasty or Lothrop (modified) primarily necessary. Three papers, two by Jacobs and the other by Kennedy (both Triologic theses) indicate that patients who had their polyps removed were markedly improved subjectively, but had visible nasal polyps in the frontal recess postoperatively [6–8] (Fig. 11.1). Guidelines for performance of frontal sinus surgery are listed in Table 11.1. While some surgeons recommend routine preservation of the middle turbinates, best success is achieved with middle turbinate reduction or removal, allowing the frontal sinus better drainage. (Table 11.2) In most cases, patients will do well.

In patients with symptoms related to the frontal sinus, the frontal sinus will often also do well once surgery has been determined to be necessary, with removal of disease from the lower sinuses and judicious irrigations. Medical therapy should obviously be initiated prior to surgical therapy in most patients (Fig. 11.2). First-line therapy in these patients who often complain of headache or severe pressure is anti-inflammatory medication. If polyps aren't medically reduced to allow for drainage, then patients will not

Table 11.1. Guidelines for frontal endoscopic sinus surgery (ESS) in the polyposis patient

1.	Patient with acute or chronic complicated frontal sinusitis invading into orbit or skull base
2.	Patients with chronic pain, marked pressure, or frontal headache with or without purulence refractory to medical therapy
3.	Failed endoscopic sinus surgery in symptomatic chronic frontal sinusitis/polyposis
4.	Mucocele and polyposis

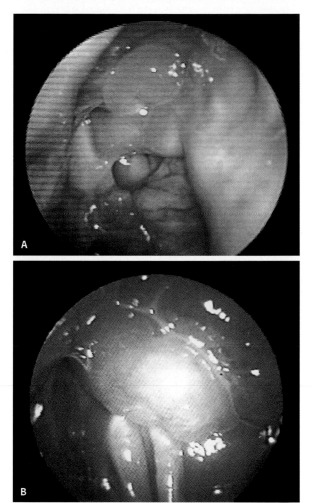

Fig. 11.1. A Postoperative persistent/recurrent nasal polyps in the frontal recess in an asymptomatic patient. B Modified Lothrop with polypoid changes in an asymptomatic patient

improve. Antibiotics alone are not sufficient. Oral and topical corticosteroids are the best medications to reduce the size of polyps. Usually a short 7–10-day burst is sufficient to improve symptoms, although prolonged steroids for up to 1 month may be necessary [9]. In patients who have fungal polyposis, corticosteroids may be necessary for 1 month or more. This treatment along with antifungals or antibiotics as necessary will control most symptomatic patients.

Aggressive medical therapy can frequently reverse symptomatic frontal disease due to polyposis.

Indications for surgical intervention include:

- Persistence of frontal symptoms
- Abnormal physical examination with purulence from the frontal sinus despite aggressive medial therapy

Often, endoscopic total ethmoidectomy and opening the frontal recess or ostia will allow for drainage of the frontal sinuses. Where polypoid and fungal de-

Table 11.2. Guidelines for extent of sinus surgery with nasal polyposis

1. Total ethmoidectomy

2. Wide maxillary antrostomy

3. Wide/large sphenoidotomy

4. If patient not asthmatic and without fungal disease
   – Consider saving middle turbinates.

5. Asthmatic patients with fungus, ASA Triad –
   – Remove middle turbinates

6. Primarily and revision surgery – asymptomatic frontal sinus
   – Conservative removal polyp frontal recess/ostium

7. Symptomatic frontal sinus patients – primary & revision
   A. Start out with ostioplasty if frontal recess/ostia dilated or widened by disease
   B. If ostia narrow remove lower polyps and irrigate sinuses
   C. Modified Lothrop or create wide ostium if frontal markedly stenotic or closed
   D. External sinus surgery – Osteoplastic flap

11

bris are anticipated in the frontal sinuses, endoscopic irrigation will often remove fungal debris unblocking the frontal ostia. Since, as earlier mentioned, polyposis will often expand the frontal ostia, endoscopic irrigation and judicious removal via a microdebrider of obstructive polyps is possible. It is important to remember that frontal ostioplasty, in patients without frontal sinus expansion, is difficult to perform due to osteitic changes. Great care must be taken to avoid causing frontal ostial stenosis. Conservative treatment around frontal recess/ostia works best in these patients. Only those patients with symp-

tomatic refractory or complicated polypoid disease require consideration for a modified Lothrop or an osteoplastic flap. Since in these patients the floor of the frontal sinus is often attenuated by disease causing expansion, a modified Lothrop is a good procedure to consider. Certainly, extensive polypoid tissue with or without fungus, mucocele, or infection unable to be cleared with a modified Lothrop should be considered for an osteoplastic flap and, in some cases, a craniofacial procedure (Fig. 11.3). It is rare that acute complicated sinusitis will occur in a patient with nasal polyposis in the frontal sinus. The goal of surgery in these patients is to drain all involved sinuses. Trephination, endoscopic frontal ostioplasty, modified Lothrop, or osteoplastic flap should be considered.

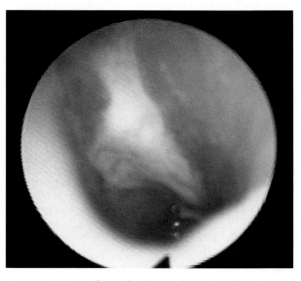

Fig. 11.2. Patient with nasal polyps and purulent frontal recess with headache/pressure

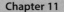

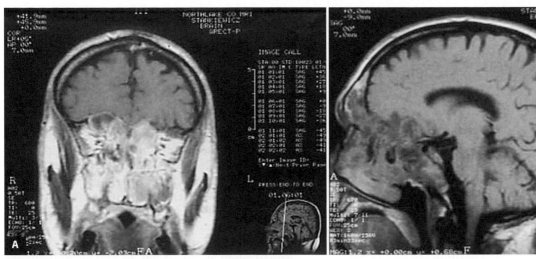

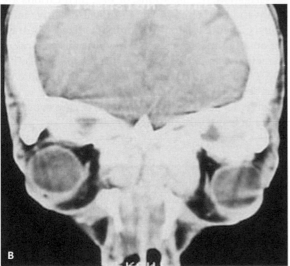

Fig. 11.3. A Markedly expanded frontal polyposis into the skull base (MRI, sagittal and coronal view) B Markedly expanded ethmoid polyposis with proptosis (CT scan, coronal)

Nasal Polyposis in the Frontal Sinus – Secondary or Revision Surgery

After endoscopic sinus surgery for nasal polyposis and chronic rhinosinusitis, very few patients are cured despite a significant improvement in their symptoms. Indeed, in most patients, endoscopic si-

nus surgery is a beginning treatment and not the end. Most patients with polyps, especially asthmatics with or without aspirin sensitivity, will require long-term medical care to control polyposis.

In our own experience, the need for revision surgery is as follows:

- Patients with nasal polyps without asthma – 30%
- Patients with polyps and asthma – 50%
- Samter's triad (aspirin triad) – about 70%–80%

Therefore, medical therapy is important for control of disease. All patients are maintained on a topical steroid spray. Oral and topical steroids are used as necessary along with antibiotics or antifungals. Each patient is individualized to a therapeutic regimen to best control their polyps. Given as noted that polyposis is a genetic disorder almost all patients will, to a certain degree, regrow polyps. Indeed, as mentioned, the frontal ethmoid area is the first area for polyps to reappear after sinus surgery. In most cases, polyps block the frontal sinus postoperatively, but patients remain asymptomatic.

Patients who become symptomatic may require revision surgery.

Symptom recurrence in these patients is most frequently due to:

- Frontal sinus blockage by polyps and infection or
- Frontal sinus ostial stenosis after frontal ostioplasty

Prior to surgical intervention, a trial of topical steroid drops (not sprays) along with oral prednisone or injection of triamcinolone (40 mg/ml) into the polyps may reduce polyp size and symptoms [3]. Topical steroid drops, which can be ophthalmic or nasal drops, placed in ether a head-back (Mygind) or head-down (Moffitt) position can be effective.

Oral prednisone can be continued for up to 1 month or used in 3–4 months bursts to control disease [2, 3, 9]. Patients with fungal disease and polyposis may benefit from antifungal irrigations, nebulization, or steroid nebulization.

Patients with persistent symptomatic frontal sinus polyposis refractory to medical therapy require revision surgery. If endoscopic sinus surgery is chosen, then the frontal ostia should be opened as widely as possible but not circumferentially. Debris is cautiously irrigated, removing all secretions and fungi. A curved microdebrider can actually remove or debulk frontal sinus polypoid disease. A modified Lothrop provides not only a wider entrance into the frontal sinus but also removal of the upper septum, causing less chance of polypoid growth below the frontal sinus. Since chronic frontal sinus polyposis can often cause thinning of the sinus floor, a modified Lothrop is made less difficult in these cases. Severe expanded sinus polypoid disease with or without a mucocele can undergo treatment with an osteoplastic flap if it is not manageable using endoscopic techniques. The frontal sinus can either be obliterated or the floor opened from above (Lothrop) into the nose. Stenting should be considered for the endoscopic modified Lothrop if the anterior-posterior width is narrow and there is marked osteitic bone thickness present. Stents should be left for at least 3 months. In a trou-blesome revision case, stents should be left in place for perhaps a year or more.

Postoperative Care After Frontal Sinus Polyp Surgery

Surgery for nasal polyposis in general requires an individualized regimen of short- and long-term care. Anti-inflammatory medications, primarily steroids, are the drugs of choice. Together with oral steroid bursts or taper, topical steroids used as a drop can help control recurrent frontal recess/ostial polyps [2]. Injection of steroids into the polyps can also control recurrent frontal recess/ostial polyps. Leukotriene inhibitors should also be considered. Antifungal irrigation, nebulizations, or oral medications are costly and help temporarily in fungal-sensitive individuals. Their use should be individualized. Not staying on a regimen of selected medications will result in recurrence of the disease. In the most sensitive ASA Triad patients, aspirin desensitization should be considered (Fig. 11.4) [1].

Table 11.3 lists short- and long-term care considerations in frontal/frontal recess polyposis.

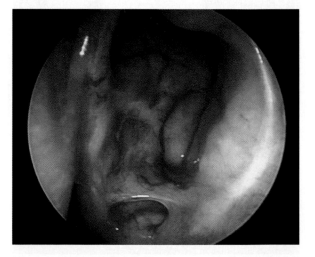

Fig. 11.4. ASA Triad (Samter's) patient controlled on topical steroids after aspirin desensitization

Table 11.3. Short- and long-term postoperative treatment for best control of nasal polyposis

Short-term

1. Oral prednisone burst, which can be repeated every 4 months.

2. Topical nasal steroid drops e.g., Dexamethasone

    – One month postoperative

3. Antibiotics which are culture directed for persistent bilateral infection

4. Saline irrigations

5. Leukotriene inhibitor

6. Antifungal (oral, topical, or irrigation) medications as needed

7. Triamcinolone injection

Long-term

1. Oral prednisone every 3–4 months

2. Topical steroid drops or nebulization

3. Leukotriene (if helpful)

4. Prednisone 5 mg qd or qod for more difficult cases, increasing to 10 mg qd with URI

5. Antifungal irrigations, nebulizations, or oral medications (as needed)

6. Select long-term regime individually

7. Triamcinolone injection

Conclusion

> Frontal sinus anatomy relative to the lower and anterior paranasal sinuses will often shield the frontal sinuses from symptomatic disease, especially with nasal polyposis. Conservative treatment with anti-inflammatory medications controls disease in most cases. Symptomatic frontal recess/sinus polyposis refractory to medical therapy requires wide osteoplasty, modified Lothrop, or external open procedures to best control disease and relieve symptoms.

References

1. Berges-Gimeno MP, Simon RA, Stevenson DD (2003) Long term treatment with aspirin desensitization in asthmatic patients. J Allergy Clin Immunol 111:180–186
2. Bonfils P, Nores JM, Halimi P et al (2003) Corticosteroid treatment of nasal polyposis with a three year follow-up. Laryngoscope 113:683–688
3. Citardi MJ, Kuhn FA (1998) Endoscopically guided frontal sinus beclomethasone instillation for refractory frontal sinus/recess edema and polyposis. Am J Rhinol 12(3):179–182
4. Del Gaudio JM (2003) Race and gender differences in frequency of skull base erosion in allergic fungal sinusitis. Am J Rhinology, publication pending. Presented at Fall 2003 ARS meeting. Orlando, Florida
5. Del Gaudio JM, Wise SK (2004) Consideration of degree of frontal sinus disease to the presence of frontal headache. Am J Rhinology, publication pending – Department of Otolaryngology-Head and Neck Surgery, Presented Spring ARS/COSM 2004 meeting, Phoenix, Arizona
6. Jacobs J (1997) One hundred years of frontal sinus surgery. Laryngoscope 100:Supp. 83:1–36
7. Jacobs J (1998) Conservative approach to inflammatory nasofrontal duct disease. Ann Otol 107:658–661
8. Kennedy DW (1992) Prognostic factors, outcomes and staging in ethmoid sinus surgery. Laryngoscope 102 (Suppl) 1–18
9. Kuhn FA, Javer AR (2002) Allergic fungal sinusitis: A four year follow-up. Am. J. Rhinology 14:149–156
10. Larsen PL, Tos, M (2004) Origin of nasal polyps: An endoscopic autopsy study. Laryngoscope 114:710–719
11. Norlander T Fukami, M Westin KM (1993) Formation of mucosal polyps in the nasal and maxillary/sinus cavities by infection. Otolaryngol-Head and Neck Surgery 109:522–529
12. Settipane GA (1987) Nasal polyps: Pathology, immunology, and treatment. Am J Rhinol 1:119–126

Chapter 12

Allergy and the Frontal Sinus

12

Berrylin J. Ferguson

Core Messages

- Allergy is an adverse reaction by a host to an otherwise innocuous agent. Allergic rhinitis is an IgE-mediated response to any of a number of allergens, including pollens, fungi, animal epidermals, insects, and dust mites

- Allergic rhinitis is typified clinically with sneezing; rhinorrhea, itching and nasal congestion

- The outflow tract of the frontal sinus is a narrowed recess
  Hypothetically, swelling of the nasal mucosa can lead to congestion of the frontal recess. Although the incidence of allergic rhinitis is only slightly elevated in patients with acute infectious frontal sinusitis, it is disproportionately elevated in patients with chronic or recurrent frontal infections and hyperplastic rhinosinusitis

- A localized allergic response to a fungal allergen, typified histologically with allergic, eosinophilic mucin and fungal hyphae present in the mucin, is characteristic of allergic fungal sinusitis (AFS). AFS may occur in any sinus, including the frontal sinus

Contents

Introduction

Approximately 20% of the population in the United States has allergy. Evaluation of allergy is an integral part of the assessment of all patients with sino-nasal complaints. In a review of 190 consecutive patients with chronic rhinosinusitis refractory to medical management (none received preoperative immunotherapy) and who subsequently underwent endoscopic sinus surgery, Emanuel and Shah found that 84% tested positive for inhalant allergies [2]. Perennial allergens, such as dust mites, were much more likely to be positive than seasonal allergens such as pollens. In patients with acute frontal sinusitis, Ruoppi and colleagues reported in a retrospective review of 91 patients that 24% had allergic rhinitis, and of five patients who went on to have a chronic course, three (60%) had allergic rhinitis [10]. Suonpaa and Antila in Sweden reported a rising incidence of acute infectious frontal sinusitis along with an increased association with allergic rhinitis and nasal polyps [14].

Rhinosinusitis is overdiagnosed by patient and physician alike, particularly for the symptom of frontal headache which in isolation from other symptoms of sinusitis, such as nasal obstruction or purulent discharge, is not suggestive of frontal sinusitis [12]. Symptoms of sinusitis include fatigue, drainage, and facial pressure. All of these symptoms can be produced by allergic rhinitis.

This chapter will review the diagnosis and treatment of allergic rhinitis as well as allergic fungal sinusitis (AFS) localized to the frontal sinus.

Allergic Rhinitis

Diagnosis

The diagnosis of allergic rhinitis is supported by a history of symptoms typical for allergic rhinitis and confirmed by skin or blood testing for allergies.

Symptoms of allergic rhinitis include:

- Nasal congestion
- Fatigue
- Postnasal discharge
- Rhinorrhea
- Sneezing

Many of these symptoms typify chronic sinusitis. If the patient can relate a history in which symptoms resolve in different localities and return with reoccupation of the home or local environment, then the diagnosis of allergic rhinitis is even more likely.

Patients with perennial allergic rhinitis (PAR) are often unaware they have an allergy, whereas patients with seasonal allergic rhinitis (SAR) have usually made the diagnosis on their own and will tell you they have "hayfever." The chronic inflammatory stimulation of PAR leads to moderate to severe nasal congestion and increased postnasal drainage and little of the classic "hayfever" symptoms such as sneezing, eye itching, or anterior rhinorrhea. Many patients have PAR with seasonal flares.

Allergy testing is valuable in the management of patients with chronic nasal symptoms and chronic noninfectious frontal sinusitis for two reasons:

- Allergy testing can identify allergens that the patient did not previously suspect so that environmental controls can be directed
- Allergy testing provides the basis for formulation of allergen vials for immunotherapy

The most frequent example of the first reason listed above is a patient with dust mite or mold allergy. The environmental control most effective for dust mite includes mattress and pillowcase covers impermeable to dust mites, combined with frequent washing of bed linens. Patients sensitive to mold should inspect their dwelling for water leaks or mold growth in their home and workplace and remove the source of fungal growth.

Indications for immunotherapy include patients who:

- Fail to achieve relief from targeted pharmacotherapy or
- Have symptoms over half of the year so that immunotherapy becomes a cost-effective alternative and the only intervention that has the potential to cure the patient

There are two major forms of allergy testing. One is a blood test (in vitro test) and the other is a skin test. There are multiple in vitro tests available for allergy testing including but not limited to, radioallergosorbent test (RAST), modified RAST, and the Pharmacia CAP system (CAP). A total IgE is not a good screen for allergy, since it can often be within normal limits and yet the patient will have significant specific IgE-mediated hypersensitivity to a few antigens.

In Vitro Screens

A mini-allergy screen of six antigens using RAST batteries of one grass (Timothy), one weed (common ragweed), one tree (oak), two molds (*Alternaria* and *Helmithosporium*), and one dust mite (*Dermatophagoides pteronyssinus*) (with epidermals, i.e. cat, horse, etc., added if indicated by history) has a predictive value of 75%. If the battery is expanded to a total of nine antigens by including a second grass (Bermuda), an additional tree (mountain cedar), and an additional mold (*Cladosporium*) then the predictive value increases to 95% compared to a 13-antigen screen. This study was performed in patients living in Southwestern Texas [4]. Practitioners in other parts of the country would need to tailor the antigens to the most prevalent and likely allergens in their particular region. Pollen maps available from many of the testing companies can help guide the selection of these antigens.

In vitro testing with modified RAST or CAP shows significant association with intradermal dilutional test (IDT) results; however, CAP appears to be more efficient than modified RAST in confirming mold (Alternaria) allergy [1].

Skin Testing

Skin testing for allergy is of two types: intradermal or prick testing. Intradermal dilutional testing (IDT), also known as skin endpoint titration (SET), is the most time-consuming and sensitive allergy test and is able to indicate a safe starting dose for immunotherapy. A common practice is to perform a screen using dust mite, cat, dog, mold mix, tree mix, and grass mix initially and only perform additional IDT within the pollens or mold subgroups if the respective mix is positive.

There is a wide variety of *prick testing* devices. One of the most popular, most reproducible, and fastest to apply is the Multitest II device that can apply up to eight antigens at one time. A negative Multitest using 14 antigens plus histamine and glycerin controls indicates that significant inhalant allergy is unlikely. A positive Multitest may require additional in vitro or skin testing [5].

The simplest screen for allergies includes either an in vitro allergen screen of 6–9 allergens (which would include perennials such as dust mite and molds) or a Multitest II prick test.

The focus of the screen test should be on the following perennial allergens, since they are most often associated with chronic rhinosinusitis:

- Dust mite
- Cockroach
- Cat (if applicable)
- Molds

If the screen is negative, then the patient probably does not have inhalant allergy. If the screen is positive, then the patient may well be allergic to multiple other allergens, and further, more detailed investigation is warranted.

Medical Therapy for Allergic Rhinitis

- The cornerstone for the treatment of allergic rhinitis is avoidance of the allergens that provoke the symptoms

When environmental controls are impractical or incompletely effective, then pharmacotherapy is instituted. A wide variety of medications is available for the treatment of allergic rhinitis. Medications selected should be targeted toward the patient symptoms.

Medications effective for allergic rhinitis include:

- Topical and oral antihistamines
- Topical and oral decongestants
- Topical and systemic steroids
- Mast cell stabilizers (cromolyn)
- Leukotriene receptor antagonists
- Anticholinergics
- Saline nasal washes

These medications and their relative efficacy toward frontal sinus symptoms are diagrammed in Table 12.1.

Nasal steroid sprays provide the most comprehensive relief of allergic rhinitis symptoms with the least

Table 12.1. Medications and their relative efficacy toward frontal sinus symptoms

	Congestion	Sneezing	Rhinorrhea	Nasal itching
Nasal steroid	+++	+++	+++	+++
Antihistamine				
Sedating	–	+++	++	++
Nonsedating	–	+++	+/–	++
Decongestant	+++	–	–	–
Ipratropium	–	–	+++	–
Cromolyn	+	+	+	+
Montelukast	++	+	+	+

morbidity. In patients with frontal sinus obstruction or narrowing, topical steroids can be directed to the frontal recess with the neck hyperextended or flexed to maximize deposition of the steroid in the frontal recess. Patients should always be educated in directing the steroid spray away from the septum and toward the lateral wall of the nose or up toward the frontal recess in order to minimize septal excoriation and bleeding and the very rare complication of septal perforation. Nasal steroid sprays may show efficacy within 12 hours, but often require several days to a week to achieve maximum efficacy. They may also be more effective, if initiated a few days to a week prior to the patient's pollen allergy season.

Azelastine is a topical antihistamine nasal spray, which has a symptom relief profile similar to that of nasal steroid sprays. Its onset of action is within a day. Its use is limited by a bad taste appreciated by approximately 30% of users and a slight sedation potential.

Oral antihistamines can be divided into sedating and nonsedating drugs. Fexofenadine, loratadine, and desloratadine at recommended doses cause no sedation and are effective for sneezing and itching symptoms, but they have little impact on nasal congestion. For this reason, antihistamines are often paired with a decongestant. Sedating antihistamines are available over-the-counter and have anticholinergic properties, which thicken sinus and nasal secretions and over-dry the nose in some patients. The utility of oral antihistamines in patients with frontal sinusitis is probably limited because of the failure of antihistamines to significantly reduce congestion.

Topical decongestants can be utilized for short periods of time to decongest the nose and to optimize drainage of the frontal recess. Prolonged use can lead to rebound swelling. This may be minimized with concurrent use of a topical nasal steroid spray [3]. Most practitioners do not recommend long-term use of oral decongestants because of associated adverse events.

If the patient needs chronic nasal decongestion, one of the following medications can be used:

- Topical nasal steroid spray
- Azelastine
- Leukotriene receptor antagonist

The most recent pharmacotherapeutic agent to receive an indication for seasonal allergic rhinitis is the cysteinyl leukotriene receptor antagonist montelukast. This drug, approved for usage in asthma in 1996, also shows efficacy in seasonal allergic rhinitis [8]. Montelukast is the only leukotriene receptor antagonist currently approved for the treatment of seasonal allergic rhinitis. It is effective for the symptoms of rhinorrhea, congestion, sneezing, and nasal itch. In general, it is less effective than a nasal steroid spray; however, there are some patients who may respond markedly well to Montelukast.

Allergic Fungal Sinusitis (AFS) and the Frontal Sinus

AFS localized to the frontal sinus is uncommon but not rare.

The diagnosis of AFS is supported by:

- Elevated total IgE
- Elevated specific IgE to the cultured fungus
- Histopathologic evidence of eosinophilic mucin with fungal hyphae

Radiologic findings in the frontal sinus include bony erosion and heterogeneity of opacification densities on computed tomography (CT). On MRI, a signal void may occur because of the proteinaceous nature of the eosinophilic plugs [5].

The surgical treatment options for frontal AFS range from a large endoscopic frontal sinusotomy with evacuation of the allergic hyphal ridden contents to frontal sinus obliteration. The latter is most appropriate in a small frontal sinus with a difficult and narrow frontal recess. Here, obliteration of the frontal sinus affected by AFS with fat or hydroxyapatite is recommended. Relative contraindications to frontal sinus obliteration include sinuses in which it is impossible to assure that the entire mucosal lining of the frontal sinus has been removed. This includes frontal sinuses with bony erosion next to dura. It is also more difficult to obliterate a large and highly aerated frontal sinus. In these cases, a nonobliterative approach is suggested. This will allow future appraisal with CT scanning to monitor for recurrence. The recidivism of AFS in a nonobliterated sinus is high, and patients should be followed closely every 3 to 6 months over the first year. If the frontal sinus cannot be adequately visualized postoperatively endoscopically, a total IgE or CT should be obtained several months postoperatively. A normal total IgE is reassurance of no current recurrence, while a highly elevated IgE, demands investigation for possible recurrence, with revision surgery or a steroid burst. An obliterated frontal sinus may fail to achieve resolution, if the frontal sinus mucosa is not entirely removed. Recurrent frontal sinusitis and mucoceles can occur many years after initial frontal sinus obliteration.

Adjunctive medical therapies for AFS include:

- Systemic and topical steroids
- Antifungal therapy
- Leukotriene modulators
- Saline rinses
- Immunotherapy
- Environmental controls which limit high airborne fungal exposure

With frontal AFS, it is unlikely that nasal steroid sprays will reach the frontal sinus; therefore systemic steroids are generally recommended. Doses of systemic steroids recommended vary in dosage and duration. In general, no additional benefit is achieved with prednisone dosage equivalents in excess of 60 mg per day, which approximate the maximal natural steroid surge in a stress response. Descending tapers over 10 –30 days are frequently employed, and some advocate a year of prednisone tapered down to 5 mg every other day [11]. Steroids should be dosed in the morning to minimize hypothalamic–pituitary suppression.

Short-term consequences of steroid usage include:

- Personality changes
- Increased hyperglycemia
- Increased risk for gastric ulcer
- Slight increase in risk for avascular necrosis of the hip

Long-term consequences of systemic steroid usage include:

- Growth retardation in children
- Osteoporosis
- Glaucoma
- Cataracts

The role of systemic and topical antifungal therapy in AFS is controversial. In the pulmonary form of the disease, allergic bronchopulmonary aspergillosis (ABPA), systemic oral itraconazole resulted in statistically significant reductions in medication usage and total IgE in a randomized placebo-controlled trial [13].

Topical antifungal therapy in chronic rhinosinusitis with Amphotericin B was shown to result in a 70% improvement in symptoms in a noncontrolled trial [9].

A subsequent randomized, blinded controlled trial with a smaller quantity of antifungal irrigation showed no significant differences in the antifungal or placebo groups [15].

Immunotherapy to fungal antigens in surgically treated AFS reduces recurrence in the initial few years; however, long-term follow-up of these patients reveals that whether or not they receive immunotherapy, most patients improve after 4 to 10 years [6].

Conclusion

Allergic rhinitis is a common comorbidity in patients with recurrent acute frontal sinusitis and chronic frontal sinusitis. The diagnosis of allergic rhinitis depends on history, and on skin and in vitro allergy testing. Optimal therapy of allergic rhinitis includes the identification and elimination of the allergen exposure. Pharmacotherapy should be targeted toward the allergic symptoms. Immunotherapy can be utilized in patients who failed to achieve adequate symptom relief with environmental controls and pharmacotherapy, or who have symptoms for the larger part of the year. Immunotherapy may reduce recurrence of allergic fungal sinusitis in the first several years following surgical extirpation.

12

References

1. Chambers DW, Cook PR, Nishioka GJ, Erhart P (1997) Comparison of mRAST and CAP with skin endpoint titration for *Alternaria tenius* and *Dermatophagoides pteronyssinus*. Otolaryngol Head Neck Surg 117:471–474
2. Emanuel AA, Shah SB (2000) Chronic rhinosinusitis: Allergy and sinus computed tomography relationships. Otolaryngol Head Neck Surg 123:67–91
3. Ferguson BJ, Paramaesvaran S, Rubinstein E (2001) A study of the effect of nasal steroid sprays in perennial allergic rhinitis patients with rhinitis medicamentosa. Otolaryngol Head Neck Surg 125(3):253–260
4. Lehr AJ, Mabry RL, Mabry CS (1997) The screening RAST: Use in a valid concept? Otolaryngol Head Neck Surg 117:54–55
5. Levine JL, Mabry RL, Mabry CS (1998) Comparison of multitest device skin testing and modified RAST results. Otolaryngol Head Neck Surg 118:797–799
6. Marple B, Newcomer M, Schwade N, Mabry R (2002) Natural history of allergic fungal rhinosinusitis: A 4- to 10-year follow-up. Otolaryngol Head Neck Surg 127(5):361–366
7. Marple BF (2001) Allergic fungal rhinosinusitis: Current theories and management strategies. Laryngoscope 111(6):1006–1019
8. Nayak AS, Philip G, Lu S, Malice MP, Reiss TF (2002) Montelukast Fall Rhinitis Investigator Group. Efficacy and tolerability of montelukast alone or in combination with loratadine in seasonal allergic rhinitis: A multicenter, randomized, double-blind, placebo-controlled trial performed in the fall. Ann Allergy Asthma Immunol 88(6):592–600
9. Ponikau J, Sherris D, Kita H, Kern E (2002) Intranasal antifungal treatment in 51 patients with chronic rhinosinusitis. Allergy Clin Immunol 110:862–866
10. Ruoppi P, Seppa J, Nuutinen J (1993) Acute to the frontal any to: Etiological factors and treatment outcome. Acta Oto-Laryngologica 113:201–205
11. Schubert MS (2004) Allergic fungal sinusitis: Pathogenesis and management strategies. Drugs 64(4):363–374
12. Stankiewicz JA, Chow JM (2002) A diagnostic dilemma for chronic rhinosinusitis: Definition accuracy and validity. Am J Rhinol 16(4):199–202
13. Stevens DA, Schwartz HJ, Lee JY et al (2000) A randomized trial of itraconazole in allergic bronchopulmonary aspergillosis. N Engl J Med 342:756–762
14. Suonpaa J, Antila J (1990) Increase of acute frontal sinusitis in Southwestern Finland. Scand J Infect Dis 22:563–568
15. Weschta M, Rimek D, Formanek M, Polzehl D, Podbielski, Riechelmann H (2001) Topical antifungal treatment of chronic rhinosinusitis with nasal polyps: A randomized, double-blind clinical trial. J Allergy Clin Immunol 113:1122–1128

Chapter 13

The Role of Fungus in Diseases of the Frontal Sinus

13

Robert T. Adelson, Bradley F. Marple

Core Messages

- Fungal disease in the nose and sinuses is classified based on clinical, radiologic, and histologic findings

- The diagnosis of invasive fungal sinusitis is based on histopathologic evidence of fungi invading sinonasal tissue

- Acute fulminant invasive fungal sinusitis (AFIFS) is almost always seen in immuno-compromised patients

- The frontal sinus is involved in 4.8% of cases with AFIFS

- Treatment of AFIFS involves management of any underlying immunosuppression and medical/surgery therapy directed against the offending pathogen

- Chronic invasive fungal sinusitis involves tissue invasion by fungi but a slower progression of disease compared to AFIFS

- Sinus fungal ball results from accumulation of dense fungal particles in a sinus cavity in the absence of mucosal invasion

- Single sinus involvement is seen in 59%–94% of sinus fungal ball cases, and a sinus CT frequently demonstrates radiodensities within that sinus

- Allergic fungal sinusitis (AFS) involves atopy against fungal particles that results in an intense inflammatory reaction perpetuated through sinus ostial obstruction

- AFS is mostly found in temperate regions with relatively high humidity

- Surgery is the basic foundation for any successful intervention in AFS

- Systemic steroids are part of the standard therapy of AFS, although no consensus on the ideal dose or duration has been reached

- The single most important component of postoperative care is institution of immunotherapy directed against multiple fungal antigens

Contents

The nose and paranasal sinuses are heir to a great diversity of disease states, of which fungal species are an increasingly well-understood etiologic agent. Over the past 25 years our enhanced understanding of the role of fungus in sinus disease and the complex interactions between host and pathogen have allowed a logical classification of disease states such that proper prognostic information can be provided and therapeutic interventions undertaken. Coincident with this same time period was the introduction and popularization of endoscopic techniques to better delineate frontal sinus anatomy and address pathologic conditions in this location. As fungal rhinosinusitis of every type requires some level of endoscopic assessment or surgical therapy, disease involving the frontal sinus is now more amenable to proper treatment than at any time in the past.

Basic Mycology

Fungi are eukaryotic organisms ubiquitous in our environment, and nearly so in our own bodies. Scientists estimate the total number of these different fungal species to be between 20,000 and 1.5 million, of which only a fraction of a percent are responsible or human illnesses, perhaps with only a few dozen species responsible for over 90% of infections [21,41,50]. Fungi can exist either as yeast or molds. Characteristically, molds produce *hyphae*, multicellular, branch-

ing tubular extensions (2–10 µm in diameter), which coalesce as a colony known as a *mycelium* [41]. Yeasts are unicellular, from 3–15 µm in diameter, and reproduce asexually via budding, though failure of buds to detach can result in a characteristic chain of fungal cells known as *pseudohyphae* [41]. The spore is fungi's evolutionary solution to the survival problems posed by unfavorable conditions. These derivatives of sexual or asexual fungal reproduction disperse easily into the environment, can withstand adverse surroundings, and retain their germinative abilities until more receptive surroundings are encountered. Inhalation of spores is the most common route by which fungal rhinosinusitis is initiated. Once the nasal mucosa has been accessed, development of a pathologic condition is determined not only by the inherent characteristics of the fungus, but by the host's immune system and the complex interaction between the two.

Classification of Fungal Rhinosinusitis

Fungal disease of the nose and paranasal sinuses can be classified based on the clinical, radiologic, and histologic manifestations of the host-pathogen relationship. Most commonly accepted classification schemes divide fungal rhinosinusitis into invasive and noninvasive diseases based solely on histopathologic evidence of fungus penetrating host tissue [11] (Table 13.1).

Table 13.1. Classification of fungal rhinosinusitis

Invasive fungal sinusitis
Acute fulminant invasive fungal sinusitis
Granulomatous invasive fungal sinusitis (GIFS)
Chronic invasive fungal sinusitis (CIFS)
Noninvasive fungal sinusitis
Saprophytic fungal infestation (SFI)
Sinus fungal ball
Allergic fungal rhinosinusitis

From [11]

13

Exacting classification of sinonasal fungal disease will allow physicians to efficiently investigate the suggestive symptoms, initiate treatment, and provide patients with an accurate prognosis. Each of these fungal conditions is addressed below, especially with regard to fungal involvement of the frontal sinus.

Invasive Fungal Sinusitis (IFS)

A diagnosis of IFS hinges upon histopathologic evidence of fungi invading nasal tissue: hyphal forms within sinus mucosa, submucosa, blood vessel, or bone, and can be further divided based on the clinical features of an affected patient's course (see Table 13.1) [9].

Acute Fulminant Invasive Fungal Sinusitis

The characteristics of acute fulminant invasive fungal sinusitis (AFIFS) are:

- A clinical time course of less than four weeks' duration

- Prominent pathologic evidence of vascular invasion [11]

- The family Mucoraceae of the order Mucorales is home to those genus responsible for virtually all cases of AFIFS, appropriately referred to as rhinocerebral mucormycosis [12]

- AFIFS is almost always seen in immunocompromised patients, though it has been rarely reported in patients with normal immune function [4]

- Conditions associated with impaired neutrophil function, such as hemochromatosis, insulin-dependent diabetes, AIDS, leukemia, or those undergoing iatrogenic immunosuppression are particularly prone to development of AFIFS [8,15]

- A high index of suspicion for invasive disease should be maintained in the immunocompromised patient with symptoms of rhinosinusitis, as early findings are often subtle

Clinical Presentation

The presenting symptoms of AFIFS are not distinctly different from those of acute bacterial rhinosinusitis (ABRS).

Patients may present with:

- Rhinorrhea

- Double vision

- Headache or facial pain

- Fever of unknown origin. This is the most frequent finding, present in 50%–90% of patients in the three days prior to diagnosis [15, 55]

- Anesthetic regions of the face or oral cavity. These are particularly concerning signs and symptoms of early invasive disease and can precede mucosal changes. Patients should be questioned specifically, and facial sensation must be tested accurately to identify subtle, though revealing, neurologic deficits [12]

Endoscopic exam and directed biopsies are indicated in any immunocompromised patient with facial anesthesia or signs and symptoms of ABRS that fail to improve despite 72 hours of appropriate medical therapy [12,15,16].

Endoscopic findings will change dramatically as the disease progresses. Alterations in the visualized nasal mucosa are understated early in the course of AFIFS; however, nasal mucosa changes are the most consistent physical finding and should always be investigated by thorough endoscopy. Mucosal abnormalities are most commonly noted at the middle turbinate (67%), followed by the nasal septum (24%) [15]. Pale mucosa that does not bleed normally and pain greater than expected based on exam findings are reflective of tissue ischemia and incipient fungal angioinvasion [7,15,16]. The natural history of AFIFS leads to extrasinus involvement and more obvious findings in later stages of the disease.

Findings seen in later stages of the disease include:

- Necrotic nasal and/or palate mucosa
- Densely anesthetic regions of the face
- Proptosis
- Ophthalmoplegia
- Decreased vision
- Mental status changes

Radiology

Diagnostic imaging of the paranasal sinuses is often performed in the work-up of patients with presumed or proven AFIFS. Fine-cut, noncontrasted CT scans of the sinuses in axial and coronal planes are required to adequately evaluate sinus anatomy and the expected extent of disease. MRI is recommended in patients who present with signs or symptoms of orbital or intracranial involvement, or in those with skull base erosion noted on CT scans. Although bone erosion and extrasinus extension are historically cited as classic findings of AFIFS, recent investigations have shown severe unilateral thickening of nasal cavity mucosa to be the most consistent CT finding suggestive of early IFS; yet this is still a nonspecific finding [7]. Others have suggested thickening of peri-antral fat planes as another early indicator of AFIFS; however, most authors have found this finding to be either nonspecific or too uncommonly encountered in AFIFS cases to assist in providing diagnostic assistance [7].

Treatment of AFIFS

Treatment of AFIFS relies on medical and surgical therapy directed against the offending fungal pathogen in addition to, and most importantly, reversal of the patient's underlying immunocompromised state. Operative debridement decreases the pathogen load, removes necrotic tissue and likely allows the patient's immune system valuable time for recovery. Intracranial and intraorbital excursions to remove extensive disease have not been rewarding. Surgeons have paid

heed to the uniformly poor outcomes of radical resections of disease beyond the confines of the sinonasal cavity, and instead favor endoscopic techniques that are limited and directed, yet completely address the sinonasal disease process [15,19]. Systemic antifungal therapy is routinely employed in AFIFS as an adjunct to surgery. New formulations of amphotericin-B, the mainstay of antifungal therapy for over 40 years, have improved safety profiles, less renal toxicity, and are effective in treating AFIFS [15,54]. The topical route of administration via nasal nebulizer may provide optimal delivery of drug within the sinonasal cavity and should be considered in every AFIFS patient [12].

The prognosis of AFIFS is heavily dependent on the patient's immune status, as those who recover neutrophil function have the greatest chance of survival [19]. Accordingly, patients in diabetic ketoacidosis survive at a rate of 60%–90%, while leukemic patients have 20%–50% survivorship, as their immune deficiency is not amenable to rapid improvement [12,15].

Frontal Sinus Disease

The frontal sinus is the most unlikely site of involvement in AFIFS, as only 4.8% of cases in a large series demonstrated the definitive histopathologic changes, and never in isolation from the other paranasal sinuses [16]. Though outcomes are not reported to any extent in the literature, the frontal sinus' proximity to the intracranial space would give AFIFS in this location tremendous potential for untoward outcomes. Endoscopic techniques, such as the Lothrop or Draf II procedures, widely expose and ventilate the frontal sinus to obtain biopsies and remove disease. Arguments could be made for an osteoplastic flap exposure of the frontal sinus; however, this approach should be considered an option of second choice, and the sinus must never be obliterated when addressing AFIFS. Wide access to the frontal sinus allows the surgeon clear access to perform postoperative surveillance with routine office endoscopy as well as deliver topical antifungal medication via irrigations or nebulized delivery systems.

Chronic Invasive Fungal Sinusitis

In contradistinction to the impressive clinical velocity of AFIFS, a second category of invasive fungal disease encompasses a more unhurried progression of illness with very similar histopathologic findings. Chronic invasive fungal sinusitis (CIFS) is a peculiar, slowly progressive fungal infection that has been further classified into two subtypes based on histopathology [8]. Granulomatous invasive fungal sinusitis (GIFS) is a rare condition, reported mainly in parts of north Africa and southeast Asia, which as been largely ascribed to infection with *Aspergillus fumigatus*. Histologic findings of noncaseating granulomas distinguish GIFS from the more common nongranulomatous CIFS [9,42]. Most authors regard GIFS and the nongranulomatous subtype, CIFS, as identical with respect to the patient's clinical course, diagnostic evaluation, and treatment options [9,53].

Typical patient presentations include standard symptoms of chronic rhinosinusitis, made remarkable by their long duration, slow progression, and refractoriness to standard antibiotic therapy. Patients are usually immunocompetent, and therefore it is not until the development of persuasive ophthalmologic or neurologic findings such as facial paresthesias, seizures, altered mental status, proptosis, or vision changes that more insidious diagnostic possibilities are explored [53].

Because of the chronicity of CIFS, coupled with concerning neurologic deficits, the differential diagnosis should include [49,53]:

- Malignant processes
- Benign neoplasms
- Autoimmune disease
- Intracranial pathology
- Orbital neoplasms
- Unusual sinonasal infectious agents

Diagnosis

Diagnostic evaluation should begin with a complete head and neck exam, including nasal endoscopy and biopsy as well as cranial nerve testing to determine the extent of imaging that will be required initially. Neurologic or ophthalmologic deficits warrant a contrast-enhanced MRI of the head to delineate involvement of the dura or orbital contents in addition to standard fine-cut axial and coronal CT scans of the sinuses to identify likely extent of disease. A diagnosis of invasive fungal disease can be provided only on histopathologic grounds, though imaging will shorten the differential diagnosis and guide biopsies [53].

Treatment

Controversial issues in CIFS begin once the diagnosis is secured. The extent of surgery necessary to control CIFS is a point of disagreement between authors, as is the need for and duration of concomitant antifungal medication. A minority of authors draw a distinction between granulomatous and nongranulomatous CIFS, treating the nongranulomatous variety with aggressive surgery and antifungals as for AFIFS, while surgery alone is prescribed for GIFS [9,42]. The majority opinion favors evaluation of the involved structures and the pace of each individual patient's infection with plans to exenterate all visible sinus disease, preserve as much normal anatomy as possible, and allow prolonged culture-guided systemic antifungal medications to arrest and eliminate the remaining fungal infection [53]. Though the literature lacks definitive recommendations for duration of systemic antifungal therapy in CIFS, it may be possible to transition some postoperative patients to topical antifungal irrigations in an effort to avoid the renal toxicity of long-term amphotericin B. We have had experience in converting a pediatric patient with CIFS despite multiple endoscopic debridements and several months of systemic amphotericin B to topical amphotericin B irrigations, preserving renal function and continuing to keep his disease in check [43].

Frontal Sinus Disease

CIFS of the frontal sinus is not a well-documented phenomenon, and as such it is not clear that diagnostic or treatment strategies would be significantly different from those described for the other paranasal sinuses. Patients with symptoms of chronic rhinosinusitis refractory to medical therapy, especially persistent headache, visual changes, or development of neurologic deficits require expeditious physical examination and appropriate imaging. Infections of the frontal sinus have an unfortunate predilection for early involvement of the intracranial space, either directly via bone erosion or in a radiographically silent manner via angioinvasion of vessels that traverse the posterior table. We recommend aggressive surgical therapy to resect all visible frontal sinus disease and establish healthy tissue margins. An endoscopic approach is favored, with a low threshold for an osteoplastic flap exposure to ensure that all disease has been cleared and adequate ventilation established. Postoperative antifungal medication is always initiated systemically, with conversion to topical irrigations as dictated by clinical response and follow-up endoscopy.

Noninvasive Fungal Sinus Infections

Three separate conditions are identified as fungal diseases of the nose and paranasal sinuses in which the fungus is entirely extramucosal. While the aforementioned invasive processes can be viewed as variants of a common process, the noninvasive processes exert harm through very different mechanisms.

Saprophytic Fungal Infestation

Saprophytic fungal infestation (SFI) is a clinical condition which is incompletely understood with regard to its natural history as well as its role in sinonasal pathology. The malady is defined by visible growth of fungus on mucous crusts within the sinonasal cavity, and not the presence of fungi demonstrable by culture alone [11]. Fungal mucocrusts are identified during nasal endoscopy and can be removed in the clinic setting. Home nasal irrigation is recommended, as is weekly examination until the condition resolves. Imaging studies are not likely to be a helpful addition. The role of antifungal irrigations in treating saprophytic infestations has not been well studied, but is probably more than is required to control this incipient stage of a noninvasive fungal disease.

Recent studies have proposed a greater role in sinonasal disease states than previously ascribed to noninvasive fungus. Though not specifically addressing SFI, a study from the Mayo clinic has added a valuable new viewpoint to our understanding of fungi in sinonasal disease. Ponikau et al., by virtue of their thorough mucous collection and sensitive culture techniques, have implicated fungi in a nonallergic eosinophilic inflammation responsible for most, if not all, forms of chronic rhinosinusitis (CRS) [46]. The etiologic role of fungi in chronic rhinosinusitis could not be solidified by this study, as 93% of CRS patients and 100% of normal control subjects were found to have positive fungal cultures from their nasal mucous samples [46].

The full spectrum of sinonasal disease attributable to fungus has yet to be illuminated, but continued research to delineate pathogenesis will allow therapy beyond the simple mechanical debridement presently recommended for cases of SFI.

Sinus Fungal Ball

Sinus fungal ball (SFB) best typifies noninvasive fungal disease of the paranasal sinuses, a condition resulting from sequestration within a sinus of densely tangled, concentrically arranged masses of fungal hyphal elements in the absence of mucosal invasion [10]. SFB (formerly, and inaccurately, referred to as "mycetoma") has been reported since the late 19th century, though all case series have been small owing to the relative infrequency of this condition. One large case series on the subject estimates 3.7% of inflammatory sinus conditions to represent SFB, while confirming other authors' assertions that SFB affects older populations (average age of 64 years) and women (62%) [14].

Clinical Presentation

Medical attention is typically sought for symptoms consistent with chronic rhinosinusitis, though the extensive duration and refractoriness to medical therapy of a patient's facial pain or headache, nasal airway obstruction, or purulent rhinorrhea may be indicative of a less common process [11, 13]. Nasal en-

13

doscopy may demonstrate polyp disease, which is found in only 10% of patients, but is more likely to reveal normal to mild mucosal inflammation without evidence of fungus or other revealing characteristics [20].

Radiology

CT scans are more revealing, yet certainly not diagnostic. Single sinus involvement is reported in 59%–94% of SFB cases, almost always with near complete opacification of the involved sinus, and frequently demonstrating radiodensities within such opacifications (41%) [14, 20]. Bony sclerosis of involved sinus walls is common, as radiographic evidence of this bony thickening is noted in 33%–62% in different case series [14, 39]. In contradistinction to the bony erosion commonly seen in allergic fungal sinusitis, similar sinus bony attrition is noted in only 3.6%–17% of CT scans of SFB patients [14, 20, 39]. The presence of isolated sinus opacification on CT scans will appropriately prompt either further imaging (MRI) or endoscopic surgery for both diagnostic and therapeutic purposes.

Treatment

Complete surgical removal of the fungal ball and thorough irrigation of involved sinuses constitutes ample treatment for this noninvasive fungal disease. Endoscopic techniques are usually sufficient to effect complete extirpation of the disease; however, trephinations for irrigation or endoscope ports as well as external approaches should be considered in more challenging cases. Despite the long history of treating SFB with external approaches, more recent studies report recurrence rates of 3.7%–6.8% in those patients treated endoscopically [14, 20]. Postoperative antifungal therapy is not necessary unless the patient suffers from comorbid conditions with predispositions to compromised immune function. Progression from SFB to AFIFS has been reported in patients with blood dyscrasias, diabetes, systemic steroids, or other similar conditions associated with immunodeficiency [13]. Antifungal selection should be guided by fungal histology and culture results to identify the least

toxic, most cost-effective agent available. Amphotericin B formulations should be restricted to cases in which culture results suggest resistance to imidazole antifungals [13].

Frontal Sinus Disease

Frontal sinus involvement with SFB is distinctly unusual. The first case of SFB isolated to the frontal sinus was reported in 1978, successfully treated solely by removal via an osteoplastic flap approach [52]. Other authors reflect the relative rarity of this condition. Ferreiro reported an incidence of 21% for SFB involving the frontal sinus, with only 7% of patients having disease isolated to that site alone [14]. A frontal sinus location was identified in only 1.8% of Klossek et al.'s series of 109 patients with SFB [20]. Difficult locations within the frontal sinus were addressed via a complete endoscopic anterior ethmoidectomy combined with irrigations through the anterior wall of the frontal sinus, successfully treating both cases of frontal sinus SFB [20]. The frontal sinus poses particular surgical challenges, as addressed in this chapter and elsewhere in the text. Those procedures that permit complete surgical access and visualization of the frontal sinus will allow the surgeon to provide a successful operation.

Allergic Fungal Rhinosinusitis

The most recently described and intensely investigated of the fungal diseases of the paranasal sinuses is certainly the condition that has come to be known as allergic fungal rhinosinusitis (AFS). Originally described in 1976, the condition was recognized as a curious combination of sinonasal polyposis, crusting, and culture evidence of *Aspergillus* that resembled the clinical and pathologic findings of allergic bronchopulmonary Aspergillosis (ABPA) [48]. Further characterization of this process as a distinct disease entity involving the paranasal sinuses culminated in Robson coining the phrase by which the condition is known today, "allergic fungal sinusitis" (rhinosinusitis) [18, 40, 47]. Though *Aspergillus* was almost exclusively associated with the disorder in early descriptions, later studies have held responsible the dematiaceous family of fungus for the substantial majority of cases of AFS, giving credence to a more generalized moniker [6, 29].

Pathogenesis

Despite an upsurge in both our understanding of the disease process and our success in treating AFS, all investigators have not accepted a single explanation of the pathogenesis of AFS. A popular theory, referred to as "the AFS cycle," offers a preliminary construct through which the multifactorial process can be understood and against which treatment strategies can be targeted. Manning's theory regards AFS as the sinonasal correlate of ABPA, and depicts a cascading inflammatory cycle resulting in the diagnostic characteristics of AFS [32, 33, 35, 37]. Disease initiation requires fungal antigens inhaled by an atopic host to generate Gel and Coombs type I (IgE) and type III (immune-complex) reactions, which evoke an intense eosinophilic inflammatory response. Patency of sinus ostia is compromised, and resultant sinus stasis engenders fungal proliferation as well as the production of viscid allergic fungal mucin. This mucin accumulates within sinuses, producing further obstruction and perpetuating the AFS cycle [17, 32, 35, 37].

Sequestered mucin collections, the hallmark of AFS, provoke changes in the effected sinuses consistent with those usually attributed to mucoceles [5, 35, 45]:

- Bony remodeling
- Decalcification
- Extension into surrounding anatomic spaces

Persistence of the disease state allows inflammatory mediators to effect slow yet deliberate damage to the sinonasal mucosa [21].

These inflammatory mediators are:

- Major basic protein
- Eosinophil cationic protein
- Eosinophil peroxidase
- Eosinophil derived neurotoxin

- Tumor-necrosis factor-β
- Interleukins 4, 5, 10 and 13

Epidemiology

AFS is more commonly diagnosed in the younger populations (average ages of 21.9–42.4 years) and may represent 5%–10% of all patients undergoing surgery for chronic rhinosinusitis [29, 35, 37, 39]. Manning has suggested a slight male preponderance (1.6 : 1), though this is not borne out in other reviews [29]. Multiple studies have depicted AFS to have a geographic variability favoring temperate regions with relatively high humidity, especially Texas, the Mississippi River basin, and portions of the American southeast and southwest [13a].

Clinical Features

The AFS cycle's unrelenting inflammation is responsible for generating a broad tableau of patient signs and symptoms. Subtle presentations consistent with nasal polyposis or the symptoms of recalcitrant chronic rhinosinusitis are the rule.

Unchecked AFS may lead to [5, 31, 33, 36, 45]:

- Blindness
- Exophthalmos
- Blatant facial dysmorphia
- Intracranial invasion
- Complete nasal airway obstruction

AFS patients are atopic (>90%) and frequently report histories of allergic rhinitis and asthma; yet a complete Samter's triad is not part of the disease process, since aspirin sensitivity is not an associated feature [35]. Typically, these patients have symptoms of sinusitis refractory to trials of antibiotics, intranasal corticosteroids, and immunotherapy, as well as attempts at prior surgical treatment if allergic fungal mucin was not noted or collected at the time of operation, thereby failing to establish the correct diagnosis [17, 33, 35].

13

Diagnosis

Despite a definitive consensus on the diagnosis of AFS, several sets of criteria have been developed to describe the common characteristics of this unique disease entity. Bent and Kuhn's criteria are generally regarded as the most well accepted diagnostic criteria for AFS (Table 13.2) [2]. We find the aforementioned criteria useful as well; however, we substitute a positive fungal stain result for their requirement of a positive fungal culture. Fungal morphology is sufficient to establish the presence of fungi, and often specific enough to identify the responsible organism at the genus level [50]. Reliance on fungal cultures for diagnosis is hindered by the variable yield of such cultures (64%–100%) as well as techniques which may merely identify a saprophytic organism within the nose and not a fungus responsible for the patient's clinical findings [29, 35].

A word must be added concerning the importance of allergic fungal mucin as a diagnostic criterion of AFS, as this is perhaps the most specific finding of the disease and deservedly occupies a central role in our understanding of the pathogenesis, histology, diagnosis, and treatment of AFS. The presence of allergic fungal mucin, absent other features of AFS, probably requires re-examination to ensure the certitude that AFS is not the correct disease to treat. Allergic fungal mucin is thick, highly viscous, tan to dark green/brown material that may be removed from the sinuses with some difficulty. Extramucosal fungi are identified microscopically with various silver stains, while hematoxylin and eosin stains accentuate the sheets of eosinophils and Charcot-Leyden crystals within a mucinous background [17, 35].

Table 13.2. Bent and Kuhn diagnostic criteria for allergic fungal rhinosinusitis

1. Gel and Coombs Type I (IgE-mediated) hypersensitivity
2. Nasal polyposis
3. Characteristic radiologic findings
4. Positive fungal stain and/or fungal culture
5. Eosinophilic mucin without fungal invasion into sinus tissue

From [2]

Imaging

Diagnostic imaging findings in AFS have been delineated in a number of retrospective reviews including both CT and MRI modalities. AFS patients demonstrate bilateral disease in 51% of cases, with asymmetric involvement in 78% of reviewed cases [42]. Complete opacification of at least one sinus was noted in 98% of reviewed cases.

Complete sinus cavity opacification in that study was associated with the following signs that have become suggestive of AFS:

- Sinus expansion (98%)
- Remodeling of the sinus walls (95%)
- Bony erosion (91%)

Our own review of radiographic imaging in AFS patients identifies bone erosion at a much lower rate (20%), but emphasizes the ability of noninvasive disease to mimic other more aggressive sinus pathology [45]. AFS can also be characterized by the nature of CT scan attenuation and MRI signal intensities. In all patients studied, opacified sinuses were found to have increased central signal attenuation on noncontrast CT, which correspond with hypointense areas on T1-MRI and signal voids on T2-MRI [30, 42]. The presence of peripheral enhancement of involved sinuses on MRI-T2, in combination with the above features, strongly favors an inflammatory process such as AFS [30].

One additional imaging characteristic that is often associated with AFS is the frequent presence of heterogeneous areas of signal intensity within opacified sinuses on soft tissue algorithms of CT scans. At the present time, these signals are thought to be the result of heavy metal accumulations and calcium salt precipitation within inspissated allergic fungal mucin [42]. Though these radiologic data have been collected in a retrospective fashion, an amalgamation of the above CT and MRI findings can be convincing, if not confirmatory, for the diagnosis of AFS.

Surgical Therapy

Though the optimal treatment strategy for AFS is still open for discussion, there can be no disagreement regarding surgery as the basic foundation for any successful intervention in this disease process. We employ functional endoscopic sinus surgery techniques to interrupt the "AFS cycle" and set the stage for postoperative immunomodulation.

The goals of sinus surgery are [35]:

- Complete extirpation of all allergic mucin and fungal debris
- Production of permanent drainage and ventilation of the affected sinuses while preserving underlying mucosa
- To provide postoperative access to the diseased areas, such that adequate adjunctive care can be performed

Our practice has been to prescribe one week of preoperative antibiotics and corticosteroids (equivalent to 0.5–1.0 mg/kg/day of prednisone) to decrease generalized nasal inflammation and polyp volume, thereby improving visualization at the time of surgery [35]. Postoperative care is rigorous. Patients complete a taper of their corticosteroids over one month and complete a several-week course of appropriate antibiotics. Clinic appointments are scheduled as frequently as needed to endoscopically examine and debride the operative sites. Topical antifungal irrigations have been suggested as adjunctive care, yet supportive date for this type of therapy are still pending [21, 35, 46]. It is in the postoperative period that adjunctive medical interventions are brought to the forefront of AFS treatment.

Medical Therapy

The similarities between ABPA and AFS play a large role in much of the current concepts of medical therapy for AFS. Successful application of corticosteroids in ABPA patients led to their introduction in AFS cases. Decreased recurrence rates in those treated with corticosteroids, and marked recidivism in those who inappropriately discontinue treatment, have made systemic steroids part of the standard therapy for AFS, though no consensus has been reached on the ideal dose or duration [3, 21, 51]. The addition of topical corticosteroids within the newly ventilated sinonasal cavity is expected to assist in alleviating local inflammation, whereas pre-operatively, this route is limited by obstructing nasal polyps [35].

Unquestionably, the single most important component of postoperative care is institution of immunotherapy directed against multiple fungal antigens. Though immunotherapy is now accepted as the standard of care, initially a leap of faith was required to surmount logical objections to this practice based on experiences in ABPA, the theoretical model for AFS. Given that immunotherapy will often worsen the condition of patients with ABPA, the prevailing notion was that introducing additional fungal antigens would similarly exacerbate AFS. Mabry challenged this convention and his work would thereafter alter the management of AFS.

Mabry postulated that surgical extirpation of the fungal antigenic load, an intervention not possible in ABPA, would then allow immunotherapy to safely produce the desired modulation of a patient's inappropriate inflammatory reaction to fungi [24, 25, 34]. Radio-allergosorbent testing (RAST) testing for multiple fungal and nonfungal antigens [which has results that parallel those of skin end-point titration (SET)] guided the immunotherapy regimen [27]. Patients receiving immunotherapy had significantly better overall outcomes than those postoperative patients who declined or discontinued immunotherapy. Dramatic symptom control and significant decreases in the use of topical and systemic steroid use, reductions in revision surgery, and improvements in both subjective quality of life scores and objective assessments of the postoperative inflammatory state of the nose were documented in retrospective reviews of disease-matched subjects [1, 23, 26]. These therapeutic benefits have been durable over several years during immunotherapy (3–5 years) and are similarly proving to be so up to 17 months after completing a full course of immunotherapy [28]. Recidivism rates as low as 10% can be achieved with the combination of medical and surgical therapy described herein [1, 28, 38].

Additional adjunctive measures in the management of AFS directly target the fungi that initiate the "AFS cycle." Systemic antifungals have not clearly demonstrated their value in treating AFS, and all are fraught with poor therapeutic indices, risks of serious medical complications, increased costs, and uncertain duration of drug therapy [35]. Given that patients may inhale up to 5.7_10^7 spores of various fungi each day, it seems more efficacious to alter the host's immune response rather than expose the patient to chronic antifungal therapy [44]. Topical antifungals likely have lower risks of complications; however, their efficacy, as in systemic therapy, is limited to conjecture.

AFS Involving the Frontal Sinus

Though it is difficult to establish the frequency with which the frontal sinus is involved in cases of AFS, one radiographic study puts the estimate as high as 71% [42]. The frontal sinus' proximity to both the anterior cranial fossa and orbit increases the precision necessary to completely address disease in this location. Accumulations of allergic fungal mucin, in a manner very similar to the pressure atrophy exerted by mucoceles, can cause dissolution and erosion of already delicate bone and invasion of the allergic fungal mucin into the orbit or intracranial space [35]. Evacuation of allergic fungal mucin from the frontal sinus coupled with permanent pathways for ventilation and drainage can be achieved by assiduously opening the frontal ostium without harming the surrounding mucosa or middle turbinate [21, 35]. Kuhn and Swain caution against frontal sinus obliteration in treating fungal disease of this location, especially in complicated cases with erosion through the posterior table or orbital roof, as frontal sinus mucosa cannot be removed completely from the underlying periorbita or dura [21].

Surgery should allow postoperative visualization of the frontal recess during clinic endoscopy for recurrence of disease. Pre- and postoperative systemic corticosteroids, postoperative topical corticosteroids, and immunotherapy against fungal and nonfungal antigens guided by RAST testing complete our approach to treatment of AFS of the frontal sinus. Postoperatively, in patients with frontal sinus AFS, a noncontrasted CT scan of the sinuses may be helpful in monitoring for recurrent disease or frontal ostial stenosis with mucocele formation.

Conclusion

The role of fungus in paranasal sinus disease has been more clearly elucidated in the past 25 years than in any prior period of investigation. Researchers have been particularly motivated to classify and define the variety of states of fungal rhinosinusitis as advances in both medical and surgical therapies have brought much of this type of disease under control. The frontal sinus is not a common location for fungal disease, and as such, most otolaryngologists will have limited experience in treating fungal pathology in this location. An understanding of fungal sinus disease states, appropriate diagnostic investigations, and perioperative medical therapy, coupled with sound knowledge of the surgical anatomy of the frontal sinus will provide patients with their best opportunity for an optimal outcome.

References

1. Bassichis BA, Marple BF, Mabry RL, et al (2001) Use of immunotherapy in previously treated patients with allergic fungal sinusitis. Otolaryngol Head Neck Surg 125: 487–490
2. Bent J, Kuhn F (1994) Diagnosis of allergic fungal sinusitis. Otolaryngol Head Neck Surg 111: 580–588
3. Bent JP III, Kuhn FA (1996) Allergic fungal sinusitis/polyposis. Allergy Asthma Proceedings 17: 259–268
4. Blitzer A, Lawson W (1993) Fungal infections of the nose and paranasal sinuses, part I. Otolaryngol Clin North Am 26: 1007–1035
5. Carter KD, Graham SM, Carpenter KM (2001) Ophthalmologic manifestations of allergic fungal sinusitis. Am J Opthalmol 127: 189–195
6. Chrzanowski RR, Rupp NT, Kuhn FA, et al (1997) Allergenic fungi in allergic fungal sinusitis. Ann Allergy Asthma Immunol 79: 431–435
7. DelGaudio JM, Swain RE, Kingdom TT, Muller S, Hudgins PA (2003) Computed tomographic findings in patients with invasive fungal sinusitis. Arch Otolaryngol Head Neck Surg 129: 236–240

8. deShazo RD (1998) Fungal sinusitis. Am J Med Sci 316: 39–45

9. deShazo RD, O'Brien M, Chapin K, Soto-Aguilar M, Gardner L, Swain R (1997) A new classification and diagnostic criteria for invasive fungal sinusitis. Arch Otolaryngol Head Neck Surg 123:1181–1188

10. deShazo RD, O'Brien M, Chapin K, Soto-Aguilar M, Swain R, Lyons M, Bryers WC, Alsip S (1997) Criteria for the diagnosis of sinus mycetoma. J Aller Clin Immunol 99: 475–485

11. Ferguson BJ (2000) Definitions of fungal rhinosinusitis. Otolaryngol Clin North Am 33:227–235

12. Ferguson BJ (2000) Mucormycosis of the nose and paranasal sinuses. Otolaryngol Clin North Am 33:349–365

13. Ferguson BJ (2000) Fungus balls of the paranasal sinuses. Otolaryngol Clin North Am 33:389–398

13a. Ferguson BJ, Barnes L, Bernstein JM, et al (2000) Geographic variation in allergic fungal rhinosinusitis. Otolaryngol Clin North Am 33:441–449

14. Ferreiro JA, Carlson BA, Cody DT (1997) Paranasal sinus fungus balls. Head Neck 19:481–486

15. Gillespie MB, O'Malley BW (2000) An algorithmic approach to the diagnosis and management of invasive fungal rhinosinusitis in the immunocompromised patient. Otolaryngol Clin North Am 33:323–334

16. Gillespie MB, O'Malley BW, Francis HW (1998) An approach to fulminant invasive fungal sinusitis in the immunocompromised host. Arch Otolaryngol Head Neck Surg 124:520–526

17. Houser SM, Corey JP (2000) Allergic Fungal Rhinosinusitis: Pathophysiology, epidemiology and diagnosis. Otolaryngol Clin north Am 33:399–408

18. Katzenstein AA, Sale SR, Greenberger PA (1983) Allergic Aspergillus sinusitis: a newly recognized form of sinusitis. J Allergy Clin Immunol 72:89–93

19. Kennedy CA, Adams GL, Neglia JP, et al (1997) Impact of surgical treatment on paranasal fungal infections in bone marrow transplant patients. Otolaryngol Head Neck Surg 116:610–616

20. Klossek JM, Serrano E, Peloquin L, et al (1997) Functional endoscopic sinus surgery and 109 mycetomas of paranasal sinuses. Laryngoscope 107:112–117

21. Kuhn FA, Swan R (2003) Allergic fungal sinusitis: Diagnosis and treatment. Curr Opin Otolaryngol Head Neck Surg 11:1–5

22. Luna B, Drew RH, Perfect JR (2000) Agents for treatment of invasive fungal infections. Otolaryngol Clin North Am 33:277–300

23. Mabry RL, Mabry CS (1997) Immunotherapy for allergic fungal sinusitis: The second year. Otolaryngol Head Neck Surg 117:367–371

24. Mabry RL, Mabry CS (2000) Allergic fungal sinusitis: the role of immunotherapy. Otolaryngol Clin North Am 33: 433–440

25. Mabry RL, Manning SC, Mabry CS (1997) Immunotherapy in the treatment of allergic fungal sinusitis. Otolaryngol Head Neck Surg 116:31–35

26. Mabry RL, Marple BF, Folker RJ (1998) Immunotherapy for allergic fungal sinusitis: Three years' experience 119: 648–651

27. Mabry RL, Marple BF, Mabry CS (1999) Mold testing by RAST and skin test methods with allergic fungal sinusitis. Otolaryngol Head Neck Surg 121:252–254

28. Mabry RL, Marple BF, Mabry CS (2000) Outcomes after discontinuing immunotherapy for allergic fungal sinusitis. Otolaryngol Head and Neck Surg 122:104–106

29. Manning SC, Holman M (1998) Further evidence for allergic fungal sinusitis. Laryngoscope 108:1485–1496

30. Manning SC, Merkel M, Kriesel K, et al (1997) Computed tomography and magnetic resonance diagnosis of allergic fungal sinusitis. Laryngoscope 107:170–176

31. Manning SC, Schaefer S, Close, L (1991) Culture-positive allergic fungal sinusitis. Arch Otolaryngol Head Neck Surg 117:174–178

32. Manning SC, Vuitch F, Weinberg A, et al (1989) Allergic aspergillosis: A newly recognized form of sinusitis in the pediatric population. Laryngoscope 108:1485–1496

33. Marple BF (1999) Allergic fungal sinusitis. Curr Opin Otolaryngol 7:383–387

34. Marple BF (2000) Allergic fungal rhinosinusitis: surgical management. Otolaryngol Clin North Am 33:409–418

35. Marple BF (2001) Allergic fungal rhinosinusitis: Current theories and management strategies. Laryngoscope 111: 1006–1019

36. Marple BF. Gibbs SR, Newcomer MT, Mabry RL (1999) Allergic fungal sinusitis induced visual loss. Am J Rhinol 13:1915

37. Marple BF, Mabry RL (1998) Comprehensive management of allergic fungal sinusitis. Am J Rhinol 12:263–268

38. Marple BF, Mabry RL (2000) Allergic fungal sinusitis: Learning from our failures. Am J Rhinol 14:223–226

39. Marple BF, Orfaly T (2001) Clinical and histopathologic comparison between allergic fungal sinusitis and sinus fungal ball. Unpublished data

40. Millar JW, Johnston A, Lamb D (1981) Allergic aspergillosis of the maxillary sinus. Thorax 36:710

41. Mitchell TG (2000) Overview of basic medical mycology. Otolaryngol Clin North Am 33:237–250

42. Mukherji SK, Figueroa RE, Ginsberg LE, et al (1998) Allergic fungal sinusitis: CT findings. Radiology 207: 417–422

43. Murray A (2004) Personal communication. University of Texas Southwestern Medical Center, Department of Otolaryngology-Head and Neck Surgery, Division of Pediatric Otolaryngology

44. Novey HS (1998) Epidemiology of allergic bronchopulmonary aspergillosis. Immunol Allergy Clin North Am 18: 641–653

45. Nussenbaum B, Marple BF, Schwade ND (2001) Otolaryngol Head Neck Surg 124:150–154

46. Ponikau JU, Sherris DA, Kern EB, et al (1999) The diagnosis and incidence of allergic fungal sinusitis. Mayo Clin Proc 74:877–884

13

47. Robson J, Hogan P, Benn R, et al (1989) Allergic fungal sinusitis presenting as a paranasal sinus tumor. Aust N Z J Med 19:351–353
48. Safirstein B. (1976) Allergic bronchopulmonary aspergillosis with obstruction of the upper respiratory tract. Chest 70:788–790
49. Sarti EJ, Blaugrund SM, Lin PT, et al (2000) Paranasal sinus disease with intracranial extension: Aspergillosis versus malignancy. Laryngoscope 98:632–635
50. Schell WA (2000) Histopathology of fungal rhinosinusitis. Otolaryngol Clin North Am 33:251–276
51. Schubert MS, Goetz DW (1998) Evaluation and treatment of allergic fungal sinusitis II: Treatment and follow-up. J Allergy Clin Immunol 103:717–723
52. Stevens MH (1978) Aspergillosis of the frontal sinus. Arch Otolaryngol 104:153–156
53. Stringer SP, Ryan MW (2000) Chronic invasive fungal rhinosinusitis. Otolaryngol Clin North Am 33:375–387
54. Wehl G, Hoegler W, Kropshofer G, Meister B, et al (2002) Rhinocerebral mucormycosis in a boy with recurrent acute lymphoblastic leukemia: Long-term survival with systemic antifungal treatment. J Ped Hem Onc 24:492–494
55. Yohia RA, Bullock JD, Aziz AA, et al (1994) Survival factors in rhinoorbital cerebral mucormycosis. Surv Ophthalmol 39:3–22

Chapter 14

Frontal Headache

14

Allen M. Seiden

Core Messages

- Frontal headache frequently accompanies obstruction and inflammation of the frontal sinuses, but may also reflect other sources of head pain not related to sinus pathology

- Focal areas of impaction and inflammation in the ostiomeatal complex may cause pain referred to the dermatomes of the first and second divisions of the trigeminal nerve

- A thorough history that defines the pattern of headache is essential to help diagnose its cause

- A diagnosis of sinus-related headache needs to be confirmed by a thorough nasal examination that should include nasal endoscopy and appropriate radiographs

- Many of the primary and secondary headache disorders may cause headache in the frontal region, and therefore need to be considered in the differential diagnosis

Contents

Introduction

Headache is a remarkably common complaint. According to the American Council for Headache Education (ACHE), 90% of men and 95% of women have had at least one headache during this past year [10]. Also, according to the ACHE, 90% of these are so-called primary headaches, i.e. migraine, tension-type, or cluster headaches, whereas 10% are secondary headaches resulting from other medical conditions, including infection.

Frontal headache is the most prevalent symptom of frontal sinus disease [13]. In the presence of other nasal symptoms, such as congestion or purulent discharge, the diagnosis is relatively straightforward. Interestingly, when patients present with frontal sinus opacification in the presence of chronic pansinusitis, they often do not complain of headache. However, disease limited to the frontal sinus typically causes severe frontal headache as the only symptom. If the frontal sinus is completely obstructed, there may be little drainage into the nose, and patients in fact may be unaware that their pain is sinus-related.

Patients with chronic headache pain will often present to a variety of specialists, looking to relieve their discomfort. Evaluation by their primary care physician or neurologist may result in a diagnosis of one of the primary headache syndromes, and an underlying sinus problem may be missed. Figure 14.1 shows the CT scan of a 16-year old girl who complained of headaches for over one year, without associated nasal obstruction or nasal discharge. She was diagnosed with migraines, but had not responded to traditional therapy. The scan demonstrates complete opacification of both frontal sinuses, and endoscopic frontal sinusotomy drained inspissated mucus that relieved her headache pain.

Likewise, patients will present to the otolaryngologist because they or their referring physician believe the headache to be related to underlying sinus pathology. The primary focus of the otolaryngologic evaluation is to exclude this possibility, but to do so requires not only an understanding of what can cause sinus-related pain, but also an ability to recognize other, more common headache syndromes. To evaluate a complaint of headache fully, the otolaryngologist must have an understanding of the common causes of headache with a working differential diagnosis that must include the primary headache syndromes.

Pathophysiology

Clinicians and patients alike recognize a relationship between nasal/sinus pathology and head pain, but this relationship is highly variable and therefore controversial. There has been little data to document irrefutably when and why it exists. In the case of acute frontal sinusitis, pressure changes occur that seem to make pain a constant symptom. However, in the setting of chronic sinusitis, pain may or may not be present, the reasons for which are difficult to discern.

Sluder was one of the first to describe frontal headache resulting from closure of the infundibulum and frontonasal opening leading to a vacuum or negative pressure, similar to that which occurs in the ear secondary to a blocked eustachian tube [29]. He observed that this phenomenon most often occurred in the frontal sinus rather than the other paranasal sinuses. Although confirmatory data is scant, several studies as cited by Stammberger and Wolf have demonstrated that hypoxia in the sinuses can give a sensation of pain [32].

Sluder was also one of the first to recognize that sinus inflammation can present with referred pain [29]. This concept was supported by a series of ex-

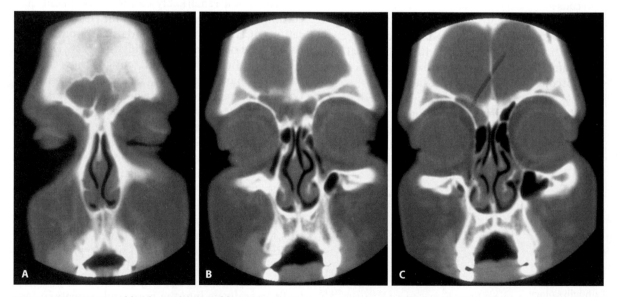

Fig. 14.1A–C. A 16-year-old girl complaining of frontal headaches for over one year was diagnosed with migraine headaches. A,B On CT scan, the frontal sinuses are completely opacified. C Prominent agger nasi cells with obstruction of the right frontal recess

periments performed by Wolff in the 1940's [39]. In a small series of human volunteers, noxious electrical stimuli were placed at various sites within the paranasal sinuses, at the sinus ostia, and within the nasal cavity. Surprisingly, the sinus mucosa was not very sensitive. Rather, the mucosa surrounding the ostia and nasal turbinates was much more pain-sensitive. In addition, the pain was often not felt locally, but was referred to dermatomes of the first and second divisions of the trigeminal nerve. Thus, whereas stimulation applied to the walls of the frontal sinus led to a mild localized pain at that site, stimulation of the frontal recess and frontonasal area produced an intense local pain and pain over the medial canthus, zygoma, and upper molars.

Wolff's experiments are considered classic and are frequently quoted [39]. However, in a recent review Blumenthal points out that these results were based on a very small sample of normal subjects, and some difficulty was encountered in actually accessing the sinus cavities [3]. Tarabichi reviewed a series of 82 patients with chronic sinusitis and headache undergoing endoscopic sinus surgery, and found no correlation between the severity and site of pain with the extent or location of mucosal disease [35]. This suggests the need for caution when trying to diagnose the etiology of headache based upon pain localization.

The ophthalmic and maxillary divisions of the trigeminal nerve innervate the nose and paranasal sinuses. Free nerve endings respond to chemical, mechanical, and caloric stimuli to prompt the release of substance P [32]. This produces an orthodromic impulse traveling along nociceptive C fibers that is interpreted centrally as pain, but may not be well localized by higher cortical centers. At the same time, Stammberger and Wolf have postulated that an antidromic impulse results in the peripheral release of substance P, causing localized neurogenic edema and hypersecretion [32]. This produces additional mucosal swelling and impaction, furthering the sensation of pain.

Based on this concept, areas of narrowing in the nose or ostiomeatal complex might be prone to impaction causing mechanical stimulation of the trigeminal nerve and thereby be associated with headache pain. It has long been recognized that a septal spur impacting the lateral nasal wall may sometimes cause atypical facial pain [5]. In addition, a number of recent studies have demonstrated a relationship between nasal contact points and headache pain [22, 36, 38]. Not uncommonly this pain may be frontal or periorbital in location. For example, the patient whose radiograph is pictured in Figure 14.2 presented with a 10-month history of persistent right frontal headaches. The CT scan demonstrates a large, obstructing agger nasi cell and secondary mucosal thickening within the frontal recess, although the frontal sinus seems to be well aerated. His headache was relieved by surgically opening the frontal recess.

Patients with persistent frontal headache are often referred to the otolaryngologist to rule out underlying nasal or sinus pathology. Considering the foregoing discussion, there are a number of situations that need to be considered. An acute frontal sinusitis almost always presents with severe frontal headache of relatively short duration, generally with associated nasal symptoms. Most patients with isolated chronic frontal sinusitis also typically present with headache, described as a dull, constant pressure, but often in the absence of nasal symptoms. Intranasal examination, including nasal endoscopy, may well be normal, making it difficult to distinguish these headaches from the more common headache syndromes.

The intracranial complications of frontal sinus infections include:

- Meningitis
- Epidural abscess
- Brain abscess
- Venous sinus thrombosis
- Subdural empyema
- Osteomyelitis of the frontal bone

The mechanisms of intracranial spread of frontal sinus infections include [4]:

- Perineural invasion
- Retrograde thrombophlebitis
- Direct extension through defects in the sinus bony walls

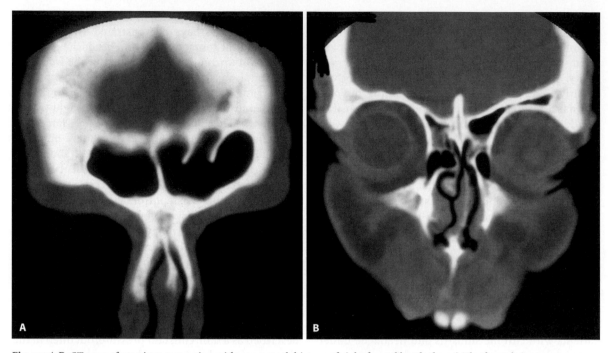

Fig. 14.2A,B. CT scan of a patient presenting with a 10-month history of right frontal headaches. A The frontal sinus appears aerated without disease. B A large, right agger nasi cell with secondary mucosal thickening within the frontal recess

Headache is the most prominent symptom should such complications develop, perhaps with focal neurologic signs.

In the absence of frontal sinus opacification, disease in the frontal recess can produce chronic frontal headache (Fig. 14.2). Similarly, abnormalities of the ostiomeatal complex and middle turbinate may cause periorbital and retro-orbital pain [14, 32]. On the other hand, it is important to remember the relatively high incidence of asymptomatic anatomic abnormalities within the ostiomeatal complex [4, 11]. Therefore, it is essential to try to verify that such findings are indeed related to the patient's symptoms [25].

Finally, osteomas of the frontal sinus may cause chronic headaches (Fig. 14.3). Although osteomas of the paranasal sinuses are not particularly common, the frontal sinus is the most frequent site of involvement [26]. Most often they are asymptomatic and are picked up incidentally on x-ray; however, continued growth may cause pressure against the anterior or posterior table, resulting in headache [26]. In addi-

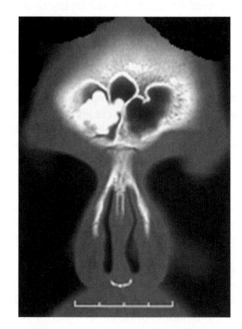

Fig. 14.3. A large osteoma within the frontal sinus in a patient presenting with frontal headaches

14

tion, formation at the frontonasal opening may impair ventilation of the sinus and result in pain [18].

Patient Evaluation

In order to determine the etiology for a patient's headache, much reliance is placed upon the history. It is a complicated problem because all aspects of the pain, including its onset, duration, location, and severity may be quite variable, no matter the cause. Nevertheless, appropriate questioning can usually delineate a pattern that is very suggestive for certain pathology. In this regard, asking the patient to keep a headache diary can be very helpful. As discussed below, the International Headache Society's (IHS) diagnostic criteria for the primary headache disorders are based exclusively on historical factors, so that proper questioning can help to rule out these types of headache [30].

The characteristics of headache associated with anterior ethmoid and frontal sinus disease are:

- The pain is localized around the [32]:
- Glabella
- Inner canthus
- Between the eyes
- Above the eyebrow
- The pain is generally described as dull, along with a sensation of pressure or fullness

In contrast, a migraine headache typically is characterized as throbbing or pulsating, although an acute frontal sinusitis may produce pain of a similar description. A tension-type headache is often described as a tight, drawing pain, whereas a sharp, lancinating pain is generally indicative of neuralgia.

The IHS criteria only recognize acute sinus headache, stating that chronic sinusitis is not validated as a cause of headache or facial pain unless associated with an acute exacerbation [3, 30]. As pointed out by Blumenthal [3], however, the IHS criteria derive from a consensus of expert opinion by a group of headache specialists, mostly neurologists. It is not validated by evidence-based studies [2]. These experts attribute the pattern of headache pain to the specific sinus involved by infection, as per Wolff's experiments from the 1940's [39] (Table 14.1).

More recently the American Academy of Otolaryngology/ Head and Neck Surgery Task Force on Rhinosinusitis defined major and minor symptoms of adult rhinosinusitis, listing facial pain as a major symptom and headache as a minor symptom [17]. These criteria, also, were based upon expert opinion, but acknowledged the frequency with which clinicians treating sinus disease have noted associated headache pain. A subsequent study has demonstrated the inconsistency of diagnosing sinusitis based upon symptoms alone [33], and a more recent modification of the task force criteria recommends the need for specific physical or radiographic findings to corroborate a diagnosis of sinus pathology [21]. Nevertheless, a number of studies have supported the relationship of head pain to chronic sinus disease [32, 35].

Table 14.1. International Headache Society criteria for acute sinus headache

Acute sinus headache
A. Purulent discharge in the nasal passage either spontaneous or by suction
B. Pathological findings in one or more of the following tests: a. X-ray examination b. Computerized tomography or magnetic resonance imaging c. Transillumination
C. Simultaneous onset of headache and sinusitis
D. Headache location a. In acute frontal sinusitis, headache is located directly over the sinus and may radiate to the vertex or behind the eyes b. In acute maxillary sinusitis, headache is located over the antral area and may radiate to the upper teeth or to the forehead c. In acute ethmoiditis headache, located between and behind the eyes and may radiate to the temporal area d. In acute sphenoiditis headache, located in the occipital area, the vertex, the frontal region, or behind the eyes
E. Headache disappears after treatment of acute sinusitis

Adapted from [18]

Head pain related to frontal sinus disease may be constant or intermittent. It is typically worse in the morning upon awakening, and is frequently exacerbated by bending over or the Valsalva maneuver. It may be affected by weather changes, and may be associated with complaints of dizziness, nausea, and photophobia, symptoms also suggestive for migraine headache [6].

If along with frontal headache patients present with active nasal symptoms such as congestion and drainage, this will usually alert the clinician to the possibility of an underlying sinus problem. Having said that, a prevalence of nasal symptoms has been reported in patients with migraine headaches [7], and patients may also have associated rhinitis that is unrelated to their head pain. Therefore, further workup is required to confirm the headache is indeed sinus-related. Similarly, patients may have no nasal complaints despite the presence of extensive inflammatory changes within the paranasal sinuses. Ultimately, a thorough nasal examination and appropriate radiographs best confirm the diagnosis.

To detect evidence of occult inflammatory sinus disease or sites of mucosal contact, anterior rhinoscopy alone is generally not adequate. To visualize the middle meatus, superior meatus, and sphenoethmoidal recess properly, nasal endoscopy is indispensable. Even posterior septal spurs may be missed when using just a nasal speculum. A variety of anatomic variations involving the nasal septum and ostiomeatal complex that predispose to both headache and recurrent sinusitis are now well described, and can usually be recognized during a routine endoscopic examination [32].

It is very important to correlate endoscopic findings with symptoms.

In patients presenting with frontal headache, findings suggestive of frontal recess/frontal sinus disease include:

- Purulent discharge from the frontal recess (Fig. 14.4)
- Polypoid change in the upper middle meatus under the attachment of the middle turbinate
- Enlarged and edematous agger nasi cell (Fig. 14.5)

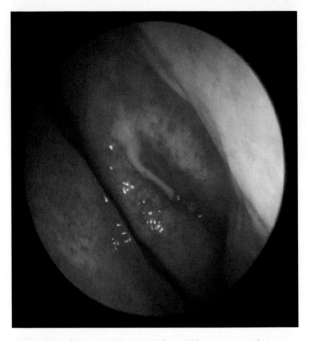

Fig. 14.4. Endoscopic view of a left middle meatus, with a purulent discharge from the upper middle meatus and frontal recess suggesting frontal sinus infection

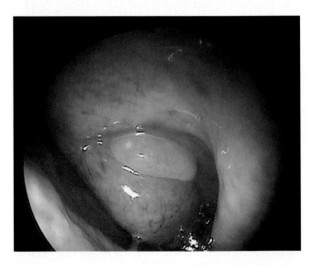

Fig. 14.5. Endoscopic view of a left middle meatus with mucosal edema over the agger nasi region and a polyp protruding from the upper middle meatus, suggesting frontal recess and frontal sinus disease

14

These findings would certainly warrant further investigation.

If a nasal endoscopic examination is unremarkable, but the history strongly suggests nasal- or sinus-related pain, radiologic study is still indicated. Plain sinus radiographs do not demonstrate the frontal recess and ethmoid sinus adequately, and as such are rarely helpful. Computed axial tomography (CT) in the coronal plane remains the procedure of choice, with appropriate bone windows [40]. In addition to frank opacification, it is important to look for areas of mucosal contact and secondary mucosal thickening, particularly in association with anatomic variations. When no mucosal inflammation at all is present but anatomic variations can be seen, the relationship of such findings to chronic headache becomes much more tenuous and controversial [8]. In these situations it is best to try to confirm this relationship by administering local anesthesia to these areas during an active headache, after which the patient should experience some relief [5, 24].

Alternatively, reducing nasal and sinus inflammation and observing a change in the patient's headache pattern may achieve some confirmation, although there is little data in this regard. Such therapy might include topical and systemic decongestants, topical and systemic steroids, antibiotics, or allergy medications as appropriate.

Differential Diagnosis

Patients with anterior facial headache pain will often assume their pain to be sinus-related, and thereby will frequently present to an otolaryngologist. Even if active sinus pathology is found, the patient's headache complaint may be unrelated. It is therefore important for the clinician to be able to consider a differential diagnosis, even though the patient may ultimately be referred elsewhere for management of these headache disorders. Many of the primary and secondary headache disorders may cause headache in the frontal region, and therefore need to be considered [25]. These headaches generally have associated symptoms that distinguish them from nasal- and sinus-related headache, and so the distinction is made largely based upon the history and ruling out any underlying nasal or sinus pathology.

Primary Headache Disorders

Migraine Headaches

Published in 1992, the American Migraine Study found that 17% of women and 6% of men had experienced a migraine headache in the previous year [34]. Since it is one of the most prevalent headache disorders, migraine headache must be considered in anyone presenting with chronic head pain.

Migraine headache is classified as occurring either with aura, formerly known as classic migraine, or without aura, formerly known as common migraine. In migraine with aura, the headache phase is preceded by symptoms likely consistent with transient cerebral ischemia, such as visual changes, hemiparesis, sensory loss, or aphasia. These symptoms can last for as long as one hour, and can also occur at

Table 14.2. International Headache Society diagnostic criteria for migraine headache [25]

With aura:
Two attacks or more fulfilling below criteria
At least three of the following:
One or more fully reversible aura symptoms
Aura symptoms gradually develop
Aura lasts less than one hour
Headache phase beginning within 60 minutes after the aura phase or simultaneously
History and physical do not suggest another disease to explain the headache disorder
Without aura:
Five or more attacks fulfilling the below criteria
Headache lasting 4–72 hours
Headache has at least two of the following
Unilateral location
Pulsating quality
Moderate to severe intensity
Aggravation with physical activity
During the headache, has one of the following:
Nausea or vomiting
Photophobia and phonophobia
History and physical do not demonstrate another disease to explain the headache disorder

the onset of headache. Migraine without aura, which accounts for 80% to 85% of migraine headaches, is not preceded with an aura, and therefore can be somewhat more difficult to diagnose [28]. However, the headache phase and its associated symptoms, such as nausea and vomiting, are identical between migraine with and without aura. The International Headache Society diagnostic criteria for migraine headache are listed in Table 14.2 [30].

A number of environmental and dietary factors can precipitate a migraine attack and thereby aid in the diagnosis.

Common migraine triggers include [20]:

- Menstruation
- Stress
- Fatigue
- Altered sleep
- Weather changes
- Exposure to bright lights
- Exposure to loud noises
- Perfume or other strong odors

Common dietary migraine triggers include:

- Red wine
- Chocolate
- Cheeses
- Aspartame
- Caffeine

14

Characteristics of migraine pain are:

- The pain tends to build over hours and lasts for hours to days
- The headache tends to be episodic
- Characterized by intense and throbbing pain
- Commonly unilateral in location although it may alternate sides

Frequenty migraine-associated systemic symptoms include:

- Nausea
- Vomiting
- Diarrhea
- Photophobia
- Phonophobia
- These symptoms are unusual in sinus-related headache.

It is not uncommon for patients with migraine headache to experience pain in the frontal region. In a study of patients with migraine without aura, the initial headache was localized solely to the frontal region in 31% and to the frontal region along with another region in an additional 25% of patients [27]. In a study of patients suffering migraine with aura, the initial headache involved the frontal region in 59% of patients [28].

In an attempt to ease the diagnosis of migraine headache, a number of investigators have explored the possibility of using screening tools generally consisting of shortened questionnaires that still maintain reasonable reliability. Lipton et al. [19] evaluated a total of 563 patients presenting with headache in a primary care setting. All patients completed a self-administered migraine screener and were then evaluated by a headache expert, the diagnosis of migraine being assigned based upon IHS criteria. They found that three variables had the strongest and most significant association with the diagnosis of migraine: nausea, photophobia, and headache-related

Table 14.3. Three-question migraine screening tool [19]

(Positive response to two out of three):
1. You feel nauseated or sick to your stomach
2. Light bothers you (a lot more than when you don't have headaches)
3. Functional impairment due to headache in last 3 months

disability, with a predictive value of 93.3%. The authors do provide the caveat that this is a screening tool and not a diagnostic instrument. Patients reporting positively to two of the three screening items should then be evaluated more thoroughly to establish a diagnosis of migraine headache (Table 14.3).

Tension-Type Headache

Tension-type headache is the most common headache disorder, with a reported lifetime prevalence of 69% in men and 88% in women [15]. In contrast to migraine headache, tension-type headache is characterized by a dull aching pain of mild to moderate severity typically in a hatband distribution. Some describe the pain as a pressure-like sensation or tightness, most commonly located in the frontal and temporal regions and less commonly in the parietal and occipital regions [25]. One review found the frontal region to be the predominant region of pain in 40% of patients [16]. Although the pain is usually bilateral, it may be unilateral in 10% to 20% of patients.

Tension-type headache is classified as either episodic, occurring less than 15 times per month, or chronic, occurring more than 15 times per month. The IHS diagnostic criteria for tension-type headache are listed in Table 14.4 [30].

Table 14.4. International Headache Society diagnostic criteria for tension-type headache [25]

Ten or more headaches fulfilling the below criteria
Less than 15 headaches per month (episodic) or greater than 15 headaches per month (chronic)
Lasting from 30 minutes to 7 days
At least two of the following:
Pressing or tightening quality
Mild to moderate intensity
Bilateral location
No aggravation with physical activity
Both of the following:
No nausea or vomiting
Photophobia and phonophobia are absent (one may be present)

Cluster Headache

Cluster headaches are not very common, but may easily be confused with sinus headaches. The pain is unilateral, localized to the periorbital, frontal, and temporal regions, and is perhaps the most extreme headache experienced by patients (hence the term *suicide headaches*). The frontal region in fact is a common site for localization of cluster headache pain, involved in as many as 77% of cluster attacks [21]. They tend to be shorter in duration than migraines, lasting 15 to 180 minutes without treatment, but may occur up to 8 times per day. A typical pattern is 1 to 3 episodes per day over a period of 6 to 8 weeks followed by a symptom-free interval of 9 to 12 months. The headaches are generally accompanied by autonomic symptoms on the same side, including lacrimation, rhinorrhea, ptosis, and miosis.

In contrast to migraine, which is three times more common in women, cluster is five times more common in men. These men often display certain physical characteristics, such as a ruddy complexion, deep furrows of the forehead, and deep folds of the glabellar and nasolabial areas. They tend to be tall and trim, usually smoke, and are more likely to consume alcohol.

A 35-year-old white male was referred because of a severe intermittent right frontal headache for one month. He described this as following an upper respiratory infection, but had no residual congestion or drainage. However, he did describe intermittent tearing of the right eye. The headache was described as throbbing retro-orbital and frontal pain. This patient had a similar headache three years previously, and at that time endoscopic sinus surgery was performed and the headache resolved. Therefore, when this current episode began, he was placed on antibiotics and steroids, but did not respond.

Figure 14.6 is an endoscopic view of the right ethmoid cavity in this patient, demonstrating postsurgical changes with an open frontal recess. His sinus scan is shown in Figure 14.7, and is clear of disease. This patient's headache was not related to sinus pathology, but rather was a cluster headache and did respond to appropriate medication. One might speculate that the headache he experienced 3 years previously also was cluster, but this demonstrates the con-

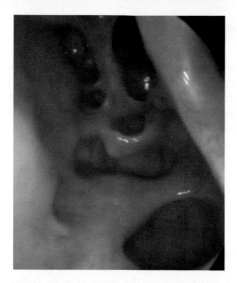

Fig. 14.6. Endoscopic view of the right ethmoid cavity in a patient who had surgery several years previously, now presenting with severe right frontal headache

fusion that might arise when evaluating these patients.

Cluster headache is classified as episodic, persisting from 7 days to 1 year, or chronic, lasting greater than 1 year. The IHS criteria for diagnosing cluster headache are listed in Table 14.5.

Table 14.5. International Headache Society diagnostic criteria for cluster headache [25]

Five attacks fulfilling below criteria
Severe unilateral orbital, supraorbital, or temporal pain lasting 15 to 180 minutes untreated

Headache associated with one of the following:
     Conjunctival injection
     Lacrimation
     Nasal congestion
     Rhinorrhea
     Facial sweating
     Miosis
     Ptosis
     Periorbital edema

Frequency: one every other day to eight per day
Examination does not suggest another neurologic disease

14

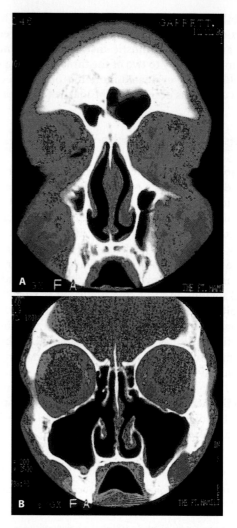

Fig. 14.7A, B. The CT scan of the patient in Fig. 14.6, demonstrating postsurgical changes but no evidence of active sinus disease

Secondary Headache Disorders

Intracranial Neoplasm

Intracranial neoplasm is the most feared cause of headache, but is not common. However, in the absence of focal neurological signs, presenting headache symptoms are usually nonspecific. Forsyth and Posner reviewed the pattern of headache in a series of 111 patients with primary (34%) and metastatic (66%) brain tumors [12]. Headache was present in 48% of these patients, with 77% resembling tension-type, 9% resembling migraine, and the remaining 14% resembling other types of headache. The pain was intermittent in 62% and constant in 36%, and generally of moderate to severe intensity. The frontal region was the most common site of headache, occurring in 68%, and was usually bifrontal although worse ipsilateral to the tumor. Only 25% of patients had unilateral headaches, always ipsilateral to the tumor. In contrast to true tension-type headache, pain was exacerbated by bending over in 32% and by a Valsalva maneuver in 23%. The headaches were worst in the morning in 36% and interfered with sleep in 32%. Nausea and vomiting were seen in 48% of patients.

Headache as the only presenting symptom in association with intracranial neoplasm is unusual, reported by one study in only 8% of patients [37]. Focal neurological symptoms were present in 57% of patients, while seizures occurred in 9%.

Patients with pre-existing headache disorders that develop headache secondary to an intracranial neoplasm can be very difficult to diagnose, as very often the headache pattern may be similar [12]. Any significant change in the quality, severity, or frequency of the patient's underlying headache should arouse suspicion, and warrants further radiological evaluation.

Temporal Arteritis

A diagnosis of temporal arteritis should be considered in any patient greater than 50 years of age with a new-onset headache, regardless of the location of that headache. Temporal arteritis is a vasculitis involving small and medium-sized vessels, and typically produces headache as its presenting symptom. The temporal location is the most common site of pain, but the frontal region has been reported as the primary site in 33% of patients [31]. Other sites include the occipital and vertex areas.

Other symptoms may include jaw claudication, fever, and visual loss. The erythrocyte sedimentation rate (ESR) is a good screening test, having been found to be greater than 50 in 89% of patients and greater than 100 in 41% [1].

Referred Headaches

Pain may occasionally be referred to the frontal region in patients with cervicogenic headaches. These are headache syndromes that arise from pathology in the cervical region, such as entrapment of the C2 nerve root or greater occipital nerve, or from a cervical facet arthropathy [23]. The headaches typically begin in the cervical region and may radiate to the frontal, temporal, or orbital regions. The pain is often precipitated or aggravated by movement of the neck or by sustained positions. Patients will often report a history of head trauma or whiplash.

Myofascial pain syndromes may also sometimes refer pain to the frontal region. These are generally associated with trigger points that refer pain to distant locations. Trigger points of the sternocleidomastoid and cervico-occipital muscles may refer pain to the frontal region [9].

Conclusion

Otolaryngologists often see patients with frontal headache for evaluation of underlying sinonasal pathology. For successful diagnosis and appropriate management, the otolaryngologist must understand the presentation and differential diagnosis of primary and secondary headache disorders that may cause headache in the frontal region.

References

1. Bengtsson BA and Malmvall BE (1982) Giant cell arteritis. Acta Med. Scand 658(suppl):1–102
2. Benninger MS, Ferguson BJ, Hadley JA et al (2003) Adult chronic rhinosinusitis: Definitions, diagnosis, epidemiology, and pathophysiology. Otolaryngol Head Neck Surg 129(3 suppl):1–32
3. Blumenthal HJ (2001) Headaches and sinus disease. Headache 41:883–888
4. Bolger WE, Butzin CA, and Parsons DS (1991) Paranasal sinus bony anatomic variations and mucosal abnormalities: CT analysis for endoscopic sinus surgery. Laryngoscope 101:56–64

5. Chow JM (1994) Rhinologic headaches. Otolaryngol Head Neck Surg 111:211–218

6. Clerico DM (1996) Rhinopathic headaches: Referred pain of nasal and sinus origin, in Diseases of the Sinuses, ME Gershwin and GA Incaudo, eds., Humana Press, Totowa, NJ 403–423

7. Cody RK and Schreiber CP (2002) Sinus headache or migraine? Considerations in making a differential diagnosis. Neurol 6:10-s14

8. Cook PR, Nishioka GJ, Davis WE et al (1994) Functional endoscopic sinus surgery in patients with normal computed tomography scans. Otolaryngol Head Neck Surg 110:505–509

9. Davidoff RA (1998) Trigger points and myofascial pain: Toward understanding how they affect headaches. Cephalalgia 18:436–448

10. Education, ACFE (2004) What You Should Know About Headache. Mt Royal, NJ

11. Flinn J, Chapman ME, Wightman AJ et al (1994) A prospective analysis of incidental paranasal sinus abnormalities on CT head scans. Clin Otolaryngol 19:287–289

12. Forsyth P and Posner J (1993) Headaches in patients with brain tumors: A study of 111 patients. Neurol 43:1678–1683

13. Friedman WH and Rosenblum BN (1989) Paranasal sinus etiology of headaches and facial pain. Otolaryngol Clin of North Am 22:1217–1228

14. Goldsmith AJ, Zahtz GD, Stegnjajic A et al (1993) Middle turbinate headache syndrome. Am J Rhinol 7p17–23

15. Kumar KL and Cooney TG (1995) Headaches. Med Clin North Amer 79:261–286

16. Langemark M, Olesen J, Poulson DL et al (1988) Clinical characterization of patients with chronic tension headache. Headache 28:590–596

17. Lanza DC and Kennedy DW (1997) Adult rhinosinusitis defined. Otolaryngol Head Neck Surg 117(pt 2):s1–s7

18. Leiberman A and Tovi F (1984) A small osteoma of the frontal sinus causing headaches. J Laryngol Otol 98:1147–1149

19. Lipton RB, Dodick D, Sadovsky R et al (2003) A self-administered screener for migraine in primary care. Neurol 61:375–382

20. Lipton RB and Rapoport AM (1996) Migraine with and without aura, in Office Practice of Neurology, MA Samuels and S Feske, eds., Churchill Livingstone, New York 1105–1111

21. Manzoni GC, Terzano MG, Bono G et al (1983) Cluster headache – Clinical findings in 180 patients. Cephalalgia 3:21–30

22. Parsons DS and Batra PS (1998) Functional endoscopic sinus surgical outcomes for contact point headaches. Laryngoscope 108:696–702

23. Pollmann W, Keidel M, and Pfaffenrath V (1997) Headache and the cervical spine: A critical review. Cephalalgia 17:801–816

24. Seiden AM (1996) Otolaryngologic evaluation and management of headache. Curr Opin Otolaryngol Head Neck Surg 4:205–211

25. Seiden AM and Martin VT (2001) Headache and the frontal sinus. Otol Clin North Am 34:227–241

26. Seiden AM and Hefny YIE (1995) Endoscopic trephination for the removal of frontal sinus osteoma. Otolaryngol Head Neck Surg 112:607–611

27. Sjaastad O, Bovim G, and Stovner LJ (1993) Common migraine ("migraine without aura"): Localization of the initial pain of attack. Funct Neurol 8:27–32

28. Sjaastad O, Fredriksen T, and Sand T (1989) The localization of the initial pain of attack: A comparison between classic migraine and cervicogenic headache. Funct Neurol 4:73–78

29. Sluder, G (1927) Nasal Neurology, Headaches and Eye Disorders. C.V. Mosby Co. St. Louis

30. International Headache Society, H.C.C. (1988) Classification and diagnostic criteria for headache disorders, cranial neuralgias and facial pain. Cephalalgia 8: Suppl 7

31. Solomon S and Cappa KG (1987) The headache of temporal arteritis. J Am Geriatr Soc 35:163–165

32. Stammberger H and Wolf G (1988) Headaches and sinus disease: The endoscopic approach. Ann Otol Rhinol Laryngol 97(suppl 134):3–23

33. Stankiewicz JA and Chow JM (2002) A diagnostic dilemma for chronic rhinosinusitis: Definition accuracy and validity. Am J Rhinol 16(4):199–202

34. Stewart WF, Lipton RB, and Celentano DD (1992) Prevalence of migraine headache in the United States. J Am Med Assoc 267:64–69

35. Tarabichi M (2000) Characteristics of sinus-related pain. Otolaryngol Head Neck Surg 122:842–847

36. Tosun F, Gerek M, and Ozkaptan Y (1999) Nasal surgery for contact point headaches. Headache 40:237–240

37. Vazquez-Barquero P, Ibanez FJ, Herrera S et al (1994) Isolated headache as the presenting manifestation of intracranial tumors: A prospective study. Cephalalgia 14:270–272

38. Welge-Luessen A, Hauser R, Schmid N et al (2003) Endonasal surgery for contact point headaches: A 10-year longitudinal study. Laryngoscope 113:2151–2156

39. Wolff HG, McAuliffe GW, and Goodell H (1942) Experimental studies on headache: Pain reference from the nasal and paranasal cavities. Trans Am Neurol Assoc 68:82–83

40. Zinreich SJ, et al (1987) CT of nasal cavity and paranasal sinuses: Imaging requirements for functional endoscopic sinus surgery. J Radiol 163:769–775

14

Chapter 15

Pediatric Frontal Sinusitis

15

Charles W. Gross, Joseph K. Han

Core Messages

- Pediatric frontal sinusitis is not common. Frontal recess disease is more common, which often needs to be addressed

- Frontal sinusitis in the pediatric population does not usually occur until the later childhood years

- Due to the infrequency of frontal sinusitis with or without complications, there may often be a delay in the diagnosis and treatment

- If frontal sinusitis is present, it is often difficult to diagnose secondary to vague complaints in children

- Medical treatment should be the first line of treatment for frontal sinusitis, and the etiology of frontal sinus disease should be determined before considering surgical intervention

- If medical treatment fails, anterior ethmoidectomy with exposure of the frontal recess should be the initial surgical approach

- Extra-sinonasal extension of the infection, though infrequent, will likely require prompt surgical intervention

Contents

Introduction

Dr. Casiano has presented detailed anatomy and embryology of the frontal sinus in Chapter 3. It is however, important to consider certain salient features when considering frontal sinusitis in the pediatric group. The reader is referred to the studies by Onodi [10] and Wolf et al. [13] for the development of the frontal sinus in Table 15.1. These developmental studies are only guidelines, as the development of the frontal sinus is the most variable of all the paranasal sinuses, and the final size of the sinus can vastly differ among patients of the same age group.

Certain information must to be considered when evaluating frontal sinusitis in children:

- Possible etiologic factors
- The possibility of response to medical therapy
- Findings of imaging studies before considering more aggressive medical or surgical therapy

Table 15.1. The dimensions of the frontal sinus in the pediatric population from two studies by Onodi [10] and Wolf et al. [13]

Investigator	Age	Frontal sinus development		
		Length (mm)	Height (mm)	Width (mm)
Onodi [10]	Newborn	3	4.5	2
Wolf [13]	Cellular ethmoidales (frontal cell)			
Onodi [10]	1–4	4.8	6.9	4.7
Wolf [13]		6.5	6	5
Onodi [10]	4–8	6–10	15–16	8–10
Wolf [13]		4–11	14–17	7–9
	8–12	Period of near-completion of pneumatization		

A classic study by Kasper [9] in which he dissected 100 pediatric cadavers remains applicable today as he noted: "Evidence is seen in the embryo at the end of the third or early part of the fourth month of a beginning extension forward and upward of the middle nasal meatus. This early extension is the forerunner of the frontal recess and, strictly speaking, is the first step in the formation of the frontal sinus and certain anterior group of ethmoidal cells."

From this extension children develop frontal sinuses at varying ages:

- In children less than 5 years old, approximately 3% of the children have frontal sinuses [2]
- Between ages 5 and 10 years, approximately 50% have frontal sinuses
- At the age of 11 years and older, 65%–75% have frontal sinuses

As previously noted, the frontal sinus development is not completed until late teenage years. However, the authors have personally seen children as young as four with a well developed frontal sinus (Fig. 15.1).

Sinusitis in children with cystic fibrosis (CF) is a frequent problem, which often poses unique and difficult management issues. It is well known that gen-

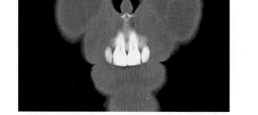

Fig. 15.1. CT scan of the frontal sinus in a coronal view of a four-year-old

eral CF patients have less well-developed sinuses. In the excellent study by Eggesbo et al. in which they analyzed 116 CF patients against controls, they found that 44% of the CF patients studied had bilateral aplasia of the frontal sinuses [3]. It should also be noted that 30% of those CF patients studied had a low ethmoid roof, which must alert the surgeon to this anatomical feature when considering surgery, as it may potentially lead to intracranial complications.

Diagnosis of Frontal Sinusitis

The diagnosis of frontal sinusitis in children is more difficult than in adults, since the symptoms are often less specific. Viral upper respiratory infection is one of the most common medical illnesses in children. It is estimated that 5%–10% of the children with these viral infections will develop acute sinusitis. Thankfully, pediatric acute sinusitis does not usually require aggressive medical or surgical therapy, since frequently it will resolve spontaneously. However, se-

15

vere cases of pediatric sinusitis require aggressive medical or surgical treatment, especially those not resolving to routine medical and supportive management.

The key elements for normal physiology of all the paranasal sinuses are:

- Patency of the sinus ostia
- Proper function of the mucociliary apparatus
- Proper quality and quantity of sinus secretions

Any impairment of these factors may lead to serious clinical consequences.

Children with recurrent sinusitis may have comorbid conditions leading to the sinusitis. These children should be evaluated for:

- Allergies
- Cystic fibrosis
- Immunodeficiency
- Impaired ciliary function

The clinical features indicating significant sinusitis in children are:

- Rhinorrhea
- Cough
- Otitis media
- Bronchitis
- Elevated temperature greater than 101° F

Children with multiple recurrent or persistent infections and unexplained continued nasal mucosal inflammation may require mucosal biopsy to evaluate for ciliary defects. If a ciliary biopsy is to be performed, it should take place at least 6 weeks from an upper respiratory infection, since viral respiratory infections have been shown to cause nasal ciliary damage that may require 6 weeks to resolve.

Appropriate treatment of acute sinusitis in children will usually lead to resolution of frontal sinusitis when present. However, when there are threatening or existing complications related to the frontal sinus, prompt (if not emergent) treatment directed to the frontal sinus is required. Evaluation of frontal sinusitis in children may be difficult because of the vagueness of symptoms and the difficulty of performing a good examination. Even though children with sinusitis may present only with persistent cough or rhinorrhea, the otolaryngologist should still perform the best examination possible. With patience (and occasionally mild sedation), most children aged 4 years and older will tolerate at least an abbreviated endoscopic examination. The endoscopic examination in the office setting can prove to be most beneficial since the quality, quantity, and often the site of origin for the secretions can be determined. If an endoscopic examination is possible, a middle meatus culture can be very valuable in the antibiotic selection process.

Imaging studies are increasingly more practical, even in young children. Newer CT scanners allow very rapid and less traumatic examination of children than those previously available. When necessary, as in severe cases, sedation or even general anesthesia may be employed. When reviewing sinus CT studies, otolaryngologists should remember that children younger than 2 years of age frequently have varying degrees of opacification even in the normal state. In a study by Hill et al., 31% of children had an incidental finding of opacification of the sinuses on a routine CT scan [8].

Medical Management

When antibiotic therapy is necessary, it should be directed toward the offending organism. Ideally, antibiotic therapy should be culture-directed, particularly after failure of prior antibiotic use. The most common pathogens for acute sinusitis are *Streptococcus pneumonia*, *Haemophilus influenzae*, and *Moraxella catarrhalis* [12]. In chronic sinusitis, involved organisms include anaerobes, *Staphylococcus aureus,* and *Streptococcus viridans.* When comorbid conditions such as allergic rhinitis, cystic fibrosis, and immune deficiency are present, they should be treated to facilitate resolution of the sinus infection. Additional supportive therapy should include hydration and moisturizing agents such as nasal saline spray. More severe nonresponding cases may require hospital admission and intravenous antibiotics, particularly when threatening complications are present.

Surgical Management

When surgery for chronic sinusitis in children is necessary, functional endoscopic sinus surgery (FESS) has proved to be very efficacious [8]. Even though surgery is effective, this should only be undertaken in recalcitrant cases. Recalcitrant cases (recurrent and chronic sinusitis) were well defined in the original thesis of Van Alyea, which has stood the test of time [11]. In his manuscript, originally published in 1946, Van Alyea stated that prolonged cases of acute frontal sinusitis imply faulty drainage with a likelihood of recurrence and progression to a chronic state. In these cases, correction of structural defects and establishment of adequate drainage channels assist in the resolution of the condition. Van Alyea also wrote that most patients with long-standing suppuration of the frontal sinus might also improve by correction of structural defects and removal of barriers to drainage.

Attention and exposure of the frontal recess is sufficient for most cases of frontal sinusitis in children requiring surgery. However, frontal sinusotomy may be required in those few cases not responding to an anterior ethmoidectomy with exposure of the frontal recess or in cases where complications are impending or present. We have not found the mini-trephination procedure in young children, other than in those with well-developed sinuses, to be a worthwhile procedure [4]. In young children who cannot tolerate office procedures, a return to the operating room for debridement and evaluation of the frontal recess as a second stage procedure is often beneficial. This is ordinarily done about 2 weeks following primary surgery. In the older patient who will allow endoscopic debridement in the office, this may not be necessary.

Complications of Pediatric Frontal Sinusitis

It is important to remember that although not frequent, frontal sinusitis in children may be a focus of spread for infection to the orbit or central nervous system.

Intracranial Complications

Despite improvements in the medical management of recurrent or chronic sinusitis, complications do continue to occur. Frontal sinusitis can often spread to the cranium due to the intimate relationship between the frontal sinus and the anterior skull base. When this occurs neurologic manifestations may be the initial presentation rather than symptoms from the frontal sinusitis.

The common intracranial complications of frontal sinusitis are:

- Meningitis
- Epidural abscess
- Subdural empyema
- Brain abscess
- Venous sinus thrombosis

When the bony confines of the sinuses are not compromised, infection can still spread to the intracranial cavity through the complex venous network that traverses this area.

In a study at the University of Virginia in which 176 cases of intracranial suppuration over a 5-year period were reviewed, 15 patients had 22 suppurative intracranial complications from sinusitis [4]. Four of the 15 patients were children. In another study by Giannoni et al., there were 18 cases of intracranial complications secondary to sinusitis over a 10-year period [5]. The same study also reports that 12% of the cerebral and 16% of the extra-axial abscesses were due to sinogenic origin. When intracranial complications are present, these patients should be managed in conjunction with a pediatric neurosurgeon. While sinusitis and intracranial complications may be initially managed medically, if a neurosurgical procedure under general is necessary, an involved frontal sinus can be drained in the same setting. Due to the resilience of children, the outcome of neurological complications is generally more favorable than in adults. Early and aggressive medical and surgical management in children often results in little or no permanent morbidity.

Orbital Complications

Pediatric frontal sinus infection can also extend into the orbit and cause periorbital cellulitis or subperiosteal abscess [1]. When an orbital subperiosteal abscess originates from the frontal sinus, the location of the abscess is generally in the lateral superior portion of the orbit. In contrast, when the subperiosteal abscess originates from the ethmoid sinuses, the abscess is usually located in the medial area of the orbit along the lamina papyracea. A specific organism in the head and neck region that has a high rate of extension and involvement of the surrounding structures in the pediatric population is *Streptococcus milleri* [7]. In their study, Han and Kerschner showed that the local extension rate of this organism with involvement of the surrounding structures was 56% [7]. Intracranial involvement was seen when *S. milleri* was cultured from infected frontal sinuses, while orbital involvement was seen when *S. milleri* was cultured from infected ethmoid sinuses.

Once periorbital extension occurs, very aggressive management is compulsory. This is most often managed in an inpatient hospital environment. Intravenous antibiotic therapy may be successful in younger patients. However, if subperiosteal abscess is present and there is no improvement with intravenous antibiotics, surgical drainage is indicated. This can often be done intranasally, but in certain circumstances external drainage may be required.

Conclusion

The majority of cases of pediatric frontal sinusitis will likely resolve with medical management and not develop complications. When complication signs become apparent, early and aggressive medical management with surgical intervention when necessary will most often result in complete recovery without permanent sequelae.

References

1. Brook I, Friedman EM (1982) Intracranial complications of sinusitis in children: a sequela of periapical abscess. Ann Otol 91 : 41–43
2. Cannon CR, McCay B, Halton JR (1995) Paranasal sinus development in children and its relationship to sinusitis. J Miss State Med Assoc 36 : 40–43
3. Eggesbo HB, Sovik S, Dolvik S et al (2001) CT characterization of developmental variations of the paranasal sinuses in cystic fibrosis. Acta Radiologica 42 : 482–493
4. Gallagher RM, Gross CW, Phillips CD (1998) Suppurative intracranial complications of sinusitis. Laryngoscope 108 : 1635–1642
5. Giannoni C, Sulek M, Friedman EM (1998) Intracranial complications of sinusitis: A pediatric series. Am Jour Rhinol 12 : 173–178
6. Gross CW, Gurucharri MJ, Lazar RH et al (1989) Functional endonasal sinus surgery (FESS) in the pediatric age group. Laryngoscope 99 : 272–275
7. Han JK, Kerschner JE (2001) *Streptococcus milleri*: An organism for head and neck infections and abscess. Arch Otolaryngol Head Neck Surg 127 : 650–654
8. Hill M, Bhattacharyya N, Hall TA, Lufkin R et al (2004) Incidental paranasal sinus imaging abnormalities and the normal Lund score in children. Otolaryngol Head Neck Surg 130 : 171–175
9. Kasper KA (1953) Nasofrontal connections. Arch Otolaryngol 322–345
10. Onodi A (1911) Die Nebenhohlen der nase beim kinde. Wurzburg: Verlag Kabitzach
11. Van Alyea OE (1946) Frontal Sinus Drainage. Ann Otol Rhinol Laryngol 55 : 267–277
12. Wald ER (1994) Sinusitis in children. Israel J Med Sci 30 : 403–407
13. Wolf G, Anderhuber W, Kuhn F (1993) Development of the paranasal sinuses in children: Implications for paranasal sinus surgery. Ann Otol Rhinol and Laryngol 102 : 705–711

Chapter 16

Frontal Sinus Fractures

16

Tanya K. Meyer, John S. Rhee, Timothy L. Smith

Core Messages

- Frontal sinus fractures can be classified into anterior or posterior table fractures with or without nasofrontal outflow tract injury

- These injuries are usually associated with other significant head and facial trauma which may require neurosurgical and ophthalmologic consultation

- High-resolution thin-cut multiplanar CT scanning is essential to accurately characterize these injuries

- Three main treatment goals include: (1) protection of intracranial structures and control of CSF leakage, (2) prevention of late complications, and (3) correction of aesthetic deformity

- Complications can be life-threatening and involve the orbit and cranium

Contents

Introduction

The treatment paradigm for the management of frontal sinus fractures has been debated for many years. Aesthetic concerns combined with minimization of acute and delayed complications have led to controversies in treatment protocols and decision-making algorithms. Mismanagement of these injuries may lead to life-threatening complications such as meningitis, brain abscess, mucopyocele, cerebrospinal fluid leak, and osteomyelitis, which can present decades after the original injury. Unfortunately, most series reported in the literature have relatively small numbers of subjects with limited follow-up periods, further contributing to the continued uncertainty about how these injuries are best managed. Although the traditional treatment paradigms were conceived before the advent of modern endoscopic and advanced imaging techniques, new studies have incorporated this technology with resultant modifications.

Problem

Frontal sinus fractures can be classified into fractures of the anterior table or the posterior table with or without associated nasofrontal outflow tract injury. Displaced anterior table fractures can cause aesthetic deformity. Anterior table fractures involving the naso-orbital-ethmoid complex or the medial supra-orbital rim can additionally involve the nasofrontal outflow tract with obstruction of the frontal sinus ostia. This can lead to mucociliary stasis, with subsequent infectious complications and potential for mucocele formation.

Characteristics of posterior table fractures:

■ Usually occur in combination with anterior table fractures
■ Frequently associated with dural or intracranial injury

Management of CSF leaks and dural tears often dictates acute treatment, although concern for dural exposure predisposing to future infectious complications must also be considered. The same concerns regarding nasofrontal outflow tract injury apply to posterior table fractures with the additional increased risk of intracranial spread of infectious complications due to loss of integrity of the anterior cranial vault. Unrecognized injury to the nasofrontal outflow tract may lead to failure of ventilation with eventual formation of mucoceles, mucopyoceles, meningitis, or intracranial abscess.

Epidemiology

Frontal sinus fractures occur in 5%–12% of maxillofacial traumas [4, 14, 15] and most commonly occur as a result of motor vehicle crashes in which the patient strikes the dashboard or steering wheel with the face [21]. Penetrating injuries to the frontal sinus are uncommon. These injuries are often associated with other maxillofacial and intracranial injury.

The force required to fracture the frontal sinus has been reported to be 800–1600 pounds, which is significantly higher than that of any other area of the skull.

Other injuries associated with frontal sinus fractures include [5, 11]:

■ Neurologic injury (76%)
■ Multiple associated facial and/or skull fractures (93%)
■ Orbital trauma (59%)

The predilection for frontal sinus fractures occurring in adults is also due to the timing of pneumatization. The sinuses begin their predominant phase of expansion from age five until adolescence, and are usually characterized by two asymmetric sinuses separated by a thin, bony septal plate. They often demonstrate variable pneumatization, with 4%–15% showing developmental failure of one of the frontal sinuses.

Diagnosis

Although plain films have been used in the past to diagnose fractures of the frontal sinus, this modality often leads to underdiagnosis of the extent of injury and inadequately assesses the posterior table and outflow tract [14]. The advent of high-resolution thin-cut multiplanar CT scanning has dramatically improved the assessment of bony facial injury. The traditional imaging planes include axial and coronal scans, although involvement of the nasofrontal outflow tract is not always definitive despite these multiplanar views. The nasofrontal outflow tract can be best visualized in the sagittal plane [10], which also provides useful information for spatial orientation in the plane of endoscopic surgical approach [8]. Although sagittal reformats can assist in further characterization of the drainage pathway (Fig. 16.1), its prognostic accuracy for eventual normal ventilation of the frontal sinus in the trauma setting is unknown. Certain findings on CT scan images strongly suggest injury to the nasofrontal outflow tract including fractures through the medial supra-orbital rim or the naso-orbital-ethmoid complex [7].

16

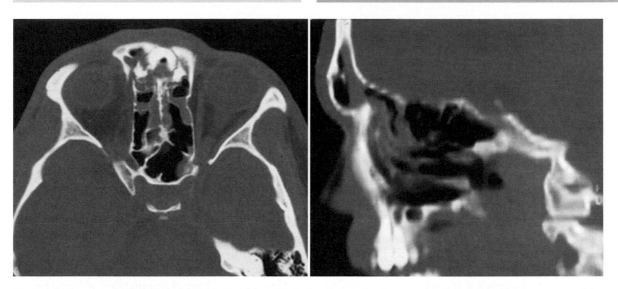

Fig. 16.1. Although not apparent in the axial view, the sagittal reformatted view demonstrates apparent anatomic patency of the frontal outflow tract despite blood and soft tissue edema

Current Management Techniques

The main goals in the treatment of frontal sinus fractures are:

- Protection of intracranial structures and control of CSF leakage
- Prevention of late complications
- Correction of aesthetic deformity

Although many classification schemes have been proposed, frontal sinus fractures can be simply classified as anterior or posterior fractures, with or without displacement, with or without outflow tract injury (Table 16.1). Displacement is defined as greater than one table width.

Anterior Table Fractures (Table 16.2)

Isolated, nondisplaced anterior table fractures do not require surgical treatment. There is minimal chance of entrapment of mucosa with subsequent mucocele formation, and aesthetic deformity is not an issue.

Table 16.1. Classification of frontal sinus fractures

Anterior table fracture
± Displacement
± Outflow tract injury
Posterior table fracture
± Displacement
± Dural injury/CSF leak
± Outflow tract injury

Table 16.2. Treatment options for fractures of the anterior table

Non or minimally displaced
No treatment necessary
Displaced
ORIF for cosmesis
Involvement of the nasofrontal outflow tract
ORIF anterior table & OPF with obliteration
Outflow tract reconstruction (not highly recommended)
Observation and medical management with future endoscopic
Ventilation if necessary

Depressed anterior table fractures can present with both of the above-mentioned problems. The fracture fragments should be reduced and fixed, with careful attention to prevent entrapment of mucosal edges. Exploration can be accomplished via an overlying skin laceration, a brow incision, or a coronal flap.

In some circumstances, noncomminuted isolated anterior table fractures can potentially be addressed endoscopically. These less severe injuries tend to occur in relatively low-energy impact settings. The fracture segments are exposed using a subperiosteal dissection under endoscopic guidance as for an endoscopic brow lift. Additional small stab incisions are made in the brow and along forehead mimetic lines. These incisions allow for bimanual fracture reduction and miniplate fixation with screws [19]. The endoscopic approach can be converted to the more traditional open approach if fracture reduction or fixation is found to be suboptimal.

Missing or severely comminuted bone fragments may present additional problems. Small areas of missing bone less than 1 cm may be left untreated, allowing the skin flap to cover the gaps and monitoring for future contour defects which can be treated in a delayed fashion. Alternatively, titanium mesh can be used to span small defects while also serving as the method of rigid fixation. Larger defects can be reconstructed with split calvarial bone grafts. If there is extensive contamination, but the fragments are of moderate size, they may be thoroughly cleansed and soaked in povidone-iodine before replacement [16]. In the setting of extensive fragmentation with gross contamination or infection, it may be best to ablate or cranialize (see discussion below) the sinus, and delay reconstruction.

Nasofrontal Outflow Tract Involvement

16

Unrecognized outflow tract injury can lead to sinus drainage failure with subsequent mucocele formation, infectious complications, and symptoms such as headache. Intraoperative assessment of patency can be unreliable secondary to traumatic mucosal edema, although some have advocated gentle probing of the outflow tract or administration of fluorescein dye with inspection for intranasal drainage. Much controversy has surrounded management of outflow tract injury, and treatment consists of reconstruction of the drainage system, obliteration of the sinus, or observation with medical management.

If the injury is unilateral, some authors have advocated removing the intersinus septum, thereby allowing drainage through the contralateral outflow tract [1]. This strategy is not widely supported, as it ignores the normal mucociliary clearance pattern and has not been supported by animal models [9]. Another option is prolonged cannulation of the frontal outflow tract as described by Luce [13], but this risks circumferential scarring with outflow tract stenosis, and is considered by many to have an unacceptable failure rate [22]. Alternatively, the outflow tract can be enlarged and relined with a flap of mucoperiosteum from the septum (Sewall-Boyden reconstruction).

Most authors have recommended obliteration of the sinus when injury to the nasofrontal outflow tract is suspected [4, 11, 14, 17, 20, 21] because this has traditionally been considered the safer option for the long-term [25]. Although most nasofrontal outflow tract reconstruction attempts have historically been plagued by stenosis and failure, new endoscopic techniques may allow delayed nasofrontal outflow tract recannulization (endoscopic frontal sinusotomy) after a trial of medical management in highly selected patients (see the "Observation with Medical Management" section below) [23].

There are three main options to obliterate or ablate the frontal sinus:

- The Reidel procedure
- Osteoplastic flap (OPF)
- Cranialization

The oldest method (Riedel) eliminates the sinus by removing the anterior wall, plugging the nasofrontal outflow tract with muscle, meticulously burring away all the mucosa from the posterior wall, and allowing the skin to collapse against the demucosalized posterior wall. This method causes a significant aesthetic deformity, and is indicated only in a grossly contaminated or infected situation.

The osteoplastic flap technique exposes the interior of the frontal sinus by creating a flap of the anterior table hinged inferiorly on pericranium. Through this exposure the mucosa of the frontal sinus can be meticulously removed, the nasofrontal outflow tracts plugged, and the sinus obliterated using adipose tissue most commonly.

Cranialization is performed in occasions involving extensive comminution of the posterior table. In this procedure, the posterior table is removed, allowing the brain to expand forward into the frontal sinus. As in the previous procedures, all mucosa must be meticulously removed from the sinus, and the nasofrontal outflow tracts must be obliterated.

Posterior Table Fractures (Table 16.3)

Many authorities advocate observation of uncomplicated nondisplaced posterior table fractures [3] (without nasofrontal outflow tract involvement, without CSF leak or dural exposure); others report serious complications resulting from this strategy. One series of five patients reports two infectious complications among nondisplaced posterior wall fractures treated nonoperatively [18]. Displacement of the posterior table has been defined as greater than one table width.

With displaced posterior table fractures, the risk of dural injury is unacceptably high. The great majority of these fractures must be explored for dural repair. To prevent late complications, these sinuses are

Table 16.3. Treatment Options for fractures of the posterior table

Nondisplaced without CSF leak
Observation
Nondisplaced with CSF leak
Conservative management of CSF leak with progression to sinus exploration if no resolution in 4–7 days
Displaced (>one table width)
Sinus exploration, repair of dura, obliteration or cranialization depending on involvement of the posterior table.
Involvement of the nasofrontal outflow tract
Obliteration or cranialization

generally obliterated. With severe comminution of the posterior table, cranialization may be the more feasible option. A pericranial flap can be used to separate the nasal and frontal cavities in patients with cribriform plate injury and thus augment the skull base and dural repair [4, 6].

Observation with Medical Management (Fig. 16.2)

Medical management has been proposed in highly selected cases: (1) isolated outflow tract injury, (2) isolated anterior table fracture with or without outflow tract injury, (3) nondisplaced uncomplicated posterior table fractures without outflow tract injury. The safety of this strategy relies on the patients' understanding of the risks of future complications and their willingness to undergo periodic follow-up. In these cases, patients are treated with a prolonged course of broad-spectrum antibiotics (4 weeks) and topical or oral steroids if there are no co-existent medical contraindications. The patients are reas-

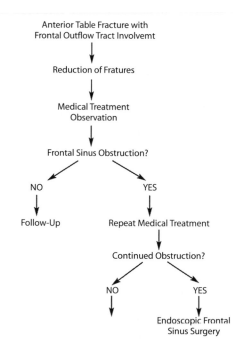

Fig. 16.2. Modified treatment algorithm for highly selected patients

sessed with serial CT scans (1 month, 3 months, 6 months, and yearly thereafter) to check for ventilation and restoration of mucociliary clearance [23]. Individuals who fail to ventilate after two courses of antibiotics or suffer an infectious complication would be evaluated for endoscopic frontal sinus surgery. In our experience, these individuals would require computer-guided surgical imaging, and undergo an extended endoscopic frontal sinusotomy (Draf type II) or endoscopic modified Lothrop procedure (Draf type III or frontal sinus drill-out) [2].

This is the preferred management protocol in this select group of patients in our institution. In 2002 we reported a series of seven patients with displaced anterior table fractures and suspected nasofrontal outflow tract injury by multiplanar CT scanning. All of these patients would have undergone OPF with obliteration under the traditional protocol. Of this group, five patients experienced spontaneous ventilation. The two patients who failed to ventilate had concomitant naso-orbital-ethmoid fractures, and were successfully treated with endoscopic frontal sinus surgery (Draf type II and modified Lothrop procedure) with four years follow-up [23].

It is important to note that medical management or endoscopic sinusotomy does not preclude the use of the time-honored obliteration procedures if these measures fail.

Drawbacks of Obliteration and Cranialization

Although obliteration has been touted as the gold standard and safest method to treat the injured frontal sinus, there are many disadvantages including:

- Facial scarring
- Frontal bone embossment
- Frontal neuralgia related to surgical trauma of supraorbital and supratrochlear sensory nerves
- Donor site associated morbidity
- The loss of physiologic ventilation of the sinuses hampers the use of radiographic studies in the evaluation of sinus disease

These individuals may also complain of chronic frontal headache, which presents a diagnostic dilemma due to our limitations in radiographic evaluation of the sinus.

Loevner et al. [12] studied 13 patients who underwent osteoplastic flap with autogenous adipose tissue obliteration. The authors concluded that partial replacement of the fat graft with soft tissue (granulation and fibrosis) occurred in most cases and ranged from 4%–85%. The imaging signals from magnetic resonance (MR) change over time, reflecting this dynamic process of remodeling such that there are no consistent MR features to distinguish recurrent sinusitis or early mucopyocele formation from expected adipose graft remodeling.

Although obliteration and cranialization are performed to prevent future mucocele formation and subsequent infectious sequelae, these procedures require meticulous attention to technical detail with regard to removing all of the sinus mucosa and permanently occluding the frontal sinus ostia.

Finally, in the acute trauma setting, the osteoplastic flap may not be raised in one continuous piece, but rather consists of multiple fracture fragments. Not only is it difficult to completely remove mucosa from these fragments, but there is a risk of bone devitalization with future resorption leading to aesthetic deformity.

Many of the same concerns regarding thoroughness of mucosa removal and future mucocele formation apply to cranialization as well. Additionally there remains the hypothetical risk of repeated frontal trauma and loss of the impact zone provided by the intact frontal sinus.

Follow-up Care

All patients, regardless of type of management, must be followed closely in the first year after injury and yearly thereafter. All of these patients must realize that they have a life-long risk for delayed complications, and must seek immediate medical attention for any complaint of frontal pressure, pain, or headache. They should receive prompt attention with an aggressive workup including appropriate imaging and medical management. These patients require long-term follow-up, as late complications have been reported more than a decade after the initial injury.

Outcome and Prognosis

Patients who have suffered frontal sinus trauma and received timely and appropriate treatment with surveillance have a good prognosis. The complication rate has been reported as 1%–3% for obliterative frontal sinus reconstructions, and as high as 10% with nonobliterative treatment [11, 21, 24]. Excellent results have been reported for delayed endoscopic ventilation of the injured frontal recess without violation of the posterior table in highly selected patient populations, and these results may influence the balance of the algorithm in the future [23]. Currently, obliteration in cases of outflow tract injury and posterior table injury remains the gold standard.

Case reports

Case 1

A 22-year-old woman presented following a motor vehicle crash in which she sustained an open, displaced anterior table frontal sinus fracture with associated NOE fracture. Fine-cut CT demonstrated these fractures and was highly suspicious for frontal sinus outflow tract fracture (Fig. 16.3). The patient underwent open reduction and internal fixation of the frontal sinus and NOE fractures using a forehead laceration for exposure. There was extensive comminution of the anterior table with small areas of bone loss. The bone fragments were meticulously reduced and fixated with miniplates. Minimal manipulation of the fragments was attempted in an effort to prevent devascularization. She was discharged home with a 4-week course of broad-spectrum antibiotics, nasal spray, and close follow-up.

At the 4-week follow-up visit, she described pressure over the frontal region. Follow-up CT demonstrated opacification of the frontal sinuses with evidence of frontal outflow obstruction. Endoscopic evaluation revealed no purulence or significant inflammation in the middle meatus. Topical nasal steroid spray, prednisone taper, and empiric antibiotic treatment was initiated for four additional weeks. Follow-up CT demonstrated no improvement.

The patient was prepared for endoscopic frontal sinus surgery. High-resolution thin-cut multiplanar CT scanning was repeated to enable use of computer guidance. An endoscopic extended frontal sinusotomy was performed (Fig. 16.4).

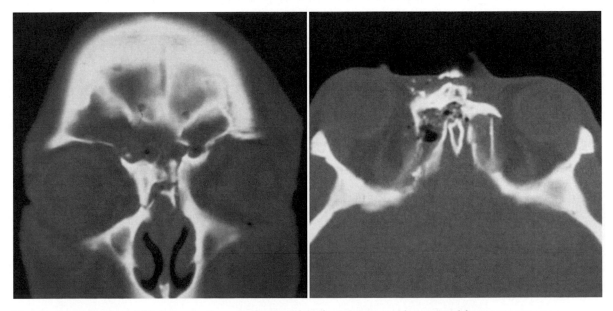

Fig. 16.3. Coronal and axial CT demonstrating opacification of the frontal sinuses with associated fractures

Clinical follow-up with endoscopic examination and debridement was performed at day 6, day 13, and then weekly for 6 weeks. Medical therapy was maximized during the initial 6-week postoperative period, which included nasal saline irrigations, topical nasal steroid sprays, perioperative tapering dose of prednisone, and culture-directed antibiotics. Endo-scopic examination at 6 months revealed a widely patent nasofrontal communication. At 2 year's follow-up, CT demonstrated excellent ventilation of the sinus with return of mucociliary clearance (Fig. 16.5). At 5 year's follow-up, no clinical evidence of frontal disease is apparent.

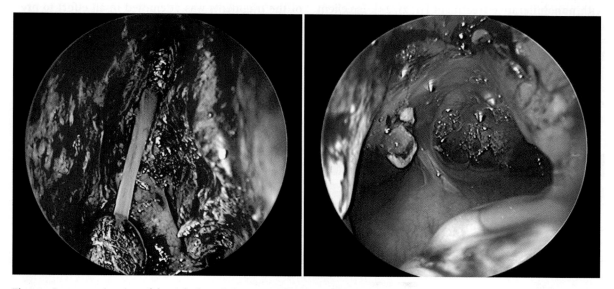

Fig. 16.4. Intraoperative view of the right frontal sinusotomy (with retained secretions) and the completed endoscopic opening. The tips of the screws used in fixation of the anterior table fracture can be seen penetrating the anterior wall of the frontal sinus

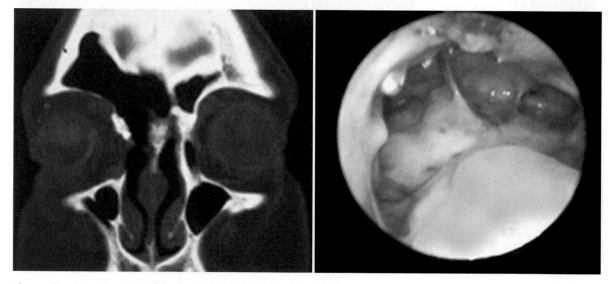

Fig. 16.5. Postoperative views of the frontal sinus, which is widely patent

16

Case 2

A 21-year-old patient presented following a motor vehicle crash in which he sustained an open, displaced anterior table frontal sinus fracture. Fine-cut CT demonstrated these fractures and was highly suspicious for frontal sinus outflow tract injury (Fig. 16.6). Displaced fractures of the nasal bones and septum were treated with closed reduction. Open reduction and internal fixation of the frontal sinus fractures was performed. There was extensive comminution of the anterior table. The bone fragments were meticulously reduced and fixated with miniplates. He was discharged home with a 4-week course of broad-spectrum antibiotics and nasal saline irrigation.

At the 8-week follow-up visit, the patient appeared to be healing without complication and denied frontal pain or pressure. At the 1-year follow-up evaluation, no symptoms related to the frontal sinus were reported, and CT evaluation revealed a well-ventilated frontal sinus and outflow tract (Fig. 16.7). At 4-1/2 year's follow-up, no clinical evidence of frontal disease is apparent.

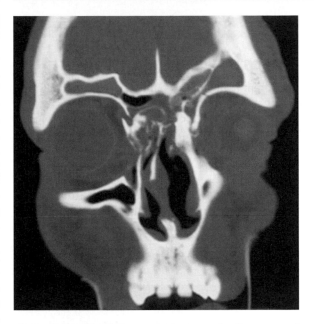

Fig. 16.6. Coronal CT demonstrating extensive fractures and soft tissue trauma in the region of the frontal sinus outflow tract

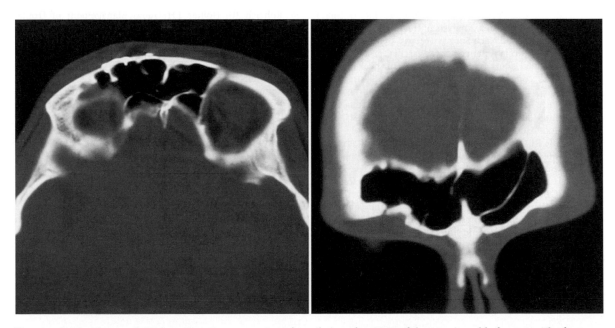

Fig. 16.7. Axial and coronal CT demonstrating restoration of ventilation after ORIF of the anterior table fractures. The fractures appear adequately reduced

Conclusions

The treatment algorithm for patients with fractures of the frontal sinus remains controversial. Proper management relies on the type and severity of the injury being treated, the patient population involved, and the experience of the managing trauma team. All of these patients must receive education about the consequences of their injury, need for continued follow-up, and attention to warning symptoms to prevent life-threatening complications.

References

1. Donald PJ (1980) Frontal Sinus and Nasofrontoethmoidal Complex Fractures: A Self-Instructional Package. Located at: American Association of Otolaryngology – Head and Neck Surgery Committee on Continuing Education
2. Draf W (1991) Endonasal micro-endoscopic frontal sinus surgery: The Fulda concept. Op Tech Otolaryngol Head Neck Surg 2:234–240
3. Duvall AJ, 3rd, Porto DP, Lyons D, Boies LR, Jr (1987) Frontal sinus fractures. Analysis of treatment results. Arch Otolaryngol Head Neck Surg 113(9):933–935
4. Gerbino G, Roccia F, Benech A, Caldarelli C (200) Analysis of 158 frontal sinus fractures: Current surgical management and complications. J Craniomaxillofac Surg 28(3): 133–139
5. Gonty AA, Marciani RD, Adornato DC (1999) Management of frontal sinus fractures: A review of 33 cases. J Oral Maxillofac Surg 57(4):372–379; discussion 380–371
6. Goodale RL, Montgomery WW (1964) Technical advances in osteoplastic frontal sinusectomy. Arch Otolaryngol 79: 522–529
7. Harris L, Marano GD, McCorkle D (1987) Nasofrontal duct: CT in frontal sinus trauma. Radiology 165(1):195–198
8. Hilger AW, Ingels K, Joosten F (1999) Sagittal computerized tomography reconstruction of the lateral nasal wall for functional endoscopic sinus surgery. Clin Otolaryngol 24(6):527–530
9. Hybels RL, Newman MH (1977) Posterior table fractures of the frontal sinus: I. An experimental study. Laryngoscope 87(2):171–179
10. Kim KS, Kim HU, Chung IH, Lee JG, Park IY, Yoon JH (2001) Surgical anatomy of the nasofrontal duct: Anatomical and computed tomographic analysis. Laryngoscope 111(4 Pt 1):603–608
11. Levine SB, Rowe LD, Keane WM, Atkins JP, Jr (1986) Evaluation and treatment of frontal sinus fractures. Otolaryngol Head Neck Surg 95(1):19–22
12. Loevner LA, Yousem DM, Lanza DC, Kennedy DW, Goldberg AN (1995) MR evaluation of frontal sinus osteoplastic flaps with autogenous fat grafts. AJNR Am J Neuroradiol 16(8):1721–1726
13. Luce EA (1987) Frontal sinus fractures: Guidelines to management. Plast Reconstr Surg 80(4):500–510
14. May M, Ogura JH, Schramm V (1970) Nasofrontal duct in frontal sinus fractures. Arch Otolaryngol 92(6):534–538
15. McGraw-Wall B (1998) Frontal sinus fractures. Facial Plast Surg 14(1):59–66
16. Nadell J, Kline DG (1974) Primary reconstruction of depressed frontal skull fractures including those involving the sinus, orbit, and cribriform plate. J Neurosurg 41(2): 200–207
17. Nahum AM (1975) The biomechanics of maxillofacial trauma. Clin Plast Surg 2(1):59–64
18. Newman MH, Travis LW (1973) Frontal sinus fractures. Laryngoscope 83(8):1281–1292
19. Onishi K, Osaki M, Maruyama Y (1998) Endoscopic osteosynthesis for frontal bone fracture. Ann Plast Surg 40(6): 650–654
20. Rohrich RJ, Hollier LH (1992) Management of frontal sinus fractures. Changing concepts. Clin Plast Surg 19(1): 219–232
21. Shockley WW, Stucker FJ Jr, Gage-White L, Antony SO (1988) Frontal sinus fractures: Some problems and some solutions. Laryngoscope 98(1):18–22
22. Shumrick KA, Smith CP (1994) The use of cancellous bone for frontal sinus obliteration and reconstruction of frontal bony defects. Arch Otolaryngol Head Neck Surg 120(9): 1003–1009
23. Smith TL, Han JK, Loehrl TA, Rhee JS (2002) Endoscopic management of the frontal recess in frontal sinus fractures: A shift in the paradigm? Laryngoscope 112(5): 784–790
24. Stanley RB, Jr (1988) Management of frontal sinus fractures. Facial Plast Surg 5(3):231–235
25. Thaller SR, Donald P (1994) The use of pericranial flaps in frontal sinus fractures. Ann Plast Surg 32(3):284–287

16

Frontal Sinus Cerebrospinal Fluid Leaks

17

Bradford A. Woodworth, Rodney J. Schlosser

Core Messages

- Identification of a CSF leak etiology; accidental trauma, surgical trauma, tumors, congenital, or spontaneous; is essential for successful repair

- Anatomically, frontal sinus CSF leaks are divided into those located adjacent to the frontal recess, within the frontal recess, or within the frontal sinus proper

- Pre-operative evaluation may include beta-2 transferrin, radioactive/CT cisternogram, high-resolution CT, MRI, or intrathecal fluorescein and should be individualized for the purposes of diagnosis and localization

- Frontal sinus CSF leaks adjacent to or within the frontal recess are typically amenable to endoscopic repair

- CSF leaks affecting the posterior table within the frontal sinus proper may require external approaches, such as frontal trephine or osteoplastic flap. Combined endoscopic and external techniques are useful for defects extending to the frontal sinus outflow tract

- Severely comminuted posterior table fractures may require craniotomy and cranialization of the frontal sinus

Contents

Introduction

Pathology of the frontal sinus represents one of the most challenging and technically demanding areas for the sinus surgeon to reach endoscopically. Cerebrospinal fluid (CSF) leaks in other parts of the sinonasal cavity have been repaired with relatively high success rates using accepted endoscopic techniques for nearly 20 years [7], yet little has been published regarding repair of frontal sinus defects. The use of 70° endoscopes and giraffe instruments allows excellent access to the frontal recess, but postoperative stenosis, anatomic variants, and CSF leaks associated with the posterior table can make repair of these defects very challenging and pushes the limits of endoscopic repairs. Pertinent frontal sinus anatomy, etiologies of CSF leaks, preoperative imaging and considerations, and the technique and type of repair will be discussed.

Anatomic Site

The complex anatomy and variability of the frontal recess is described in great detail elsewhere in this text, but in the most basic sense, the broadest boundaries of the frontal recess are the internal nasofrontal beak anteriorly, the orbit laterally, the attachment of the middle turbinate medially, and the face of the ethmoid bulla (if present) and ethmoid roof posteriorly. This anatomy is highly variable, and a number of cells may alter this and encroach upon the frontal outflow tract if present, such as an agger nasi cell anterolaterally or a suprabullar cell posteriorly.

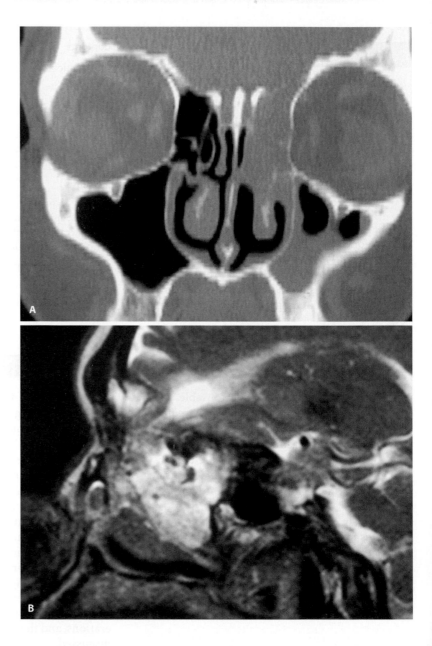

Fig. 17.1.
Coronal CT (A) and sagittal T2 weighted MRI (B) of patient with meningoencephalocele involving the posterior aspect of the frontal recess that was repaired endoscopically

17

CSF leaks affecting the frontal sinus can be divided anatomically into three general categories:

- Those adjacent to the frontal recess
- Those with direct involvement of the frontal recess
- Those located within the frontal sinus proper

While most leaks are limited to one of these distinct sites, some defects encompass multiple anatomic areas.

Skull base defects located in the anteriormost portion of the cribriform plate or the ethmoid roof just posterior to the frontal recess do not directly involve the frontal sinus or its outflow tract, but by virtue of their close proximity, the frontal recess must be addressed as described in the Surgical Methods section of this chapter. Endoscopic repairs may cause iatrogenic mucoceles or frontal sinusitis if graft material, packing, or synechiae formation obstructs the frontal sinus outflow tract.

A CSF leak that directly involves the frontal recess is one of the most difficult sites to approach surgically, because the superior extent of the defect may be difficult to reach endoscopically and the inferior/posterior extension of the defect may be difficult to reach from an external approach (Figs. 17.1–17.3). If long-term frontal patency is questionable, then an osteoplastic flap with thorough removal of all mucosa and obliteration is recommended. On the other hand, if the surgeon feels that frontal patency can be maintained, repair of the skull base defect without obliteration can be performed (Fig. 17.4).

The final anatomic site for frontal sinus CSF leaks is within the frontal sinus proper involving the posterior table above the isthmus of the frontal recess. The limits of endoscopic approaches continue to expand with improved equipment and experience. However, defects located superiorly or laterally within the frontal sinus may still require an osteoplastic flap with or without obliteration. Frontal trephination and an endoscopic modified Lothrop procedure are adjuvant techniques that are useful for unique cases (Fig. 17.5). The specific approach depends upon the site and size of the defect, the equipment available, and surgical experience.

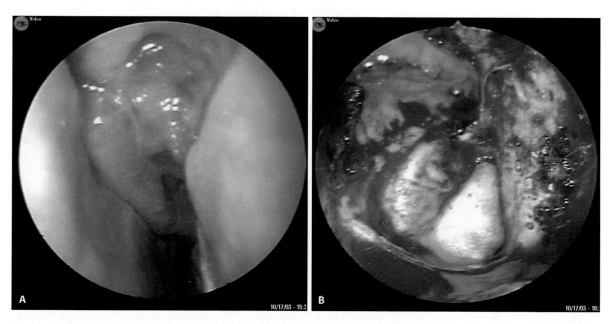

Fig. 17.2. Endoscopic view of meningoencephalocele (from patient in Fig. 17.1) highlighted by fluorescein (**A**). Mucosa stripped from posterior aspect of frontal recess and septal bone graft placed into epidural space (**B**)

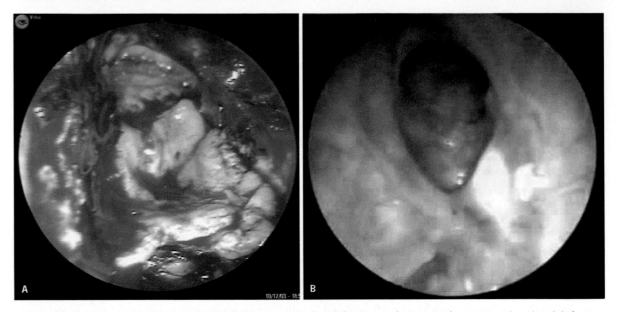

Fig. 17.3. Overlay mucosal graft (A) placed. Sialastic stent was placed for one week. Six month postoperative view (B) demonstrates successful repair and widely patent frontal sinus

17

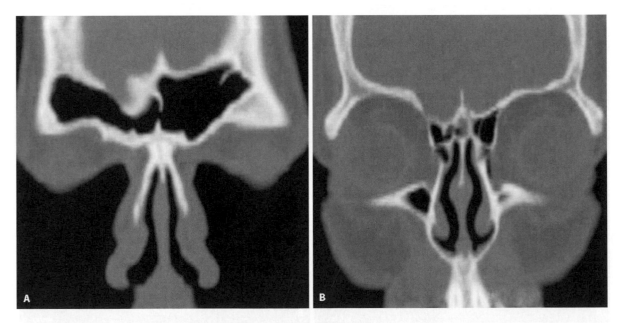

Fig. 17.4. Coronal (A, B) and sagittal (C) CTs demonstrate a traumatic skull base defect that involved the posterior table, frontal recess, and ethmoid roof (*arrows* in C depict the extent of the defect). This required a combined endoscopic and osteoplastic approach

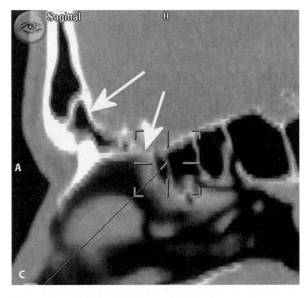

Fig. 17.4C

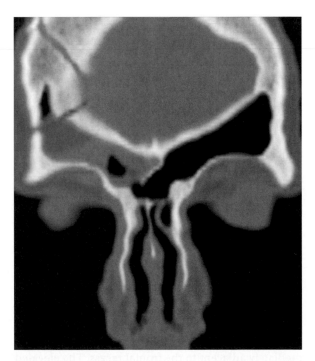

Fig. 17.5. Isolated skull base defect in the lateral aspect of the frontal sinus without involvement of the frontal recess. Such defects can be repaired via trephine while maintaining patency of the frontal recess

Surgical Goals for Frontal CSF Leaks

- Goal #1 – Successful repair of the skull base defect and cessation of the CSF leak.

- Goal #2 – Long-term patency of the frontal sinus or a successful obliteration with meticulous removal of all mucosa within the frontal sinus.

- Always be cognizant of both goals when deciding upon a specific surgical approach and repair for each skull base defect.

Etiology

The underlying cause of a CSF leak will affect the management of the subsequent repair.

CSF leaks are broadly classified into:

- Traumatic (including accidental and iatrogenic trauma)
- Tumor-related
- Spontaneous
- Congenital

These etiologies influence the size and structure of the bony defect, degree and nature of the dural disruption, associated intracranial pressure differential, and meningoencephalocele formation. These factors greatly influence medical and surgical treatment and help predict long-term success.

Trauma

Frontal sinus fractures represent approximately 5%–12% of craniofacial injuries and have a high potential for late mucocele formation, intracranial injury, and aesthetic deformity [5, 8, 10]. Traumatic disruption of the posterior table of the frontal sinus or frontal recess with a dural tear can create an obvious CSF leak or present years later with meningitis, delayed leak, or encephalocele. Projectile injuries from bullets, shotgun blasts, or shrapnel can result in significant comminution of the skull base, and are more likely to involve intracranial injury. CSF leaks usually begin within 48 hours, and 95% of them manifest within 3 months of injury [15]. Although over 70% of traumatic CSF leaks close with observation or conservative treatment, a 29% incidence of meningitis has been reported in long-term follow-up when managed nonsurgically [1].

Conservative, nonsurgical measures are often adequate for injuries limited to the frontal recess and/or posterior table, but severe fractures may require operative intervention due to a high risk of subsequent mucocele formation. Here, operative intervention addresses both the CSF leak and the potential for future mucocele development, depending upon the anatomic site of the defect. Other considerations include the overall health of the patient, associated intracranial or intraorbital injuries, and other skull base or facial fractures. These additional issues influence surgical treatment and approach.

Functional endoscopic sinus surgery (FESS) and neurologic surgery are the two most common surgeries leading to iatrogenic skull base defects. Significant defects can result from powered instrumentation if they occur during bone resection near the skull base. A CSF leak can occur in the posterior table of the frontal sinus or frontal recess during routine frontal sinusotomy. The posterior table may be less than 1 mm thick, and is much thinner than the anterior table. An expansile mucocele or tumor can create dehiscences along the posterior table that are more susceptible to iatrogenic CSF leak during instrumentation. More aggressive surgical techniques for managing frontal sinus disease, such as the endoscopic Lothrop/Draf procedures and osteoplastic flaps, carry a risk of iatrogenic CSF leak as high as 10% [13].

CSF leak following neurological surgery can occur during frontal craniotomy if the superior or lateral recess of the frontal sinuses are entered with removal of the bony plate. Individuals with extensive pneumatization are at higher risk. CSF leaks in the lateral recess are often impossible to repair endoscopically and may require an osteoplastic flap or trephine approach. Placement of grafts over defects limited to the lateral recess via a frontal trephine may preserve the frontal recess and avoid the need for frontal obliteration.

Tumors

Anterior skull base and sinonasal tumors can create frontal sinus CSF leaks directly through erosion of the posterior table or frontal recess, or indirectly secondary to therapeutic treatments for the tumor. Persistent tumor following resection and repair will continue to erode the skull base and contribute to frontal sinus CSF leaks. Creating a watertight seal between the sinonasal and intracranial cavities after tumor removal can be difficult. If the tumor is approached intracranially, a pericranial flap is often used to create a barrier. CSF leaks may still occur due to tears in the flap that occur during elevation, devascularization, and necrosis, or from inadequate coverage. Posterior table defects and frontal sinus floor defects (after cranialization) may still be present and contribute to CSF leak. Prior chemotherapy or radiation creates significant healing difficulties due to poor vascularity of the wound bed.

Congenital

Since the frontal sinus is not present at birth, congenital leaks of the frontal sinus proper do not exist. However, CSF leaks may develop within or adjacent to the frontal recess, and congenital defects often arise from the foramen cecum [14]. These patients often have a low, funnel-shaped skull base that can make repairs more challenging.

Spontaneous

Patients with no other recognizable etiology for their CSF leak are deemed spontaneous. Most frequently these leaks occur in obese, middle-age females who demonstrate elevated intracranial pressure (ICP) [12]. In the frontal sinus, spontaneous leaks rarely occur through the posterior table itself and are more likely to occur at weaker sites of the skull base, such as the ethmoid roof or anterior cribriform plate immediately adjacent to the frontal recess. The elevated CSF pressures seen in this subset of patients leads to the highest rate (50%–100%) of encephalocele formation, and the highest recurrence rate following surgical repair of the leak (25%–87%), compared to less than 10% for most other etiologies [4, 6, 11]. We recommend adjuvant therapies to treat documented elevation of the ICP as described in the Adjuncts Section of this chapter.

Diagnosis

Establishing the diagnosis and identifying the location of a CSF leak in a patient with intermittent clear nasal drainage and no history of head trauma can be difficult. Pre-operative tests should be based upon the clinical picture and the precise information needed, rather than following a rigid algorithm. In addition, the invasiveness of the test and risks to the patient should be considered. The reported sensitivity and specificity of any test should be interpreted with caution, as these statistics are highly dependent upon the patient population studied, size of the defect, flow rate of the leak, and the individual interpreting the test.

Techniques for Diagnosing and Localizing CSF Leaks

- *Beta-2 Transferrin*
  - Advantages: Accurate, noninvasive
  - Disadvantages: Nonlocalizing

- *High-resolution coronal and axial CT scan*
  - Advantages: Excellent bony detail
  - Disadvantages: Inability to distinguish CSF from other soft tissue; bony dehiscences may be present without a leak

- *Radioactive cisternograms*
  - Advantages: Localizes side of the leak, identifies low volume or intermittent leaks
  - Disadvantages: Localization imprecise

- *CT cisternograms*
  - Advantages: Contrast may pool within frontal sinus; good bony detail
  - Disadvantages: Invasive, may not detect intermittent leaks

- *MRI/MR cisternography*
  - Advantages: Excellent soft tissue (CSF/brain vs. secretions) detail, noninvasive
  - Disadvantage: Poor bony detail

- *Intrathecal fluorescein*
  - Advantages: Precise localization, blue light filter can improve sensitivity
  - Disadvantages: Invasive; skull base exposure required for precision localization

Surgical Technique

Endoscopic Approaches

Defects located inferiorly in the posterior table, within the frontal recess itself, or those immediately adjacent to the frontal recess are generally amenable to endoscopic repair, thereby minimizing the potential complications of other extracranial or intracranial procedures. The technique for endoscopic management generally outlines those previously described [12]. We typically inject intrathecal fluorescein (0.1 cc of 10% fluorescein in 10 cc of CSF injected over 10 minutes) and place a lumbar drain at the beginning of each case. This aids with intra-operative localization of the defect and confirmation of a watertight seal at the conclusion of the case. To obtain adequate exposure, a total ethmoidectomy, maxillary antrostomy, and frontal sinusotomy, as well as partial middle turbinectomies or an endoscopic modified Lothrop may be indicated. The extent of dissection should be limited to that required for each individual defect.

Using 0°, 30°, and 70° nasal endoscopes, any encephalocele present is ablated with bipolar cautery to the skull base. If the encephalocele extends under surrounding mucosa or nasal bones, dissection of the entire encephalocele is unnecessary and may lead to potential complications such as nasal stenosis. We have shown that these submucosal extensions atrophy and the mucosa returns to normal after ablation of the intracranial communication and repair of the bony skull base defect [14].

Once the skull base defect is identified, the graft site is prepared by removing a cuff of normal mucosa around the bony defect. This not only provides an area of adherence for the graft but also contributes to osteoneogenesis and osteitic bone formation. This thickens the bone around the defect and aids bony closure, if a bone graft is used, between the graft and recipient bed [2].

The choice of grafts is often of personal preference, but may include alone or in combination the following:

- Bone
- Cartilage
- Mucosa
- Fascia
- Alloplastic materials

These grafts are typically free grafts, rather than pedicled. Bone (or cartilage in select cases) grafts for large skull base defects can provide structural support for herniating dura or brain that may displace the overlay fascia or mucosa graft. Bone grafts are also useful in smaller defects when the patient has a spontaneous leak and elevated intracranial pressures. This elevated pressure contributes to disruption of the soft tissue graft and is responsible for the higher failure rates in this category. Mastoid cortex, parietal cortex, septal, and turbinate bone are all acceptable bone grafts. We prefer to use septal bone for small, flat defects and mastoid cortical bone for larger, curved defects. Otolaryngologists are more familiar with the temporal bone than the parietal bone, and this can be harvested at the time of temporalis fascia harvest if needed. If a mucosal graft is used, septal or turbinate bone may be a more suitable option. This spares an external incision and can easily be harvested from the operative field.

Regardless of the choice of graft, the bone is shaped to match the bony defect and placed in an underlay fashion in the epidural space. Care must be taken to avoid enlargement of the existing bony defect or entrapment of mucosa in the epidural space that may lead to an intracranial mucocele. A fascia or mucosal graft is then placed in an overlay fashion over the skull base defect and supported with gel-foam and intranasal packs. The graft at the skull base may be augmented with fibrin glue if desired. Nonabsorbable packing is typically removed 5–7 days postoperatively.

Even with meticulous dissection and wide exposure of the frontal recess, the potential for obstruction of the frontal recess by grafts or packing material is high. To avoid this, we often will place a soft Silastic frontal stent for one week. Careful debridement and cleaning every week for several weeks will lessen the incidence of scarring and make future surveillance easier (Fig 2 and 3).

Extracranial Repair

Defects in the posterior table of the frontal sinus are often not amenable to a strict endoscopic approach. Leaks that are particularly difficult to repair are those that extend to the isthmus of the frontal sinus outflow tract. It is this site where the skull base transitions from the horizontal (axial) orientation of the ethmoid roof/cribriform plate to the vertical (coronal) orientation of the posterior table. This area often requires a combined approach, since it is at the limit of an external osteoplastic approach from above and an endoscopic approach from below (Fig 4). A frontal trephine can provide access to the superior limits of the defect, and endoscopes may be utilized through the trephine as well as from below, but if meticulous removal of mucosa from the entire frontal sinus with subsequent obliteration is needed, an osteoplastic flap, rather than a trephine, is recommended.

Posterior table defects that are superior to the sinus outflow tract can be repaired with an external, extracranial approach using a traditional osteoplastic flap with or without frontal sinus obliteration. Attempts at repairing a posterior table defect without obliteration is not recommended for defects in the frontal sinus, unless the defect is sufficiently superior or lateral to the sinus outflow tract to allow repair without compromising the frontal recess. A well-pneumatized frontal sinus with a defect in the lateral recess can be repaired via an osteoplastic flap or trephine without compromising the frontal recess (Fig 5).

The specific technique for raising osteoplastic flaps is described elsewhere. After elevating the osteoplastic flap with direct access to the frontal sinus, preparation of the recipient bed and grafting is performed in a similar fashion as endoscopic management if the surgeon feels the frontal sinus outflow tract is not compromised, and the frontal drainage pathway will be left open. Fat obliteration should be performed if there is a question about the feasibility of a patent drainage pathway after repair. After all mucosal remnants are stripped and meticulously drilled with a diamond burr, underlay bone and overlay fascia grafts are placed as needed to close the defect. Bilateral obliteration for relatively small frontal sinuses or involvement of both posterior tables is recommended. Finally, the mucosa of the frontal recess is stripped and abdominal fat packed in the sinus.

Intracranial Repair

Large defects in the posterior table, as seen in severe facial trauma or tumors, may benefit more from repair via a craniotomy with cranialization of the frontal sinus and pericranial flap. This approach provides excellent exposure of the defect and allows better access for removal of the mucosa, but does require a craniotomy and retraction on the frontal lobe with possible sequelae such as anosmia, intracranial hemorrhage or edema, epilepsy, and memory and concentration deficits [9].

Adjuncts and Postoperative Care

Lumbar drains are a useful adjunct in the management of frontal sinus CSF leaks. They can aid a questionable diagnosis with the preoperative injection of intrathecal fluorescein and allow lowering elevated intracranial pressure in patients with a spontaneous etiology. These patients will have increased pressure postoperatively due to overproduction against a closed defect. We prefer to use a lumbar drain in select patients who will have elevated ICPs postoperatively, and we generally leave the drains in place for 2–3 days.

Acetazolamide (Diamox) is a diuretic that can be a useful adjunct in patients with elevated CSF pressures. It can decrease CSF production up to 48% [3].

The optimal timing, dosing, and long-term benefits of this approach have not been proven, but it may reduce the risk of developing subsequent skull base defects in patients with elevated CSF pressures. We periodically monitor electrolytes in any patient placed on long-term diuretic therapy.

Conclusion

Frontal sinus CSF leaks are a difficult entity to manage. When possible, endoscopic repair will provide the least morbidity, but the location and size of the defect as well as the etiology often dictate customized management. Achieving the best possible results for patients with CSF leaks depends on a thorough understanding of the underlying pathophysiology and fundamental principles of medical and surgical treatment.

References

1. Bernal-Sprekelsen M, Bleda-Vazquez C, Carrau RL (2000) Ascending meningitis secondary to traumatic cerebrospinal fluid leaks. Am J Rhinol 14(4):257
2. Bolger WE, McLaughlin K (2003) Cranial bone grafts in cerebrospinal fluid leak and encephalocele repair: A preliminary report. Am J Rhinol 17(3):153–158
3. Carrion E, Hertzog JH, Medlock MD, Hauser GJ, Dalton HJ (2001) Use of acetazolamide to decrease cerebrospinal fluid production in chronically ventilated patients with ventriculopleural shunts. Arch Dis Childhood 84(1):68–71
4. Gassner HG, Ponikau JU, Sherris DA, Kern EB (1999) CSF Rhinorrhea: 95 consecutive surgical cases with long term follow-up at the Mayo Clinic. Am J Rhinol 13:439–447
5. Gerbino G, Roccia F, Benech A, Caldarelli C (2000) Analysis of 158 frontal sinus fractures: Current surgical management and complications. J Craniomaxillofac Surg 28(3):133–139
6. Hubbard JL, McDonald TJ, Pearson BW, Laws, ER Jr (1985) Spontaneous cerebrospinal fluid rhinorrhea: Evolving concepts in diagnosis and surgical management based on the Mayo Clinic experience from 1970 through 1981. Neurosurgery 16:314–321
7. Mattox DE, Kennedy DW (1990) Endoscopic management of cerebrospinal fluid leaks and cephaloceles. Laryngoscope 100:857–862

8. May M, Ogura JH, Schramm V (1992) Nasofrontal duct in frontal sinus fractures. Arch Otolaryngol 1970 Dec; 92(6): 534–538

9. McCormack B, Cooper PR, Persky M, Rothstein S (1990) Extracranial repair of cerebrospinal fluid fistulas: technique and results in 37 patients. Neurosurgery 27: 412–417

10. McGraw-Wall B (1998) Frontal sinus fractures. Facial Plast Surg 14(1): 59–66

11. Schick B, Ibing R, Brors D, Draf W (2001) Long-term study of endonasal duraplasty and review of the literature. Ann Otol Rhinol Laryngol 110: 142–147

12. Schlosser RJ, Bolger WE (2002) Management of multiple spontaneous nasal meningoencephaloceles. Laryngoscope 112: 980–985

13. Schlosser RJ, Zachmann G, Harrison S, Gross CW (2002) The endoscopic modified Lothrop: Long-term follow-up on 44 patients. Am J Rhinol 16(2): 103–108

14. Woodworth BA, Schlosser RJ, Faust RA, et al (2004) Evolutions in management of congenital intranasal skull base defects. Arch Otolaryngol Head Neck Surg 130: 1283–1288

15. Zlab MK, Moore GF, Daly DT, et al (1992) Cerebrospinal fluid rhinorrhea: A review of the literature. ENT J 71: 314–317

17

Chapter 18

Benign Tumors of the Frontal Sinuses

18

Brent A. Senior, Marc G. Dubin

Core Messages

■ Benign tumors of the frontal sinuses with their propensity to recur and cause local injury present unique challenges to the otolaryngologist

■ Fibro-osseous lesions may be managed expectantly, or may be removed in the setting of symptomatic pathology such as cosmetic or functional deformity

■ Inverted papillomas with their high rate of associated malignancy should be completely removed

■ Tumors that in the past required open approaches may now be managed successfully with endoscopic approaches alone or with combined approaches, lowering overall morbidity while not sacrificing outcome

■ Cases must be individually assessed in order to determine the appropriate management approach

Contents

Introduction

Management of disease of the frontal recess and frontal sinus is one of the greatest challenges in rhinology. Despite advances in the understanding of the anatomy and physiology of this area along with increased comfort with endoscopic techniques, management of this area remains difficult due to its tight rigid bony anatomic constraints. As treatment of inflammatory disease of this area continues to pose a therapeutic challenge, it is of no surprise that frontal sinus tumors are particularly difficult to manage.

Many of the benign tumors that occur in this area have the potential to recur and spread into adjacent structures and compartments. Anterior extension to the skin of the face can lead to significant cosmetic deformity, whereas posterior extension into the anterior cranial fossa can lead to dural erosion, brain compression, and increased intracranial pressure. Inferior growth can lead to orbital symptoms including diplopia, proptosis, and decreased visual acuity. In all cases, tumor growth may lead to postobstructive frontal sinusitis with the possibility of spread to adjacent regions including the orbit, intracranially, or subcutaneously.

For the purposes of this chapter, benign frontal sinus tumors will be primarily classified into:

- Fibro-osseous tumors
- Inverted papilloma
- Mucoceles (discussed in Chapter 9)

The fibro-osseous lesions will then be subdivided into the three most common lesions involving the frontal sinus:

- Osteoma
- Ossifying fibroma
- Fibrous dysplasia

Each of these tumors varies with regard to risk of recurrence, degree of aggressiveness, and potential for malignant degeneration. Therefore, the primary management of each lesion will take these factors into consideration.

Fibro-osseous Tumors

Osteoma

Fibro-osseous tumors are the most frequent tumors arising in the frontal sinus and frontal recess (Fig. 18.1). Of these, the most common is the osteoma. In 1941, Wallace Teed credited Veiga with the first description of a frontal sinus osteoma in 1506, whereas

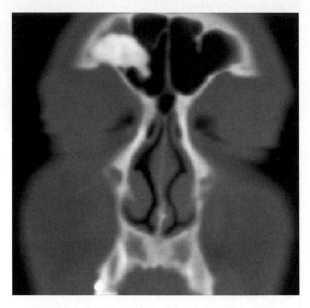

Fig. 18.1. Coronal CT through the frontal sinus illustrating typical appearance of a frontal sinus osteoma in a patient presenting with complaints of head pain

Vallisnieri was credited with detailing their bony origin [4]. The frequency of frontal sinus osteomas has been known for many years as Childrey, in 1939 cited an incidence of 0.43% in 3510 skull radiographs [24, 27]. More recently, osteomas were found in 1% of frontal sinus radiographs in symptomatic individuals [24, 27].

These bony tumors typically present in the third to fourth decade of life with a male to female ratio of 1.5:1 to 2:1 [1]. In patients of Middle Eastern or West Indian descent they may present earlier [1]. The most common presenting symptoms are headache and pain in the frontal area; however, many tumors are asymptomatic and are detected on imaging obtained for other reasons [34]. Symptoms consistent with frontal sinusitis due to outflow obstruction are also common. With larger tumors, facial cosmetic deformity may result from anterior growth, while proptosis, diplopia, and visual changes may result from inferior extension. Posterior extension may lead to intracranial complications [34]. with descriptions of meningitis, seizures, and hemiparesis all found in the literature, as well as a report by Cushing of pneumocephalus in 1938 [7,34] (Fig. 18.2).

18

cancellous bone. Both histologic types are well localized, rarely recur, and arise from the subperiosteal or endosteal surfaces of bone [6]. Neither has the potential to degenerate into osteosarcoma [6].

Fibrous Dysplasia and Ossifying Fibroma

Polyostotic fibrous dysplasia was first described by Albright in 1937, and ossifying fibroma was distinguished from it in 1963 by Reed [22,29]. In contrast to osteomas, these lesions tend to occur in a younger population. Both fibrous dysplasia and ossifying fibroma are less frequently found in the region of the frontal recess, and they tend to be less well localized. It is for this reason that resection of a focus of fibrous dysplasia tends to require multiple attempts. Ossifying fibroma has a tendency to recur more so than osteomas but less so than fibrous dysplasia [11]. Furthermore, pain tends to be less common whereas facial asymmetry and cosmetic deformity are more common (Fig. 18.3). Of note, radiation is avoided in the treatment of fibrous dysplasia due to the risk of malignant transformation.

Histologically, fibrous dysplasia is composed of highly cellular fibrous tissue with uniform spindle-shaped fibroblasts. Irregular trabeculae of woven bone without lamellar bone or osteoblastic rimming may also be found. Multifocal or polyostic disease is well recognized with associated involvement of long bones, cranial bones, mandible, or maxilla. In contrast, ossifying fibroma is nearly uniformly monostotic and lacks the osteoid and osteoblastic rimming of fibrous dysplasia. *Psammomatoid ossifying fibroma* is a variant that tends to occur in the ethmoid region of younger children and exerts more destructive growth [21].

Inverted Papilloma

Inverted papilloma was first described in 1854 and is one of the most common lesions of the nose and sinuses [38]. Classified by the World Health Organization as a type of Schneiderian (respiratory) papilloma (including cylindrical cell papilloma and exophytic papilloma), it has been alternatively called villiform cancer, papillary sinusitis, Ewing's papilloma,

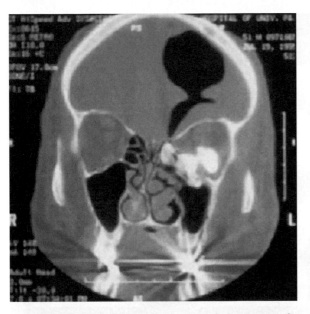

Fig. 18.2. Coronal CT illustrating pneumocephalus as a complication of a fibro-osseous tumor of the left ethmoid. Patient originally presented with change in mental status following a sneeze

Osteomas are also a common feature of Gardner's syndrome, an autosomal dominant disorder. This disorder is characterized by multiple osteomas, soft tissue tumors (subcutaneous fibrous tumors or epidermal/sebaceous cysts), and colonic polyposis [34]. As the true morbidity of this disease stems from the 40% malignant degeneration of the colon polyps, the diagnosis must at least be entertained in a patient presenting with an osteoma [34].

Osteomas are assumed to grow in a slow but continuous fashion, as was first noted in 1951 by Gibson and Walker [12]. Exact rates of growth will vary from case to case, though their growth is theoretically greatest during puberty with maximal skeletal growth [1]. The etiology of osteomas is now believed by most investigators to be developmental [34]. (Previous theories included trauma and infection; however, few patients with osteomas present with a history of trauma, and only a minority (approximately 30%) have an antecedent history of infection [34]. These lesions occur in two histologic variants: ivory and mature. The ivory lesions are formed by mature dense bone, whereas the mature variant contains

Fig. 18.3.
Triplanar imaging of a fibrous dysplasia lesion of the right maxillary sinus in an 11-year-old girl. Note the bulging of the cheek on the right side on the reconstructed facial image

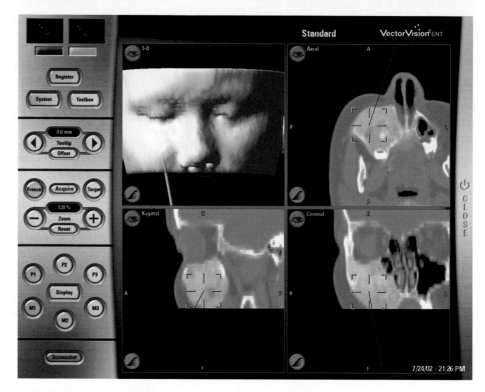

18

and transitional cell papilloma. Inverted papillomas are characterized by a high rate of recurrence and potential for transformation to squamous cell carcinoma. Rates of malignant transformation have been reported to range from less than 2% to 53%, with most authors agreeing on a rate of approximately 10% [32]. Histologically they have an inverted growth pattern with an inflammatory infiltrate of neutrophils and microcysts.

Although inverted papilloma of the paranasal sinuses is relatively common, the most common site of origin is the lateral nasal wall resulting in involvement of the ethmoid and maxillary sinuses, and thus isolated involvement of the frontal sinus is rare [37]. Frontal sinus involvement has been reported to occur in 1.1%–16%, although most reports cite a rate of 1%–5% [33]. Occurring in all age groups, this tumor most commonly occurs in the fifth to seventh decades of life. The male to female predominance ranges from 3:1 to 5:1 [11,16]. Caucasians appear to be affected more commonly than African-Americans. Presenting symptoms include nasal obstruction (87%), nasal drainage, facial pain/pressure (31%), epistaxis (17%), frontal headache (14%), and epiphora (7%) [37]. Various etiologic factors have been cited, although none proven. These include chronic inflammation, allergy, viral infection, and environmental carcinogens [9]. Recently, numerous reports have shown the presence of Human Papilloma Virus (HPV) in inverted papilloma using polymerase chain reaction (PCR) and in situ hybridization (ISH) techniques, though prevalence has varied wildly from 0%–100%. Subtypes 6, 11, 16, and 18 have all been identified, although correlation with malignant transformation is even less clear [5, 23].

Surgical resection is the treatment of choice, with procedures that provide "adequate exposure" being advocated. Radiation is reserved for patients who are poor surgical candidates, malignant lesions, or unresectable disease with associated morbidity. Recurrence rates have been cited at 25%–50% and are usually attributed to incomplete surgical removal [2,17].

Management of Benign Lesions of the Frontal Sinus

Preoperative Evaluation

In all tumors of the frontal sinus and skull base, careful preoperative evaluation is critical. Preoperative high-resolution computed tomography (CT) is the study of choice to delineate the bony anatomy and any associated distortion, the extent of the tumor within the sinus cavity, as well as extension of tumor beyond the confines of the sinus. Coronal and axial images are mandatory, though sagittal images are also of great value for frontal sinus lesions. Magnetic resonance imaging (MRI) with enhancement is also useful for delineating tumor from retained secretions (typically bright on T2-weighted images) but is less helpful in the management of bony and fibro-osseous lesions. With any dehiscence of the skull base including the posterior table of the frontal sinus, however, MRI is essential to evaluate for the possibility of meningocele or meningoencephalocele. Patients with involvement of the orbit should have a thorough preoperative visual assessment, and patients with intracranial extension should be evaluated by a neurosurgeon. Furthermore, the possibility of a CSF leak must be discussed with the patient, and plans for a lumbar drain should be made pre-operatively when appropriate. A thorough endoscopic examination is also critical to delineate anatomy and to fully evaluate for active infection. Any acute infection should be treated aggressively with broad-spectrum antibiotics due to the risk of postoperative intracranial extension.

Surgical Treatment of Bony and Fibro-osseous Tumors of the Frontal Sinus: Open Approaches

Controversy surrounding the treatment of these lesions centers on the timing of resection as well as the approach utilized. As stated previously, due to the delicate anatomy of the frontal recess and the tendency for stenosis following circumferential mucosal damage, the potential for postoperative complications is significant.

The first decision is whether to resect or observe a lesion. Although the indications for resecting a lesion that is causing frontal sinusitis from obstruction or has intracranial extension are clear, the timing of addressing smaller lesions is more controversial. Arguments have been made that small osteomas should be resected when found due to their inevitable growth, while others advocate a more conservative approach [35, 36]. Smith and Calcaterra have suggested that a lesion that occupies more than 50% of the sinus volume or obstructs the frontal outflow tract should be resected [34]. With this in mind, the conservative management with close observation and imaging at regular (i.e. 6-month) intervals may be appropriate in the reliable patient. This conservative approach is perhaps best suited for the asymptomatic lesions that are laterally located. However, lesions that have a high likelihood of causing obstruction of the frontal infundibulum should be managed more aggressively. Management decisions must be based on the individual circumstances, taking into account the patient's age, comorbidities, and the potential morbidity of the procedure required to remove the lesion.

Approaches to these lesions are divided into endoscopic, open, or a combination of both. Key considerations in deciding an approach are the exact location and size of the lesion.

Historically, trephination procedures as well as Lynch procedures have been commonly used to manage these lesions [4, 35, 36]. These techniques are often well suited for small, inferior-medial lesions due to limited visualization provided by these approaches. Visualization may be inadequate in osteomas with a broad attachment to the posterior table of the frontal sinus, where a greater risk of intracranial penetration and subsequent CSF leak exists [1]. Additionally, there is a well documented risk of frontal stenosis that exists after performing the Lynch procedure [8, 11, 30], a risk that increases with time.

Osteoplastic flaps have been presented as an alternative and were popularized by Goodale and Montgomery [13, 14]. Via a brow, mid-brow, or coronal incision, the lesion may be approached in a unilateral or bilateral manner [25]. This may be combined with frontal sinus obliteration in lesions that are very large, where significant mucosal disruption of the sinus occurs with tumor removal, or when involvement of the frontal infundibulum raises concern about postoperative frontal stenosis. Additionally, obliteration may be useful if CSF leak is encountered. In most cases, however, obliteration is not necessary, and, indeed, is avoided in order to provide for restoration of function to the sinus while preserving the ability to monitor for tumor recurrence either radiographically or by endoscopy [25]. Overall, the osteoplastic flap approach offers excellent exposure and the ability to preserve the native frontal recess anatomy, however, at the expense of surgical morbidity in the form of blood loss, scar, need for a hospital stay, and the risk of frontal numbness, frontalis weakness, and late frontal bossing.

The craniofacial resection has also been advocated for extremely large lesions with significant extrasinus extension. This technique was first advocated by Dandy in 1922 and later by Cushing in 1938 [7]. A report of eight patients with massive lesions was presented by Blitzer, who resected residual and recurrent tumors [3]. In his series with four years of follow-up, he had no recurrences.

Surgical Treatment of Bony and Fibro-osseous Tumors of the Frontal Sinus: Endoscopic Approaches

The first reported endoscopic excision of a bony tumor was provided by Menezes and Davidson in 1994 [26]. This spheno-ethmoid tumor was removed without complication and without recurrence at 1-year follow-up [26]. Seiden and Hefny then reported on a combined trephination and endoscopic approach to remove a frontal sinus osteoma via a brow incision [31]. Later, in 1996, Kennedy's group reported on the extension of endoscopic techniques for the management of bony tumors with intracranial or intraorbital involvement [18]. Additionally, Senior and Lanza reported on the use of endoscopic techniques in isolation and in combination with open approaches to remove tumors with frontal sinus involvement [32]. Intra-operatively, an emphasis on techniques that minimize bleeding is critical. Nuisance bleeding decreases visualization and can be avoided by minimizing trauma to adjacent nasal structures by utilizing

precise, meticulous technique. Bleeding which obscures the operative field will also be decreased by carrying out dissection in a posterior to anterior direction. Similarly, performance of adequate injections of vasoconstrictor agents cannot be underestimated. One percent lidocaine with 1:100,000 parts epinephrine is injected over the uncinate, into the sphenopalatine foramen and into the greater palatine foramen bilaterally. If middle turbinate resection is planned, the head of the turbinate is also injected. For tumors extending into the frontal recess, cautery of the anterior ethmoid vessels is sometimes also necessary using endoscopic bipolar forceps and angled endoscopes.

Early identification of the lamina papyracea and the skull base is critical to safely identifying and opening the frontal recess. Thorough dissection of normal tissue around the tumor is performed to widen the surgical field. Once adequate exposure of the tumor has been achieved, small tumors can be easily removed. With large tumors, a drill is often required to debulk the tumor before it can be removed transnasally (Fig. 18.4). Newer microdebriders with simul-

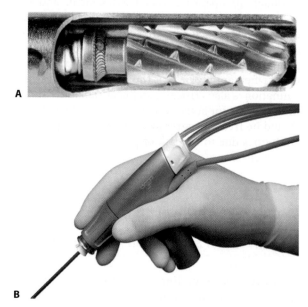

A

B

Fig. 18.4A, B. Example of a cutting drill with simultaneous suction and irrigation for use with debrider handpiece (Diego, Gyrus ENT, Memphis, TN)

18

taneous suction and irrigation coupled with angled drill burrs at 45°–70° can greatly increase the speed of the tumor debulking. As with mastoid surgery, however, care must be taken to switch to diamond burrs at the perimeter of the dissection in order to minimize potential trauma to the orbital periosteum or the dura. Once the tumor is sufficiently debulked, it may be teased from adjacent structures using angled frontal curettes and probes. Often, despite the large size of these tumors, they are only loosely attached to the adjacent bone and can be separated from their base using a rocking motion. Generally, frontal sinus stents are not utilized unless the resulting recess is exceptionally narrow or significant mucosal disruption of the frontal infundibulum has occurred. Additionally packing is not employed unless a CSF leak has occurred. If a CSF leak is encountered, it is repaired primarily in a fashion similar to that described elsewhere in this text. Large leaks, or leaks unexpectedly occurring high or lateral in the frontal sinus may require obliteration of the sinus via osteoplastic flap.

These techniques may be combined with a modified Lothrop as described by Gross et al. [15] or similarly, a trans-septal frontal sinusotomy as described by Lanza et al. [19] in order to increase frontal sinus exposure with removal of the sinus floor, intersinus septum, and superior nasal septum. They may also be used in combination with open techniques (i.e. osteoplastic flap) to increase postoperative visualization of the frontal recess for monitoring for tumor recurrence. Furthermore, trephination may be employed allowing for manipulation of the tumor from both "above and below" while providing overall improved visualization.

Cases: Fibro-osseus Lesions of the Frontal Sinus

Case 1: Endoscopic Resection of Tumor in the Frontal Recess

A 54-year-old man presented with 3 years of right-sided headache with recurrent episodes of sinusitis.

Headache was described as dull and constant, located over the right brow. Intensity of the pain seemed to increase with episodes of sinusitis. Drainage and congestion were not significant complaints.

CT scan was obtained (Fig. 18.5) with findings of a small fibro-osseous lesion of the right frontal recess with associated mucosal thickening in the ethmoid and frontal sinuses. The lesion was closely related to the right cribriform plate.

Surgery was performed via an endoscopic approach. Preoperative discussions of possible CSF leak and possible injury to the anterior ethmoid neurovascular bundle were had in addition to possible recurrence of tumor. Intraoperatively, the tumor was rocked from adjacent structures with a curette under direct vision (Fig. 18.6) and removed transnasally. Because of the small size of the tumor, no drilling was performed. No CSF was encountered, and no injury to the neurovascular bundle occurred.

Postoperatively, the patient experienced resolution of his headaches.

Pathology confirmed the tumor to be benign osteoma.

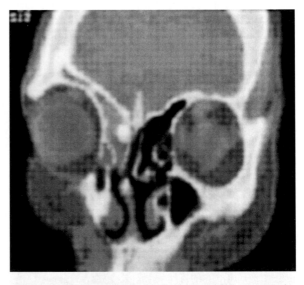

Fig. 18.5. Coronal CT illustrating presence of fibro-osseous lesion in the region of the right frontal recess with adjacent mucosal thickening of the frontal sinus and ethmoid sinus. Note proximity of the lesion to the cribriform plate

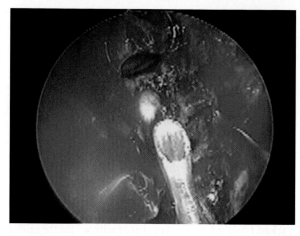

Fig. 18.6. Endoscopic view showing curetting of the fibro-osseous lesion shown in Fig. 18.5. The lesion was gently rocked free of its attachments

Case 2: Open Resection of Tumor of the Frontal Sinus

A 21-year-old woman presented with recurrent pain in the right frontal region following resection of frontal sinus fibrous dysplasia via osteoplastic flap 3 years earlier. At the time of the original procedure, frontal sinus stent was placed to maintain integrity of the frontal sinus. New CT imaging reveals recurrence of tumor encapsulating the previously placed stent (Fig. 18.7).

Surgery was performed via an osteoplastic flap. Tumor was drilled down to the roof of the orbit and posterior table of the sinus (Fig. 18.8). The intersinus septum and the floor of the sinus were removed to maintain sinus aeration.

Postoperatively, pain resolved, and the patient remains asymptomatic 2 years following surgery with a patent frontal sinus.

Considerations in Endoscopic Approaches to Fibro-osseous Lesions

- Complete sinus surgery with wide exposure to allow for careful inspection of the skull base and lamina papyracea

- Cautery of the anterior ethmoid artery and vein using bipolar forceps if risk of injury is high

- Use of endoscopic drills (Diego, GyrusENT, Memphis, TN) to debulk tumors to ease removal and delivery out of the nose (Fig. 18.4)

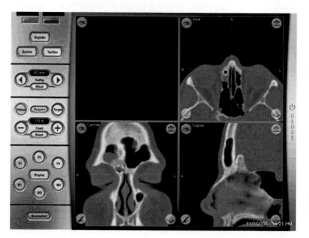

Fig. 18.7. Triplanar imaging of recurrent monostotic fibrous dysplasia of the right frontal sinus managed previously via osteoplastic flap with placement of frontal sinus stent. Previously placed stent is clearly visible

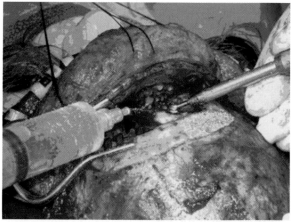

Fig. 18.8. Recurrent monostotic fibrous dysplasia of right frontal sinus. Access is being provided with an osteoplastic flap frontal sinusotomy, and the tumor has been drilled down to the posterior table. The intersinus septum is being drilled down to facilitate drainage to the contralateral side

18

■ After the tumor has been shelled out and debulked, it may be gently rocked and teased away from adjacent structures with a Lusk maxillary ostium seeker or the Kuhn-Bolger curette (Karl Storz Endoscopy, Culver City, CA)

Surgical Management of Inverted Papilloma: Open and Endoscopic

Traditionally, management of inverted papilloma without involvement of the frontal sinus involved lateral rhinotomy or midface degloving with an "en bloc" resection of the lateral nasal wall and maxilla. In 1990, Phillips reported on recurrence rates in 112 cases of inverted papilloma resection from 1944–1987, cases in which a variety of approaches were performed. The recurrence rate with each technique were: medial maxillectomy (14%), transnasal with sinus exenteration (35%), and transnasal alone (58%) [28]. Subsequently, the increased visualization and surveillance associated with endoscopic techniques led to the increased, albeit controversial, use of endoscopic resection by many authors [35, 36].

Extension of inverted papilloma into the area of the frontal recess or frontal sinus presents a unique challenge. Because endoscopic techniques provide limited access to much of the frontal sinus, inverted papillomas that extend into this area often require an open or combined open/endoscopic approach via an osteoplastic flap or fronto-ethmoidectomy. The osteoplastic approach provides excellent exposure and allows for an en bloc resection of a papilloma with a cuff of normal mucoperiosteum. Obliteration after resection makes postoperative surveillance difficult both clinically and radiographically and is therefore avoided if at all possible.

Despite the limitations of endoscopy in the resection of frontal sinus inverted papillomas, regardless of the surgical approach employed, the endoscope remains a critical tool in evaluation and treatment. The careful examination both intra-operatively and postoperatively of the surrounding mucosa can increase a surgeon's ability to remove all neoplastic disease and rapidly identify recurrent tumor. Emphasis at the time of surgery should also be placed on creating a cavity that can easily be monitored postoperatively in the clinic with angled endoscopy. Case series of endoscopic resection of inverted papillomas of the frontal sinus were recently reported [10, 20].

Endoscopic management of inverted papilloma that either primarily or secondarily involves the frontal sinus can be considered in select cases [10]. Lesions that do not involve the lateral or anterior frontal sinus may be managed endoscopically if the frontal recess is large enough. Regardless, endoscopic assessment of inverted papilloma of the frontal sinus at the same time as endoscopic resection of ethmoid/maxillary disease can accurately assess the need for open approaches and can open the recess from below to facilitate postoperative surveillance [10]. Furthermore, as with removal of fibro-osseous tumors, endoscopic resection can be combined with open approaches to ensure complete resection. Although a majority of patients may ultimately require an open resection of inverted papilloma that involves the frontal sinus, a select few may be managed entirely endoscopically [10]. This may be facilitated by extended endoscopic techniques in the form of a modified Lothrop or a trans-septal frontal sinusotomy [20].

Cases: Inverted Papilloma of the Frontal Sinus

Case 1: Recurrent Inverted Papilloma of the Frontal Sinus

A 46-year-old woman presented with pain, pressure, proptosis, and diplopia. Her history was significant for having undergone medial maxillectomy via lateral rhinotomy for an inverted papilloma of the right side 7 years earlier. Endoscopic examination revealed a polypoid mass of the right ethmoid with extension into the right frontal sinus. CT revealed opacification of the right frontal sinus (Fig. 18.9), and MRI suggested the opacification to be soft tissue and not inspissated secretions.

Surgical pathology from the earlier resection was reviewed, confirming benign inverted papilloma. Endoscopic approach was performed. Preoperative counseling focused on orbital injury with tumor

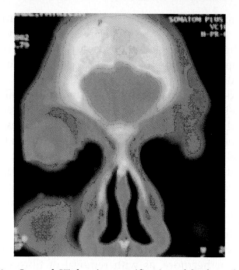

Fig. 18.9. Coronal CT showing opacification of the frontal sinus from recurrent inverted papilloma

overlying the dehiscent orbit, in addition to recurrence and need for further surgery in light of the frontal tumor extension. Intraoperatively, tumor was freed from its attachments at the frontal ostium, without necessitating an open approach. No stenting was performed, the tumor having dilated the frontal ostium. Tumor was safely removed from the dehiscent lamina papyracea. Post-operatively, patient remains tumor free at 2 years post-op with a patent frontal sinus (Fig. 18.10).

Postoperative Considerations

Regardless of the technique used, all patients are treated with antibiotics in the postoperative period. Typically, a broad-spectrum antibiotic with good CSF penetration is chosen.

If a CSF leak was encountered and repaired, a lumbar drain may be placed and the patient kept on bedrest for 3–4 days. After this time period, the drain is clamped for 24 hours and then removed if no leak is present. Great care must be utilized, however, as large skull base defects may result in greater likelihood of pneumocephalus with lumbar drainage. Headache not responsive to pain medications should prompt a lateral brow plain radiograph and neurosurgical

evaluation if necessary. Packing is only placed if a leak is encountered and is removed 1–3 days following the lumbar drain. As with any CSF leak, a high level of suspicion for meningitis must be maintained, and the patient must be appropriately educated as to the signs and symptoms. Vaccination against *S. pneumoniae* should be considered.

If diplopia occurs postoperatively, early consultation with an ophthalmologist is essential. Trauma to the trochlea or extra-ocular muscles must be considered and addressed.

Any orbital pain or change in vision is considered an orbital hematoma until proven otherwise. Increased orbital pressure from an arterial bleed is managed with a canthotomy with cantholysis and an emergent ophthalmology consultation.

For osteomas, recurrence is rare with complete removal, so follow-up surveillance is less important; however, with other fibro-osseus lesion and inverted papillomas, regular and long-term surveillance is essential. The ability to identify residual or recurrent disease endoscopically is, arguably, the most significant advantage provided by the endoscope.

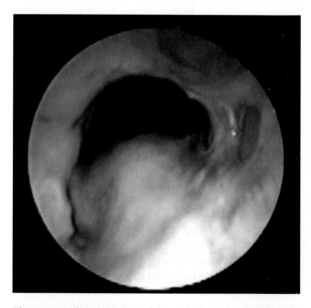

Fig. 18.10. Endoscopic view of the right frontal sinus illustrating patency 2 years following endoscopic removal of recurrent inverted papilloma of the frontal sinus shown in Fig. 18.9

Conclusions

Benign neoplasms of the frontal sinus present a unique challenge to the otolaryngologist. While certain fibro-osseous lesions with their slow rates of growth may be successfully observed, inverted papilloma should be removed completely. Traditionally, open approaches have been the mainstay for all these tumors; however, now, with advances in endoscopic instrumentation and availability of computer-aided surgery, more and more may be removed endoscopically or in combined approaches, reducing patient morbidity, and speeding recovery without sacrificing outcome. However, the exact approach to each of these tumors needs to be tailored to the individual situation, taking into consideration the nature of the tumor including its size and extent, the patient's co-morbidities, and the technical comfort of the surgeon.

References

1. Atallah N and Jay MM (1981) Osteomas of the paranasal sinuses. J Laryngol Otol 95(3):291–304
2. Batsakis JG (1979) Tumors of the head and neck (2nd ed). Williams and Wilkins, Baltimore. 132–137
3. Blitzer A, Post KD, and Conley J (1989) Craniofacial resection of ossifying fibromas and osteomas of the sinuses. Arch Otolaryngol Head Neck Surg 115(9):1112–1115
4. Broniatowski M (1984) Osteomas of the frontal sinus. Ear Nose Throat J 63(6):267–271
5. Buchwald C, et al (1995) Human papillomavirus (hpv) in sinonasal papillomas: A study of 78 cases using in situ hybridization and polymerase chain reaction. Laryngoscope 105(1):66–71
6. Cotran R, Kumar, Vinay, Collins, Tucker, Robbins, Stanley, (1994) Robbins pathologic basis of disease. 5th ed, ed. Stanley LR. 1994, WB Saunders, Philadelphia
7. Cushing H (1938) Experiences with orbito-ethmoidal osteomata having intracranial complications. Surgery, Gynecology, and Obstetrics 44:721
8. Dedo HH, Broberg TG, and Murr AH (1998) Frontoethmoidectomy with Sewall-Boyden reconstruction: Alive and well, a 25-year experience. Am J Rhinol 12(3):191–198
9. Dolgin SR, et al (1992) Different options for treatment of inverting papilloma of the nose and paranasal sinuses: A report of 41 cases. Laryngoscope 102(3):231–236
10. Dubin M, Sonnenburg RS, Melroy CT, Ebert C, Couffey C, Senior BA (2004) Staged endoscopic and combined open/endoscopic approach in the management of inverted papilloma of the frontal sinus. In American Rhinologic Society. New York
11. Fu YS and Perzin KH (1974) Non-epithelial tumors of the nasal cavity, paranasal sinuses, and nasopharynx. A clinicopathologic study. Ii. Osseous and fibro-osseous lesions, including osteoma, fibrous dysplasia, ossifying fibroma, osteoblastoma, giant cell tumor, and osteosarcoma. Cancer 33(5):1289–1305
12. Gibson T and Walker FM (1951) Large osteoma of the frontal sinus: A method of removal to minimize scarring and prevent deformity. Br J Plast Surg 4(3):210–217
13. Goodale RL and Montgomery WW (1961) Anterior osteoplastic frontal sinus operation. Five years' experience. Ann Otol Rhinol Laryngol 70:860–880
14. Goodale RL and Montgomery WW (1964) Technical advances in osteoplastic frontal sinusectomy. Arch Otolaryngol 79:522–529
15. Gross WE, et al (1995) Modified transnasal endoscopic lothrop procedure as an alternative to frontal sinus obliteration. Otolaryngol Head Neck Surg 113(4):427–434
16. Hallberg OE and Begley JW (1950) Origin and treatment of osteomas of the paranasal sinuses. Arch Otolaryngol 51:750–760
17. Hyams VJ (1971) Papillomas of the nasal cavity and paranasal sinuses. A clinicopathological study of 315 cases. Ann Otol Rhinol Laryngol 80(2):192–206
18. Kennedy DW (1996) Endoscopic approach to tumors of the anterior skull base and orbit. Otolaryngol Head Neck Surg 7:257–263
19. Lanza DC, McLaughlin RB, Jr, and Hwang PH (2001) The five year experience with endoscopic trans-septal frontal sinusotomy. Otolaryngol Clin North Am 34(1):139–152
20. Loehrl T and Smith TL (2004) Options in the management of inverting papilloma involving the frontal sinus. Oper Tech Otolaryngol–Head Neck Surg 14(1):32–34
21. Margo CE, Weiss A, and Habal MB (1986) Psammomatoid ossifying fibroma. Arch Ophthalmol 104(9):1347–1351
22. Marvel JB, Marsh MA, and Catlin FI (1991) Ossifying fibroma of the mid-face and paranasal sinuses: Diagnostic and therapeutic considerations. Otolaryngol Head Neck Surg 104(6):803–808
23. McLachlin CM, et al (1992) Prevalence of human papillomavirus in sinonasal papillomas: A study using polymerase chain reaction and in situ hybridization. Mod Pathol 5(4):406–409
24. Mehta BS and Grewal GS (1963) Osteoma of the paranasal sinuses along with a case report of an orbito-ethmoidal osteoma. J Laryngol Otol 77:601–610
25. Melroy CT, Dubin MG, and Senior BA (2004) Management of benign frontal sinus tumors with osteoplastic flap without obliteration. Oper Tech Otolaryngol–Head Neck Surg 15(1):16–22
26. Menezes CA and Davidson TM (1994) Endoscopic resection of a sphenoethmoid osteoma: A case report. Ear Nose Throat J 73(8):598–600

27. Michaels L and Young M (1995) Histogenesis of papillomas of the nose and paranasal sinuses. Arch Pathol Lab Med 119(9):821–826

28. Phillips PP, Gustafson RO, and Facer GW (1990) The clinical behavior of inverting papilloma of the nose and paranasal sinuses: Report of 112 cases and review of the literature. Laryngoscope 100(5):463–469

29. Reed RJ (1963) Fibrous dysplasia of bone. A review of 25 cases. Arch Pathol 75:480–495

30. Schenck NL (1975) Frontal sinus disease. Iii. Experimental and clinical factors in failure of the frontal osteoplastic operation. Laryngoscope 85(1):76–92

31. Seiden AM and el Hefny YI (1995) Endoscopic trephination for the removal of frontal sinus osteoma. Otolaryngol Head Neck Surg 112(4):607–611

32. Senior BA and Lanza DC (2001) Benign lesions of the frontal sinus. Otolaryngol Clin North Am 34(1):253–267

33. Shohet JA and Duncavage JA (1996) Management of the frontal sinus with inverted papilloma. Otolaryngol Head Neck Surg 114(4):649–652

34. Smith ME and Calcaterra TC (1989) Frontal sinus osteoma. Ann Otol Rhinol Laryngol 98(11):896–900

35. Thaler ER (1999) Inverted papilloma: An endoscopic approach. Oper Tech Otolaryngol–Head Neck Surg 10:87–94

36. Tufano RP, et al (1999) Endoscopic management of sinonasal inverted papilloma. Am J Rhinol 13(6):423–426

37. Vrabec DP (1994) The inverted schneiderian papilloma: A 25-year study. Laryngoscope 104(5 Pt 1):582–605

38. Ward N (1854) A mirror of the practice of medicine and surgery in hospitals of London: London hospital. Lancet 2:480

18

Chapter 19

Frontal Sinus Malignancies

Christine G. Gourin, David J. Terris

Core Messages

- Primary neoplasms arising from the frontal sinuses are rare; more often the frontal sinus is involved secondarily from tumors arising from other paranasal sinuses

- Squamous cell carcinoma and adenocarcinoma account for the majority of cases of frontal sinus carcinoma

- The majority of frontal sinus tumors present at an advanced stage and are associated with a poor prognosis

- For most tumors of the frontal sinuses, surgical resection followed by postoperative radiation results in superior local control and survival rates compared with single modality therapy alone

Contents

Introduction

Malignant neoplasms originating from the paranasal sinuses account for 3% of all malignances arising from head and neck sites [21]. Within the paranasal sinuses, the maxillary sinus is the primary site of 60%–70% of malignancies, followed by the nasal cavity in 20%–30% and the ethmoid sinuses in 10%–15% [26, 35]. The frontal sinus is the primary site of malignancy in less than 2% of cases, more often being involved by extension of a tumor arising elsewhere [3, 25, 36, 48]. Because of their rarity, institutional experiences with malignancies arising from the frontal sinus remain largely anecdotal, with no large series reported to date.

Malignancies arising from the frontal sinus are not included in the staging system for paranasal sinus neoplasms promoted by the American Joint Committee on Cancer (AJCC) [2]. The most commonly used staging system currently applied to cases of frontal sinus malignancies was developed at the University of Florida for tumors of the nasal cavity, sphenoid, and frontal sinuses [25].

The University of Florida Staging System

- Stage I: tumors limited to the site of origin
- Stage II: extension to adjacent sites (orbit, paranasal sinuses, skin, nasopharynx, pterygomaxillary fossa)
- Stage III: base of skull or pterygoid plate destruction and/or intracranial extension

The majority of frontal sinus malignancies are stage II or III at presentation. The lymphatic drainage of the frontal sinus occurs via lymphatic channels that drain the skin and the anterior nasal vault. As a result, metastases are rare without tumor involvement of the overlying skin or extension into the anterior nasal mucosa. Regional metastases occur in 10%–15%, and distant metastases are present at the time of diagnosis in 10% of patients with frontal sinus malignancies [36]. Despite advances in anterior craniofacial surgery and in multimodality therapy, local recurrence remains the most significant cause of treatment failure and death. The histologic grade and the extent of disease appear to be the most important factors associated with prognosis of tumors of this region [3, 48].

Pathology

The frontal sinus is lined by an epithelium often termed the Schneiderian membrane, which is derived from ectoderm and consists of pseudostratified columnar epithelium and seromucinous salivary glands. Not surprisingly, the most common neoplasms arising in the frontal sinus are epithelial tumors arising from the pseudostratified columnar epithelium (squamous cell carcinoma) and adenocarcinomas arising from the minor salivary seromucinous glands.

Frontal sinus malignancies are seen more commonly in men, with a male:female preponderance of 5:1 and a peak incidence in the 5th and 6th decades of life [43]. Both tobacco smoke and certain occupational exposures are associated with an increased risk of developing malignancy of the sinonasal tract, which presumably holds true for the frontal sinus as well. The latter group includes nickel workers, in whom the incidence of squamous cell carcinoma is 28-fold greater than that of the general population; leather workers, who are exposed to tannins and chromate; and wood workers, who are exposed to formaldehyde-based adhesives, wood dust, and preservatives such as creosote, and have been reported to have a 500-fold increased risk for the development of adenocarcinoma [34, 44, 50].

An increased incidence of paranasal sinus malignancy has been reported in textile workers, petroleum refinery workers, welders, blast furnace operators, and individuals exposed to ionizing radiation [49, 50].

Exposure to Thorotrast (thorium dioxide), a radioactive contrast agent that was commonly instilled into the maxillary sinuses until 1950, has been associated with the development of maxillary and frontal sinus cancer after a mean latent period of approximately 15 years [49].

The most common types of sinonasal malignancies are [36]:

- Squamous cell carcinoma (60%)
- Minor salivary gland malignancies (adenocarcinoma, adenoid cystic carcinoma, and mucoepidermoid carcinoma) (20%–30%)
- Esthesioneuroblastoma (10%)
- Lymphoma (5%)
- Sarcoma (5%)
- Other less common malignancies including sinonasal undifferentiated carcinoma, melanoma, plasmacytoma, malignant meningioma, and infraclavicular metastases

19

Table 19.1. Malignant tumors reported to arise from the frontal sinuses.

Histology
Squamous cell carcinoma
Verrucous carcinoma
Malignant transformation of inverted papilloma
Minor salivary gland malignancies
Adenocarcinoma
Mucoepidermoid carcinoma
Sarcoma
Lymphoma
Other
Plasmacytoma
Hemangiopericytoma
Malignant melanoma
Malignant meningioma
Metastases (infraclavicular primary)

Based on [1, 3, 5, 10, 11, 17, 25, 36, 42, 43, 47]

In most cases, involvement of the frontal sinus occurs secondary to tumor spread, usually from the ethmoid sinuses, rather than occurring primarily.

The most common types of sinonasal neoplasms arising primarily from the frontal sinus are (Table 19.1) [1, 3, 10, 11, 15, 17, 25, 42, 43, 47]:

- Squamous cell carcinoma, accounting for 90% of cases
- Adenocarcinoma
- Rare reports of lymphoma, sarcoma, meningioma, and infraclavicular metastases

Epithelial Malignancies

Squamous cell carcinoma is the most common malignancy reported to arise from the frontal sinuses, accounting for 90% of all cases [5]. Bone erosion with hyperostosis has been reported in 48% of cases, and the true incidence of bone involvement may be underestimated, as the majority of cases described in the literature predate the use of CT scanning [5, 11]. The clinical presentation may mimic that of a mucocele with swelling of the overlying skin, but evidence of infection is usually absent and the degree of bone destruction and hyperostosis has been described as out of proportion to sinus expansion [43]. The 5-year actuarial survival for patients with squamous cell carcinoma of the paranasal sinuses ranges from 25% to 50%, but the prognosis for patients with squamous cell carcinoma of the frontal sinus is poor, and the majority of patients present at an advanced stage [3, 4, 23, 30]. Combined modality treatment consisting of radical surgery with postoperative radiation is most commonly employed, with irradiation alone reserved for patients with inoperable disease [25]. There is limited data to support the use of adjuvant chemotherapy in the management of sinus carcinoma, but because of favorable results seen with the use of adjuvant chemotherapy in other head and neck sites, consideration should be given to the use of chemotherapy concurrent with irradiation [11, 25].

Basaloid squamous cell carcinoma and verrucous carcinoma have both been reported to arise from the sinonasal tract. Basaloid squamous cell carcinoma is a rare tumor of the paranasal sinuses, with only 14 cases reported to date, none of which have been reported to arise from the frontal sinus [52]. A histologically distinct variant of squamous cell carcinoma, basaloid squamous carcinoma is an aggressive, high-grade tumor that is deeply invasive, multifocal, and often metastatic: the prognosis is poor because of advanced stage at presentation secondary to the tumor's aggressive characteristics. In contrast, verrucous carcinoma is a low-grade variant of squamous cell carcinoma that is associated with a more favorable prognosis and outcome when aggressive treatment is employed [37]. There have been two reports of verrucous carcinoma involving the frontal sinus, and despite low-grade histology, intracranial extension was present in both cases, which underscores the need for aggressive treatment in such cases despite the presence of more favorable histology [37]. As for squamous cell carcinoma, irradiation alone is used for patients with inoperable disease or who refuse surgery.

Inverted papilloma may involve the frontal sinus in 11%–16% of patients and is associated with malignant transformation to squamous cell carcinoma in 5%–15% [19]. Rarely, inverted papilloma may originate from the frontal sinus [36]. While inverted papilloma of the frontal sinus may be treated using an endoscopic modified Lothrop approach, the presence of malignancy mandates an external, en bloc resection [28].

Minor Salivary Gland Tumors

Adenocarcinoma is the second most common malignancy of the frontal sinus, accounting for approximately 10% of reported cases, and is associated with a better prognosis than squamous cell carcinoma. There is a known association between the development of sinonasal adenocarcinoma and exposure to the wood, leather, and textile industries as mentioned previously. The 5-year actuarial survival rate for patients with adenocarcinoma of the paranasal sinuses ranges from 40% to 60%, with the best prognosis seen in patients with papillary histology [23, 30, 48]. Multimodality therapy employing surgery and irradiation is most often used in treatment. Adjuvant chemotherapy appears to have a beneficial effect on disease control, with impressive local responses, and the 5-year disease-free survival for paranasal sinus adenocarcinoma is reported to be as high as 65%–87% [1, 27]. The prognosis for patients with disease limited to the frontal sinus is unknown because of small numbers.

Adenoid cystic carcinoma of frontal sinus origin has not been reported, but may involve the frontal sinus as a result of direct extension from the ethmoids. Adenoid cystic carcinoma of the paranasal sinuses is associated with an increased incidence of local recurrence compared to other head and neck sites and poor long-term survival rates due to the development of distant metastases. The 5-year survival rates range from 17% to 53%, with local recurrence occurring in 50%, regional recurrence in 20%, and distant metastasis in 30% [30, 40]. Histologically, adenoid cystic carcinoma may manifest as cribriform, tubular, or solid variants: the solid variant has been reported to have an increased incidence of local recurrence, but the majority of tumors have a mixed histologic pattern [40, 41]. Aggressive surgical resection combined with postoperative irradiation improves local control rates but has no effect on survival, because of the high incidence of distant metastatic disease [40]. Perineural invasion is a hallmark of this tumor and has been reported to occur in as many as 91% of paranasal sinus lesions: the presence of perineural invasion does not correlate with local control for sinonasal disease [40, 41]. Fast-neutron radiotherapy has been shown to provide higher local control rates than mixed beam or photon irradiation and can provide excellent palliation, but does not influence survival [14, 22].

Mucoepidermoid carcinoma of the paranasal sinuses is rare, and only one case arising from the frontal sinus has been reported to date [3, 25, 43, 47, 48]. While there is a paucity of data regarding paranasal sinus mucoepidermoid carcinoma, aggressive surgical treatment followed by irradiation is generally employed.

Sarcoma

Sarcomas comprise approximately 5% of paranasal sinus malignancies with a variety of histologic types described, including rhabdomyosarcoma, fibrosarcoma, angiosarcoma, leiomyosarcoma, chondrosarcoma, and osteosarcoma [47]. Occurrence in the frontal sinus is rare, with four cases reported to date: two represented osteosarcomas, one chondrosarcoma, and one unspecified [18, 45, 47]. The treatment of sarcomas is primarily surgical, with postoperative irradiation reserved for high-grade lesions, inadequate surgical margins, or inoperable recurrences [45]. Radiation therapy is often required in the postoperative setting because of the difficulty in obtaining clear margins at the skull base. Because sarcomas are relatively radioresistant, there is no role for preoperative radiation therapy, which has been shown to be of no benefit [45]. Fast-neutron radiotherapy may improve locoregional control [29]. The role of chemotherapy in conjunction with radiation therapy is unproven but may improve local control rates: regimens used include cyclophosphamide, vincristine, methotrexate, doxorubicin, and actinomycin D [45].

Lymphoma

Lymphomas arising from the paranasal sinuses are most commonly found in the nasal cavity (68%), followed by the maxillary sinus (21%), ethmoid sinuses (9%), and least often in the frontal sinus (2%) [20].

These represent extranodal non-Hodgkin's lymphomas, with survival dependent on the immunologic subtype [15, 20]:

Diffuse B-cell lymphomas are reported to have a 55% 5-year survival in comparison to T-cell lymphomas, which have a 33% 5-year survival.

Treatment is non-surgical, consisting of combined chemotherapy and irradiation. It has been suggested that sinonasal non-Hodgkin's lymphomas may be less responsive to traditional chemoradiation regimes [6]. The role of surgery is confined to biopsy for tissue diagnosis and can often be accomplished endoscopically, although an external approach may be required to obtain adequate tissue [16].

Miscellaneous Tumors

A variety of unusual tumors have been described originating from the frontal sinuses in rare instances. Mucosal melanoma of the sinonasal tract is rare and most commonly arises from the lateral nasal wall, although origin in the frontal sinus has been described [24]. Long-term survival is rare, with most patients succumbing to disease within 5 years. Prognosis appears unrelated to the site of origin, size of the primary, local recurrence or treatment [9]. Most morbidity is due to distant disease. Treatment consists of radical surgery with adjuvant irradiation if an initial metastatic workup is negative.

Meningiomas may arise in the frontal sinus as either a direct extension of intracranial disease, or be truly extracranial, resulting from entrapment of arachnoid cells outside of the cranial cavity during bone fusion or in association with arterial sheaths that extend through the dura and the bone [39]. Surgical excision is the mainstay of treatment, and unlike most sinonasal malignancies, the prognosis is favorable for extracranial meningiomas. Intracranial meningiomas are associated with a high recurrence rate. Radiation therapy is not effective [39].

Plasmacytoma and metastases from infraclavicular primary sites including the breast, lung, and kidney have been reported in the frontal sinus [12, 33, 51]. Plasmacytoma responds to either surgery or radiation therapy, and disseminated disease is treated with chemotherapy. The overall 10-year survival is reported to be 50% [51]. Metastases to the frontal sinus from infraclavicular neoplasms are poorly understood, but are associated with distant metastases at other sites and a poor prognosis.

Diagnosis

The frontal sinus is a relatively sequestered and quiescent location and as a result, early lesions of the frontal sinus may be asymptomatic or associated with vague, nonspecific complaints.

Early signs associated with frontal sinus neoplasms include: a sensation of sinus pressure or discomfort and nasal discharge (which may or may not be bloody).

Early diagnosis is uncommon. In most reported cases, patients present with soft tissue swelling of the forehead or medial upper eyelid secondary to tumor erosion through bone, and may be misdiagnosed as having frontal sinusitis with osteomyelitis of the frontal bone. (Fig. 19.1) Absence of cellulitis, fever, and purulent discharge may aid in distinguishing infection from neoplasm, although an infectious component may exist secondary to tumor obstruction of sinus drainage. Proptosis, blepharoptosis, epiphora, and diplopia are signs of orbital involvement.

The presence of the following symptoms should alert the physician to the possibility of neoplasia:

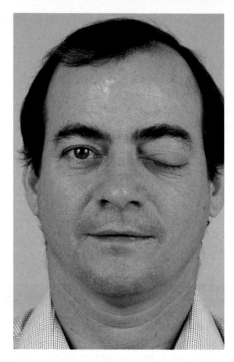

Fig. 19.1. Medial left upper eyelid swelling and proptosis secondary to medial and downward displacement of the globe by tumor

- Unilateral nasal obstruction
- Anosmia
- Intranasal mass
- Proptosis

Imaging studies assist in making a correct diagnosis. Axial and coronal computed tomography (CT) scans will demonstrate the degree of sinus aeration as well as any soft tissue or bony erosion. CT scanning is the diagnostic modality of choice to assess for bone involvement. CT is inferior to magnetic resonance imaging (MRI) in delineating soft tissue characteristics of tumor, particularly in large lesions in which the tumor margin can be difficult to distinguish from the fascia of adjacent orbital and scalp musculature, and in determining the presence and extent of intracranial extension. MRI with gadolinium enhancement and fat suppression can distinguish between inspissated secretions and soft tissue masses, differentiate

between postsurgical changes and tumor, and demonstrate perineural enhancement associated with tumor spread (Fig. 19.2). The information obtained from both CT and MRI are complementary, and both should be obtained in the evaluation of extensive lesions or when there is suspicion of malignancy.

Biopsy of tumors of the frontal sinus usually requires trephination of the floor of the frontal sinus for access in the absence of extension of disease into the ethmoid sinuses or nasal cavity. This can be attempted endoscopically but may require an external approach.

Treatment

Surgical resection is the most successful primary therapeutic modality for cancer involving the frontal sinuses [26]. The aggressive application of craniofacial approaches for tumor resection has significantly improved survival and local control rates. Surgery alone may be adequate treatment for early-stage sinonasal cancer but is most commonly combined with postoperative irradiation because of the high incidence of advanced stage disease at presentation. The addition of postoperative radiation to craniofacial resection results in improved survival rates that are comparable to less advanced stage tumors and superior to single-modality treatment alone [4, 48]. The use of radiation as a sole initial treatment modality been described but is associated with poorer 5-year disease-specific survival rates of approximately 21%–40% [3, 25]. Salvage surgery after initial radiation failure is associated with a 5-year disease-specific survival rate of 28% [13].

Regional metastases are uncommon for tumors of the paranasal sinuses, and elective treatment of the neck does not affect the survival or regional recurrence rate and is therefore not indicated [25]. The application of concurrent chemotherapy with irradiation in the management of head and neck cancer arising from other sites suggests that the use of adjuvant chemotherapy should be considered in the treatment of sinonasal cancer, particularly in the treatment of epithelial malignancies [25]. However, there is inadequate data to support the routine use of adjuvant chemotherapy in the management of frontal sinus malignancies.

19

Fig. 19.2.
Coronal T1 (A), T2 (B), gadolinium
contrasted fat suppression T2 (C),
and T1 (D) MRI images distinguish
between secretions and tumor. Note
tumor enhancement with gadolinium

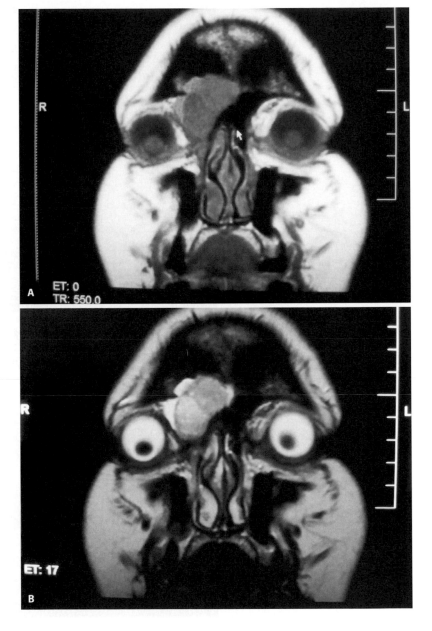

Fig. 19.2C,D

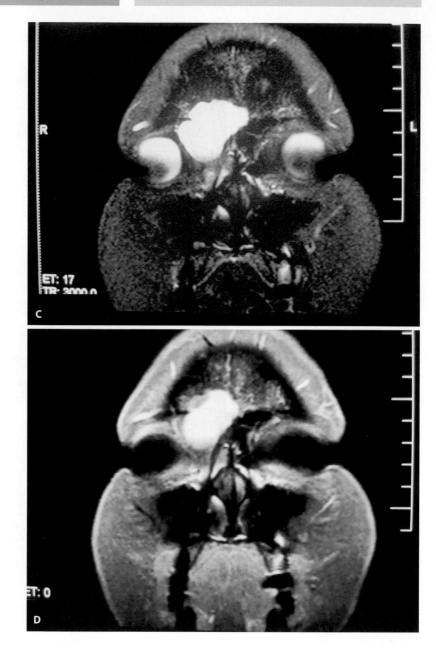

Surgical Approaches

Endoscopic approaches to the frontal sinus have been successfully used in the treatment of benign disease. There is a lack of data regarding the efficacy of endoscopic approaches to the frontal sinus in the treatment of malignant disease. An endoscopic approach can be used for biopsy of inferiorly- or medially-based tumors or tumors involving the nasofrontal duct, but an open approach is indicated for surgical extirpation of malignancy. The extent of resection required dictates the surgical approach that is used.

19

The rare case of an early tumor confined to the frontal sinus with intact bony walls or located in the most inferior aspect of the frontal sinus or nasofrontal recess can be approached through a limited external incision [36]. Access is accomplished with a 2–3-cm incision made above the medial aspect of the upper eyelid, just below the eyebrow and medial to the supraorbital nerve in the superomedial aspect of the orbit to expose the floor of the frontal sinus. The periosteum is elevated and the floor of the frontal sinus can then be entered with a cutting burr. When exposure of the anterior ethmoids or nasofrontal recess is required, a Lynch frontoethmoidectomy incision can be utilized, which extends the infrabrow incision medially and inferiorly to the level of the medial canthus and can be extended laterally to the lateral aspect of the brow. Attempts are made to preserve the integrity of the supraorbital neurovascular bundle when the anterior wall or floor of the frontal sinus is intact. When the intersinus septum has been penetrated by tumor and access to the contralateral frontal sinus is required, a gull-wing incision can be utilized, which involves a horizontal incision across the nasion connecting the incision to a contralateral Lynch incision. A major disadvantage of the gull-wing incision is the sequelae of bilateral forehead anesthesia when both supraorbital nerves are divided. A Silastic drainage tube is inserted at the completion of the procedure from the frontal sinus into the middle meatus and confirmed endoscopically. The tube is sutured in place and removed after normal drainage is restored, usually in 2–3 months. Prophylactic dacrocystorhinostomy is indicated when the lacrimal gland and/or duct is involved.

Larger tumors or those with involvement of the walls of the frontal sinus require a coronal approach for exposure, which can be combined with a bifrontal craniotomy and if needed, a lateral rhinotomy. If bifrontal craniotomy is not required, a 6-foot Caldwell-Luc x-ray of the frontal sinuses is helpful for use as a template in determining the location of the frontal sinus prior to making cuts in the frontal bone, to avoid inadvertent entry into the anterior cranial fossa. The coronal incision extends from the level of the zygoma, in the preauricular crease anterior to the tragus and extends over the vertex of the scalp above the hairline. The preauricular incision is extended vertically to the level of the vertex of the scalp to avoid division of the anterior branch of the superficial temporal artery. The lateral aspect of the incision is carried down to the level of the deep temporal fascia: staying deep to this plane avoids injury to the superficial temporal artery, which travels within the temporoparietal fascia above the deep temporal fascia, as well as the temporal branches of the facial nerve which travel in the superficial muscular aponeurotic system (SMAS). Medially, the incision is usually carried down to the level of the pericranium, which is elevated with the scalp flap to prevent desiccation and tearing of the flap in the event it is needed for reconstruction. The blood supply to the pericranial flap is based on the supraorbital and supratrochlear vessels, and its availability for reconstruction is dependent on the ability to preserve these vessels during tumor ablation.

The coronal flap is elevated to the level of the supraorbital rims, leaving the periosteum on the bone, with care taken to avoid injury to the supraorbital and supratrochlear vessels which exit at the level of the supraorbital rim. The periorbita can then be elevated from the superior, lateral, and medial walls of the orbit. At this point the frontal sinus can be entered if craniotomy is not planned (Fig. 19.3). When the posterior wall of the frontal sinus is suspected preoperatively to be involved by tumor, a unilateral

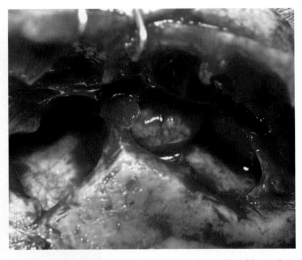

Fig. 19.3. Exposure of anterior and posterior walls of frontal sinus with a coronal approach. Note tumor obstructing the right nasofrontal duct

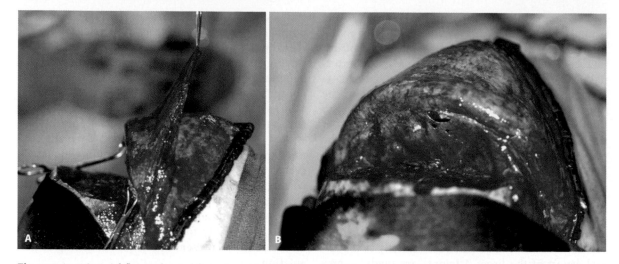

Fig. 19.4. A pericranial flap is elevated from the scalp flap (A) and used for reconstruction of a dural defect following bifrontal craniotomy (B)

or bifrontal craniotomy results in excellent exposure of the posterior wall of the frontal sinus and assessment of dural invasion. Frontal lobe dura is elevated from the posterior wall of the frontal sinus or resected if involved; the extent of resection is dictated by the extent of disease. The dura can be reconstructed with a pericranial flap, which is elevated from the scalp flap, rotated into position, and sutured to the dural defect (Fig. 19.4). When pericranium is not available, other options include pericardium, cadaveric dura, or a tensor fascia lata graft. Posterior frontal bone defects require cranialization of the remaining sinus. The nasofrontal ducts must be obliterated with muscle plugs to prevent cerebrospinal fluid leakage. Anterior wall defects can be reconstructed using split calvarial bone grafts, titanium mesh, methylmethacry-

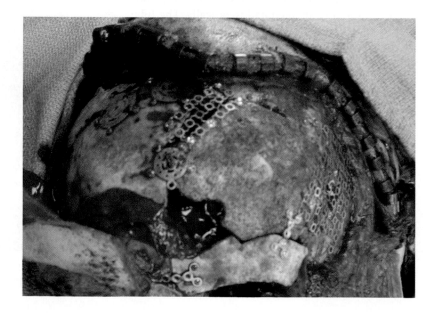

Fig. 19.5.
Reconstruction of an extensive frontal bone defect with split thickness calvarial grafts

late, or a free flap (Fig. 19.5). When tumor involvement necessitates resection of the overlying forehead skin, the resulting defect can be closed with a rotational flap if small (less than 2 cm), but larger defects usually require free flap reconstruction because of the limited mobility of the scalp skin.

Management of the orbit is a topic of some debate, largely because of the emotional issues surrounding the loss of an eye versus the oncologic safety of preserving the orbit and the functional outcome of a preserved eye [23]. The presence of orbital involvement, including invasion of the periosteum alone, adversely affects survival compared with patients without orbital or periosteal involvement [8, 30]. However, when survival of patients undergoing periosteal resection with preservation of the eye is compared with that of patients undergoing exenteration, preservation of the eye is not associated with a poorer outcome, suggesting that the orbit can be preserved in such cases [8, 30]. Tumors that invade periorbita have higher potential for invasion and a more dismal prognosis [8]. Involvement of the periorbita has traditionally been considered an indication for orbital exenteration, but several studies have suggested that limited involvement of the periorbita can be resected with orbital preservation, using frozen section control to achieve negative margins without compromising outcome [23, 31, 38]. Extensive periorbital involvement, defined as unresectable full-thickness invasion of the periorbita, or extension into the ocular fat, muscles, or orbital apex are indications for exenteration [23].

Preservation of the eye has been reported to result in preservation of functional vision postoperatively in 91% of patients; however, 41% developed ocular sequelae, the most common of which were due to abnormalities of globe position (enopthalmous) particularly if rigid bony reconstruction was not performed [23]. Ocular function is adversely affected by extent of resection of supporting structures, particularly the floor of the orbit [8]. Rigid reconstruction of the walls of the orbit is recommended for subtotal or total floor defects, defined as greater than 80% of the surface area, or multisegment defects. The function of a preserved eye is significantly worsened when postoperative radiation is used. In one large series of patients who underwent orbital preservation, radiation-induced blindness occurred in the ipsilateral eye in 35% and in the contralateral eye in 8% [25]. Overall, radiation-induced functional ocular sequelae occur in more than 50% of patients treated with postoperative irradiation with complications that include ectropion, conjunctivitis, exposure keratitis, epiphora, blindness, and cataract formation. [23]. However, the sequelae related to orbital preservation may be acceptable to patients given the aesthetic value of a preserved eye, particularly when some functional vision can be preserved. Bilateral orbital exenteration is considered by many surgeons to be a contraindication to surgical resection.

Complications

Complications arising from surgical ablation of frontal sinus carcinoma are related to the approach and extent of resection and range from wound infection to meningitis and death. Both intracranial and extracranial approaches are associated with a good cosmetic result, particularly when bony reconstruction

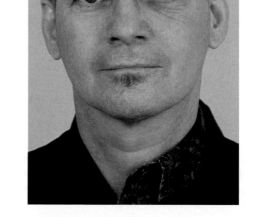

Fig. 19.6. Same patient depicted in Fig. 19.1, 3 months after bifrontal craniotomy with left lateral rhinotomy and irradiation

is employed for defects of the anterior frontal sinus wall and orbit (Fig. 19.6). Extracranial approaches are associated with a low incidence of complications, with wound infection and cerebrospinal fluid leak most common. Intracranial resection is associated with a higher incidence of complications, with meningitis and cerebrospinal fluid leak most commonly reported [30, 47]. The overall complication rate is less than 20%, with perioperative mortality following intracranial approaches ranging from 0% to 13% [3, 4, 30, 32, 36]. The postoperative complication rate following preoperative irradiation is significantly higher, ranging from 24% to 100% [13, 36]. Mental status changes may result from significant frontal lobe resection or excessive retraction.

Outcomes

The overall disease-specific 5-year survival rates for patients with paranasal sinus malignancy range from 24% to 69% [3, 4, 26, 30, 32, 48]. Local recurrence is the major cause of mortality in patients with sinonasal malignancy and occurs in 38%–89% of patients [3, 4, 32]. Results of salvage resection following failure of initial treatment are poor [36]. The incidence of local recurrence appears to be independent of the status of surgical margins following craniofacial resection and is similar in patients with both positive and negative margins [32, 46]. More than 50% of patients with negative surgical margins experience local recurrence, likely because of the difficulty in achieving wide en bloc resections and evaluating resection margins at this site, particularly when disease has spread to involve the adjacent ethmoid sinuses, orbital walls, and cranial vault [32, 47, 48].

Advanced tumor stage, histology, skull base and dural involvement, and orbital involvement are associated with a poor prognosis [3, 4, 30, 32, 48]. Squamous cell carcinoma in particular has been associated with diminished 5-year survival rates of 10%–32% compared to other histologic tumor types [30, 32]. Dural and orbital involvement similarly are associated with reduced 5-year survival rates of 23%–29% compared with 48%–69% in patients without invasion of these structures [30, 48].

Conclusion

The development of craniofacial approaches to sinonasal malignancies has resulted in improvement in local control rates, and significant palliation can be achieved with acceptable morbidity and mortality [26]. However, with improved local control, a greater proportion of patients succumb to distant metastatic disease, which is reported to develop in as many as one-third of patients [30]. As is true for cancers of the head and neck involving other sites, disease-specific survival for frontal sinus cancer is unlikely to improve without innovations in novel systemic therapies.

References

1. Abrahao M, Goncalves APV, Yamashita R et al (2000) Frontal sinus adenocarcinoma. San Paulo Med J 118: 118–120
2. AJCC Cancer Staging Manual, Sixth Edition (2002) Springer-Verlag, New York
3. Alvarez I, Sudrez C, Rodrigo JP et al (1995) Prognostic factors in paranasal sinus cancer. Am J Otolaryngol 16: 109–114
4. Bridger GP, Kwok B, Baldwin M et al (2000) Craniofacial resection for paranasal sinus cancers. Head Neck 22: 772–780
5. Brownson RJ, Ogura JH (1971) Primary carcinoma of the frontal sinus. Laryngoscope 81:71–89
6. Burres SA, Crissman JD, McKenna J et al (1984) Lymphoma of the frontal sinus. Arch Otolaryngol 110:270–273
7. Cantu G, Solero CL, Mariani L et al (1999) Anterior craniofacial resection for malignant ethmoid tumors–A series of 91 patients. Head Neck 21:185–191
8. Carrau RL, Segas J, Nuss DW et al (1999) Squamous cell carcinoma of the sinonasal tract invading the orbit. Laryngoscope 109:230–235
9. Carter TR (1986) Malignant melanoma. Arch Otolaryngol Head Neck Surg 112:450:452–453
10. Chaturvedi VN, Chauhan AN, Gode D et al (1978) Primary carcinoma of the frontal sinus. Ear Nose & Throat J 57: 47–49
11. Chowdry AD, Ljaz T, El-Sayed S (1997) Frontal sinus carcinoma: A case report and review of the literature. Australasian Radiol 41:380–382

12. Clarkson JHW, Kirkland PM, Mady S (2002) Bronchogenic metastasis involving the frontal sinus and masquerading as a Pott's puffy tumor: A diagnostic pitfall. Br J Oral Maxillofacial Surg 40:440–441

13. Curran AJ, Gullane PJ, Waldron J et al (1998) Surgical salvage after failed radiation for paranasal sinus malignancy. Laryngoscope 108:1618–1622

14. Douglas JG, Koh W, Austin-Seymor M et al (2003) Treatment of salivary gland neoplasms with fast neutron radiotherapy. Arch Otolaryngol Head Neck Surg 129:944–948

15. Duncavage JA, Campbell BH, Hanson GA et al (1983) Diagnosis of malignant lymphomas of the nasal cavity, paranasal sinuses and nasopharynx. Laryngoscope 93:1276–1280

16. El-Hakim H, Ahsan F, Wills LC (200) Primary non-Hodgkin's lymphoma of the frontal sinus: How we diagnosed it. Ear Nose & Throat J 79:740–743

17. Frew I (1969) Frontal sinus carcinoma. J Laryngol Otol 83:383–396

18. Gupta D, Vishwakarma SK (1990) Osteogenetic sarcoma of the frontal sinus. Ann Otol Rhinol Laryngol 99:489–490

19. Han JK, Smith TL, Loehrl T et al (2001) An evolution in the management of sinonasal inverting papilloma. Laryngoscope 111:1395–1400

20. Hatta C, Ogasawara H, Okita J et al (2001) Non-Hodgkin's malignant lymphoma of the sinonasal tract- treatment outcome for 53 patients according to REAL classification. Auris Nasus Larynx 2855–2860

21. Hoffman HT, Karnell LH, Funk GF et al (1998) The National Cancer Data Base Report on cancer of the head and neck. Arch Otolaryngol Head Neck Surg 124:951–962

22. Huber PE, Debus J, Latz D et al (2001) Radiotherapy for advanced adenoid cystic carcinoma: Neutrons, photons, or mixed beam? Radiotherapy Oncol 59:161–167

23. Imola MJ, Schramm VL (2002) Orbital preservation in surgical management of sinonasal malignancy. Laryngoscope 112:1357–1365

24. Jayaraj SM, Hern JD, Mochloulis G et al (1997) Malignant melanoma arising in the frontal sinuses. J Laryngol Otol 111:376–378

25. Katz TS, Mendenhall WM, Morris CG et al (2002) Malignant tumors of the nasal cavity and paranasal sinuses. Head Neck 24:821–829

26. Ketcham AS, Van Buren JM (1985) Tumors of the paranasal sinuses: A therapeutic challenge. Am J Surg 150:406–413

27. Knegt PP, Ah-See KW, Velden LA et al (2001) Adenocarcinoma of the ethmoidal sinus complex: Surgical debulking and topical fluorouracil may be the optimal treatment. Arch Otolaryngol Head Neck Surg 127:141–146

28. Krouse JH (2000) Development of a staging system for inverted papilloma. Laryngoscope 110:965–968

29. Laramore GE, Griffith JT, Boespflug M et al (1989) Fast neutron radiotherapy for sarcomas of soft tissue, bone, and cartilage. Am J Clin Oncol 12:320–326

30. Lund VJ, Howard DJ, Wei MI et al (1998) Craniofacial resection for tumors of the nasal cavity and paranasal sinuses–A 17-year experience. Head Neck 20:97–105

31. McCary SW, Levine PA, Cantrell RW (1996) Preservation of the eye in the treatment of sinonasal malignant neoplasms with orbital involvement. Arch Otolaryngol Head Neck Surg 122:657–659

32. McCutcheon IE, Blacklock JB, Weber RS et al (1996) Anterior transcranial (craniofacial) resection of tumors of the paranasal sinuses: Surgical technique and results. Neurosurg 38:471–480

33. Myers EN (1968) Metastatic carcinoma of the breast occurring in the frontal sinus. J Laryngol Otol 82:485–487

34. Nunez F, Suarez C, Alvarez I (1993) Sinonasal adenocarcinoma. Epidemiological and clinicopathological study of 34 cases. J Otolaryngol 22:86–90

35. Osguthorpe JD, Patel S (2001) Craniofacial approaches to tumors of the anterior skull base. Otolaryngol Clin N Am 34:1123–1142

36. Osguthorpe JD, Richardson M (2001) Frontal sinus malignancies. Otolaryngol Clin N Am 34:269–281

37. Paleri V, Orvidas LJ, Wight RG et al (2004) Verrucous carcinoma of the paranasal sinuses: Case report and clinical update. Head Neck 26:184–189

38. Perry C, Levine PA, Williamson BR et al (1988) Preservation of the eye in paranasal sinus cancer surgery. Arch Otolaryngol Head Neck Surg 114:632–634

39. Perzin KH, Pushparaj N (1984) Nonepithelial tumors of the nasal cavity, paranasal sinuses, and nasopharynx. A clinicopathologic study. XIII: Meningiomas. Cancer 1860–1869

40. Pitman KT, Prokopakis EP, Aydogan B et al (1999) The role of skull base surgery for the treatment of adenoid cystic carcinoma of the sinonasal tract. Head Neck 21:402–407

41. Prokopakis EP, Snyderman CH, Hanna EY et al (1999) Risk factors for local recurrence of adenoid cystic carcinoma: The role of postoperative radiation therapy. Am J Otolaryngol 20:281–286

42. Reddy KTV, Gilhooly M, Wallace M et al (1991) Frontal sinus carcinoma presenting as acute sinusitis. J Laryngol Otol 105:121–122

43. Robinson JM (1975) Frontal sinus cancer manifested as a frontal mucocele. Arch Otolaryngol 101:718–721

44. Roush GC (1979) Epidemiology of cancer of the nose and paranasal sinuses. Curr Concepts Head Neck Surg, 2:3–8

45. Ruark DS, Schlehaider UK, Shah JP (1992) Chondrosarcomas of the head and neck. World J Surg 16:1010–1016

46. Shah JP, Kraus DH, Bilsky MH et al (1997) Craniofacial resection for malignant tumors involving the skull base. Arch Otolaryngol Head Neck Surg 123:1312–1317

47. Spiro JD, Soo KC, Spiro RH (1995) Nonsquamous cell malignant neoplasms of the nasal cavities and paranasal sinuses. Head Neck 17:114–118

48. Suarez C, Liorente JL, Fernandez De Leno R et al (2004) Prognostic factors in sinonasal tumors involving the anterior skull base. Head Neck 26:136–144

49. Vianna NJ, Ulitsky G, Shalat SL (1982) Epidemiologic patterns of frontal and maxillary sinus cancer. Laryngoscope 92:1300–1303

50. Voss R, Stenersen T, Oppedel BR (1985) Sinonasal cancer and exposure to soft wood. Acta Otolaryngol 99:172–178

51. Waldron J, Mitchell DB (1988) Unusual presentations of extramedullary plasmacytoma in the head and neck. J Laryngol Otol 102:102–104

52. Wieneke JA, Thompson LDR, Wenig BM (1999) Basaloid squamous cell carcinoma of the sinonasal tract. Cancer 85:841–854

Chapter 20

The Endoscopic Frontal Recess Approach

20

Boris I. Karanfilov, Frederick A. Kuhn

Core Messages

- The endoscopic frontal recess approach is the primary procedure for management of chronic frontal sinusitis

- The frontal recess is an inverted funnel-shaped structure that best describes the anatomy; *a naso-frontal duct does not exist*

- Removal of frontal recess cells will achieve patency and function of the frontal sinus

- Specialized instruments and angled telescopes are imperative for complete procedures

- Inadequate or incomplete frontal recess cell removal is the primary cause of persistent disease or "recurrence"

- Preservation *at all costs* of frontal recess mucus membrane will avoid osteoneogenesis and scarring

- Diligent postoperative care and debridement are imperative

Contents

Introduction

Surgical management of chronic frontal sinusitis continues to be challenging and difficult despite the widespread acceptance of functional endoscopic sinus surgery principles. External versus intranasal approaches were first introduced and debated at the end of the 19th century [21]. The intranasal techniques, although successful in a small group of patients, more often resulted in persistent chronic frontal sinusitis requiring more radical external or obliterative approaches.

The first published reference to intranasal frontal sinus drainage was by Schaeffer in 1890. Several other surgeons contributed to this technique, and then in 1893 Jansen reported the need for "cleaning out" the anterior ethmoid cells to relieve frontal sinus obstruction. In 1917, Ingalls described the use of a "spring-gold tube" to stent the internal frontal sinus ostium [7]. Poor outcomes and the lack of proper instrumentation led to external and obliterative procedures becoming the standard of care in the 1930's and 1940's [1, 2, 14]. Advances in endoscopic techniques, knowledge of anatomy, and specialized instrumentation in the last 15 years have allowed for minimally invasive techniques to be employed as the primary treatment for chronic frontal sinusitis. This chapter will describe the frontal recess approach as the initial treatment option for medically resistant chronic frontal sinusitis.

Anatomy

One of the most difficult hurdles in surgical management of chronic frontal sinusitis is understanding the anatomical relationships in the frontal recess. Killian

20

was the first to use the term "frontal recess" in 1898 [9]. Traditional training taught that the frontal sinus was connected to the anterior ethmoids by a tubular, duct-like structure termed the "naso-frontal duct" despite Mosier's work in 1912 and Van Alyea's from 1934–1943. In order to conceptualize the endoscopic frontal recess approach, one must change his or her perception of this connection. *A naso-frontal duct does not exist!* This fact was recognized by Mosher as he described the connection between the frontal sinus and anterior ethmoid as a recess: a potential, inverted, funnel-shaped space with the narrow end at the internal frontal ostium and the lower bell-shaped end blending into the anterior ethmoid sinus walls [18]. Figure 20.1 is a schematic of lateral nasal wall anatomy demonstrating the frontal recess and internal frontal ostium. In 1939, Van Alyea's extensive cadaver dissections further clarified that the connection be referred to as the *frontal recess*, and this space is subject to narrowing by numerous anterior eth-

moid cells [24]. Unfortunately most of Van Alyea's work was either forgotten or overlooked by the time most modern otolaryngology training programs were established.

Van Alyea performed 247 lateral nasal wall dissections and described several cells that could potentially obstruct the frontal recess, leading to chronic frontal sinusitis [23]. He warned that inadequate removal of these cells could lead to iatrogenic chronic frontal sinusitis. These cells include the agger nasi cell, supraorbital ethmoid cells, frontal cells (Types I–IV), frontal bulla cells, suprabullar cells, and the interfrontal sinus septal cell. Details regarding these cells have been described by Kuhn and are summarized in Table 20.1 [11].

The agger nasi cell is the most anterior and constant of the frontal recess cells. This cell plays a significant role in frontal recess obstruction. Often, the agger nasi cell will fill the frontal recess, and any degree of edema will cause frontal sinus obstruction.

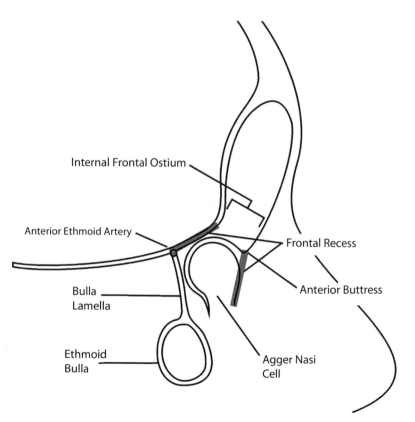

Fig. 20.1.
The frontal recess is a potential inverted funnel-shaped space with the most narrow portion being the internal ostium

Table 20.1. Frontal recess cells

1. Agger nasi cell
2. Supraorbital ethmoid cells
3. Frontal Cells
   a. Type I
   b. Type II
   c. Type III
   d. Type IV
4. Frontal bulla cells
5. Suprabullar cells
6. Interfrontal sinus septal cells

The medial and posterior agger nasi cell walls are the only two which are free-standing and require dissection to prevent postoperative scarring. Additionally, in a previously operated patient, if the cap or dome of the agger nasi cell is not removed, it can produce iatrogenic chronic frontal sinusitis. Removal of the agger nasi cell cap is well described in a paper by Kuhn [12]. The same theory of thorough dissection and a wealth of anatomical knowledge can be applied to all cells occupying the frontal recess.

Pathogenesis

In 1967, Professor Messerklinger described the mucociliary clearance pattern of the frontal sinus. He described mucus flow as up the interfrontal sinus septum, lateral across the frontal sinus roof, medially along the frontal sinus floor, out the ostium, and down the lateral frontal recess [16]. Approximately 60% of the mucus recirculates, while 40% is swept down the lateral frontal recess into the middle meatus.

■ *The lateral frontal recess is a critical area easily destroyed by drilling.*

The knowledge of the physiologic frontal sinus mucous clearance allows the endoscopic surgeon to focus on restoring normal frontal recess function, solving the cause of chronic frontal sinusitis.

The pathogenesis of chronic frontal sinusitis is similar to that of the maxillary or ethmoid sinuses. The seemingly endless combinations of frontal recess cells often produce very narrow and convoluted pathways for mucus clearance from the frontal sinus. Any inciting event which causes edema in this region halts ciliary activity. As mucociliary clearance is halted, mucus stasis results in increased edema, pH changes, and eventually the creation of an ideal medium for bacterial overgrowth. If the disease does not resolve after maximal medical therapy, the frontal recess obstruction must be removed before the health of the frontal sinus can be restored. Failures with external approaches and/or obliteration can be traced back to inadequate intranasal frontal recess dissections. These external approaches frequently irreparably damage the delicate ciliary mechanism [17]. Consequently, a thorough dissection of the frontal recess is imperative before resorting to obliterative or external techniques.

Instrumentation

In addition to a strong appreciation of frontal recess anatomy, the modern endoscopic frontal recess approach requires specialized instrumentation. The surgery is performed using a high-quality camera/video monitor and angled telescopes. In our practice, 30° and 70° telescopes are the standard; however, some endoscopic surgeons find a 45° telescope easier to manipulate in the frontal recess. Although the 45° telescopes afford adequate views of the frontal recess, there are situations that necessitate the use of a 70° telescope for complete visualization.

A set of frontal sinus instruments was developed in conjunction with Karl Storz to enable the surgeon to operate utilizing the angled telescopes and "see around the corner". The set consists of angled curettes, frontal ostium seekers, frontal sinus giraffe cup forceps, and frontal sinus through-cutting punches. The instruments are bent at 55° and 90° angles. The instruments are designed to work below the telescope; consequently, the 55° instruments work well with the 30° telescope, and the 90° instruments are designed to function best with the 70° telescope. The curettes are used to reach behind bony cell walls to pull them forward and inferiorly. The various frontal

20

recess giraffe forceps and through-cutting punches are used to cut or gently remove bony cell walls from the frontal recess. The ostium seekers are precision instruments that can retrieve small bone flakes at or above the level of the internal frontal sinus ostium.

Powered instrumentation has a limited role in primary endoscopic frontal sinus dissections. Mucosal preservation is critical to promote fast healing and avoid iatrogenic scarring of the frontal recess; therefore, microdebriders are only used in cases to reduce polyp bulk in the frontal recess or large amounts of crushed bone and mucosa from cells in the frontal recess. The 45° and 60° angled debrider blades are most frequently utilized in short on/off bursts to avoid mucosal stripping and injury. The speed advantage of powered instrumentation does not apply to modern and careful frontal recess dissection, because the risk of mucosal injury is high.

Stereotactic computer-assisted image-guided functional endoscopic sinus surgery (FESS) is now recognized as state of the art care for primary or revision frontal sinus procedure and is employed in all of our cases. Retrospective reviews have demonstrated increased surgeon confidence when operating in the frontal recess and significantly higher identification rates when utilizing a image-guided system [20].

Computer image-guided FESS is a highly accurate and reliable modality to utilize in frontal recess dissections; however, this technology will not serve as a substitute for a thorough understanding of the anatomy and availability of specialized equipment.

Technique

After performing a standard uncinectomy with maxillary antrostomy, anterior ethmoidectomy, and posterior ethmoidectomy (if indicated), the location of the anterior ethmoid artery is identified. The most common anatomic landmark to identify the artery is the insertion of the middle turbinate basal lamella at the skull base. This site marks the sharp upward slope of the skull base and is the posterior entrance to the frontal recess. The angled curettes are passed up the posterior frontal recess wall behind the cells, such as agger nasi cells or frontal cells. The cell walls are fractured forward and inferiorly (Fig. 20.2). The bony fragments can then be removed with through-cutting punches (Fig. 20.3) if attached to mucosa or with giraffes forceps if free of bony attachments (Fig. 20.4). If bone fragments are pushed into the

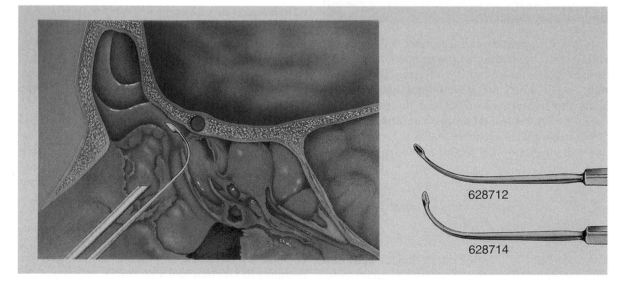

Fig. 20.2. The 90° frontal sinus curette is inserted above the roof of the agger nasi cell. The curette is then pulled anteriorly breaking down the posterior and superior agger nasi cell walls

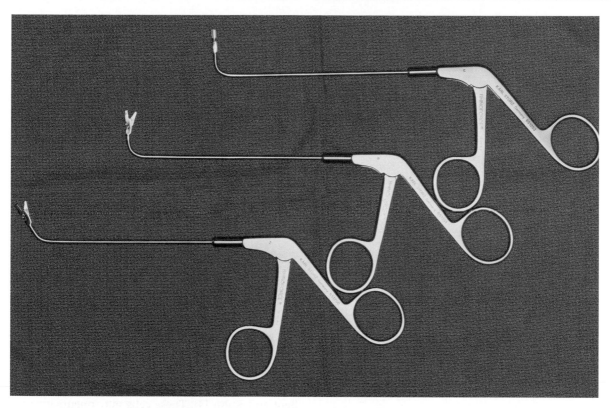

Fig. 20.3. Karl Storz 55° and 90° Kuhn through-cutting frontal sinus punches are utilized to precisely cut without stripping delicate mucosa

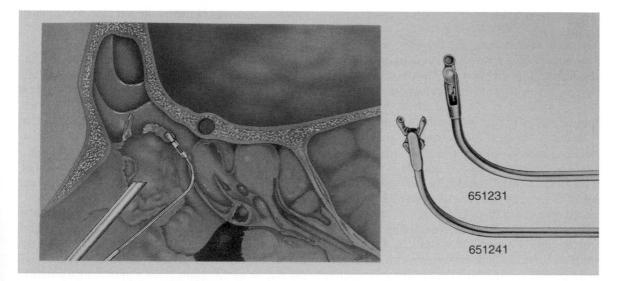

Fig. 20.4. The 90° frontal recess forceps remove the agger nasi cell roof. A bone fragment has been pushed into the frontal sinus

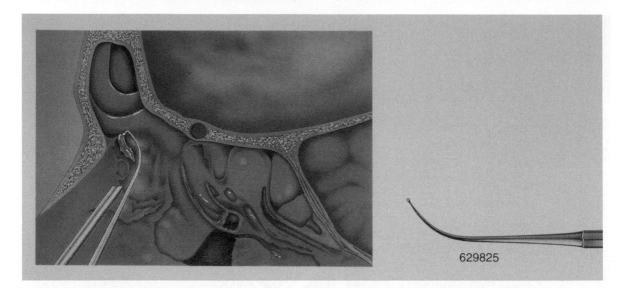

629825

Fig. 20.5. The frontal ostium seeker as pulled the bone fragment into the frontal recess where it can be grasped

frontal sinus, the different frontal ostium seekers facilitate easy removal (Fig. 20.5). This process is repeated until the internal frontal ostium is visualized.

> ■ *The key to this procedure is preservation of the frontal recess mucosa, because inadvertent removal will lead to osteoneogenesis, scarring, and frontal sinus stenosis.*

Instrument movement in the frontal recess is dictated by surrounding structures. Forward movement is the safest because there are no vital structures anteriorly, only the dense anterior buttress bone. Medial to lateral movement is the next safest, because the superior medial orbital wall tends to be thicker than the lamina papyracea. The instruments should not be used in an anterior-to-posterior direction or lateral-to-medial, because of risk of skull base penetration or injury to the thin lateral cribriform plate lamella. Both of these bony walls are thin and highly prone to fracture with subsequent CSF leak.

The agger nasi cell has been described as the most common and constant cell which can obstruct the frontal sinus [12]. Failure to recognize this cell or leaving the posterior wall or cell cap can result in scarring to the skull base or ethmoid bulla lamella. These cells must be removed by passing either the standard angled curettes or image-guided instruments to fracture the cell wall down into the frontal recess.

Frontal cells consist of four types as defined by Bent and Kuhn [5]. These cells may pneumatize far into the frontal sinus and cause obstruction of frontal sinus drainage. The principles of removal are the same as with the agger nasi cell; however, in certain cases the location of these cells can push the limits of current instrumentation, thus necessitating a combined approach.

The supraorbital ethmoid cell opens into the frontal recess posterior to the internal frontal ostium. It is important to recognize this cell so as not to mistake it for the internal ostium of the frontal sinus [19]. Computer image-guided FESS is particularly beneficial in distinguishing the two on axial sections. If a supraorbital ethmoid cell is present, both ostia should be dissected and the common wall between them resected. The goal is to create a large common frontal recess into which both cells can empty.

A cell between the two frontal sinuses is defined as an interfrontal sinus septal cell (IFSSC). Its pneumatization pattern is highly variable, and it may pneumatize into the lower interfrontal sinus septum or all the way to its top. Some IFSSCs pneumatize partially into a frontal sinus; others occupy a large volume, while rare situations present with a connection to a pneumatized crista galli. Regardless of the pneumatization pattern, this cell usually empties into one frontal recess or the other. The ostium of this cell is typically found anterior and medial to the internal frontal ostium [15].

The suprabullar cell occurs in the ethmoid bulla lamella near the attachment of the bulla to the skull base and potentially closes the frontal recess from behind. Thin axial CTs with sagittal reconstructions are essential to make the diagnosis, while computer image-guided FESS makes the dissection easier.

Frontal sinus imaging with thin-cut axial CT sections, coronal and sagittal reconstructions are necessary to completely evaluate the 3D anatomy of the frontal recess. The sagittal reconstructions provide the most data to interpret cells in the anterior-posterior plane and the relationship to the internal frontal ostium. Sillers et al. reported that corneal radiation exposure from 1-mm axial sections is only 4 rads,

whereas cataracts may develop only with a minimum acute radiation dose of 200 rads [22]. The benefits of thin axial CT sections extend beyond the detailed anatomical information; they can also be utilized in computer image-guided surgery.

Figure 20.6 is a coronal CT of a patient with chronic frontal sinusitis despite a well-performed uncinectomy and ethmoidectomy. He was offered an obliterative procedure at another institution and sought a second opinion. The intranasal endoscopic frontal recess approach was used to dissect out the obstructing Type III frontal cell demonstrated in the sagittal CT section (Fig. 20.7). The endoscopic preoperative view is demonstrated in Figure 20.8. There are several bony lamella in the frontal recess including an undissected frontal recess cell. After a thorough frontal recess dissection, the patient's 2-year postoperative intranasal endoscopic view of the internal frontal ostium demonstrates a functional and patent frontal sinus (Fig. 20.9).

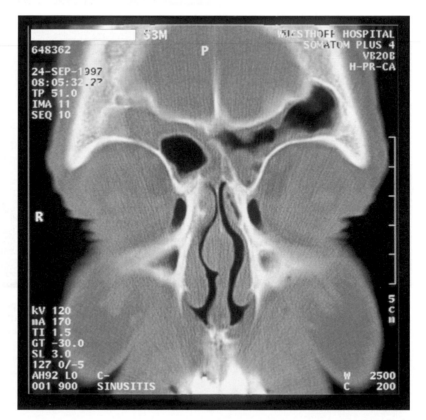

Fig. 20.6.
Coronal CT scan depicting chronic frontal sinusitis secondary to an obstructing Type III frontal cell

20

Fig. 20.7.
Sagittal CT scan of same patient with
the Type III frontal cell pneumatized
into the frontal sinus obstructing the
internal frontal ostium

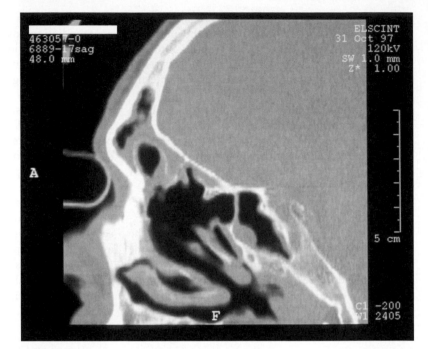

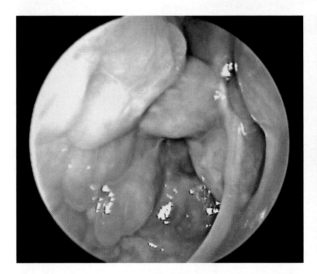

Fig. 20.8. Preoperative intranasal endoscopic view of the right
frontal recess demonstrating several undissected bony lamella
and Type III frontal cell

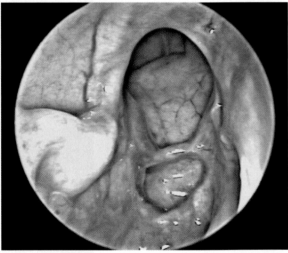

Fig. 20.9. Two-year postoperative intranasal endoscopic view
of the same patient after a standard endoscopic approach with
dissection of the frontal cell demonstrating a patent and functional frontal sinus

Postoperative Care

Postoperative care is crucial to achieving good functional results. Postoperative outcomes are influenced by intraoperative decisions which include the degree of mucosal preservation, the management of the middle turbinates, and the judicious use of frontal sinus stents or spacers.

The most important factors in achieving patent frontal sinusotomies are:

- Prevention of scar formation
- Avoiding collapse of the middle meatus

Intraoperative removal of mucous membrane results in healing by secondary intention with resultant granulation tissue followed by scar formation. Additionally, denuded bone stimulates osteoneogenesis, and the regenerated mucous membrane demonstrates poor ciliary function and decreased overall cilia counts [3, 4].

The different ways to prevent middle meatal collapse are:

- Preserve middle turbinate attachments
- Middle meatal spacers may be utilized in the ethmoid sinus
- If the turbinates are found to be unstable, a controlled synechiae technique is performed as described by Bolger et al. [6].

When the endoscopic frontal sinusotomy approach is performed with a complete ethmoidectomy, a standard glove-finger middle meatal spacer is placed in the ethmoid cavity to prevent collection of fibrin clot and subsequent scar tissue. This technique was described by Kuhn and Citardi [13]. Our intraoperative management of the frontal sinus is dependent on the degree of mucosal preservation and dimensions of the internal frontal ostium. Routine spacers or stents are not utilized for primary frontal sinusotomies with appropriate mucosal preservation, minimal bleeding, or internal frontal ostia that comfortably accept a malleable 9 French frasier suction. If a stent is required, we employ either a custom-designed glove-finger merocele spacer with a 2–0 silk tail to facilitate postoperative removal in the office or a 0.01-inch-thick piece of silastic designed with superior wings to line the delicate frontal recess. If mucosal integrity has been compromised, the Kuhn-designed silastic stent is the first choice. Stents remain in place for a minimum of 6 weeks and up to 6 months. If a stent becomes infected, immediate removal is the standard. We do not utilize commercially available stents, as our experience has demonstrated frequent failures. The key factors to a successful stent are the ability to line the variable anatomy of the frontal recess and maintain patency of the frontal sinus with appropriate placement.

Proper equipment is essential for adequate postoperative debridement in the office. Instrumentation includes 0°, 30°, and 70° telescopes, straight and malleable curved suctions to 45° and 90°, pediatric straight, 45°, and 90° forceps, and a wide selection of frontal sinus instruments. Frontal sinus instruments include 45° and 90° frontal sinus curettes, frontal ostium seekers, 45° and 90° frontal sinus giraffe forceps, and through-cutting punches. If the endoscopic frontal sinusotomy approach is planned, 70° telescopes and frontal sinus instruments must be available for postoperative debridements [8].

Adequate visualization of the internal frontal ostium is crucial after debridement to assure patency. Removal of fibrin clot is accomplished with the curved malleable suctions and made easier with the postoperative instruction for hypertonic saline irrigations. All patients are instructed to use a disposable 60-cc irrigating syringe with a hypertonic saline irrigation. Table 20.2 is a summary of the postoperative irrigation solution and schedule. Our routine schedule of postoperative visits for debridements is to see patients on day 7, then again on day 14, and a third visit between 4 and 6 weeks after surgery. With careful mucosal preservation, patients can expect excellent results and near healed frontal recesses within 2 weeks.

The need for postoperative antibiotics and steroids is assessed intraoperatively but are not part of the routine. Oral and intranasal steroids are particularly important if the patient has polypoid disease secondary to allergic fungal sinusitis or aspirin-sen-

Table 20.2. Postoperative hypertonic saline irrigations

1. Mix 2 to 3 teaspoons of pickling or canning salt and add 1 teaspoon of baking soda to 1 quart of boiled or distilled water.

2. Irrigate each nostril with a 60-cc irrigation syringe using approximately 2 cups of irrigation solution per side.

3 Bend over the sink or in the shower and irrigate with the mouth open. Irrigate a minimum of three times daily or more frequently if desired.

sitive asthma. If a patient develops a postoperative infection, endoscopically guided cultures with a calgi-swab are obtained.

Favorable surgical results are achieved not solely by postoperative debridement but also by preoperative and intraoperative decisions. Preoperative decisions include the use of antibiotics, steroids, and availability of computer image-guided surgical navigation. Intraoperative choices regarding mucous membrane preservation, through-cutting punches, and middle turbinate preservation play a crucial role in postoperative healing. Frontal sinus stents or spacers are utilized in situations where the frontal recess mucosa is damaged or the internal ostium is unusually small. Office debridement requires specialized instrumentation, and the adjuvant role of hypertonic nasal saline irrigations cannot be underestimated. Consequently, achieving frontal sinus function and patency is complicated and influenced by multiple factors.

Conclusions

To summarize, the frontal recess is an inverted funnel-like space that describes the drainage pathway from the frontal sinus to the anterior ethmoids. The frontal recess is a potential space that is routinely occupied by a number of different frontal recess cells which can act like a "cork in a bottle" to cause frontal sinus obstruction. The intranasal endoscopic approach should be considered as the primary surgical treatment for chronic frontal sinusitis. This pro-

cedure has proven highly efficacious and avoids the significant morbidities associated with open or obliterative approaches in the management of chronic frontal sinusitis. To achieve success, the endoscopic surgeon must have an exhaustive understanding of frontal recess anatomy, the frontal recess mucosa must be preserved at all costs, and proper instrumentation is required.

References

1. Anderson DM (1932) External operation of the frontal sinus: Causes of failure. Arch Otolaryngol 15:739–745

2. Anderson DM (1935) Some observations on the intranasal operation for frontal sinusitis. Minnesota Med 18:744–747

3. Benninger MS, Schmidt JL, Crissman JK, et al (1991) Mucociliary function following sinus mucosal regeneration. Otolaryngol Head Neck Surg 105:641–648

4. Benninger MS, Sebek BA, Levine HL (1989) Mucosal regeneration of the maxillary sinus after surgery. Otolaryngol Head Neck Surg 101:33–37

5. Bent JP, Cuilty-Siller C, Kuhn FA (1994) The frontal cell in frontal sinus obstruction. Am J Rhinol 2:31–37

6. Bolger WE, Kuhn FA, Kennedy DW (1999) Middle turbinate stabilization after functional endoscopic sinus surgery: The controlled synechiae technique. Laryngoscope 109:1852–1853

7. Ingals EF (1917) Intranasal drainage of the frontal sinus. Ann Otol Rhinol Laryngol 26:656–668

8. Karl Storz GmbH & Co., Tuttlingen, Germany and Karl Storz Endoscopy, America. Kuhn-Bolger Frontal Sinus/Recess Instruments – New Instruments Improve Results in Frontal Sinus Surgery. EndoWorld, ORL, No. 10-E, 1993

9. Killian G (1903) Die Killian'sche radicaloperation chronischer Sternhohleneiterungen: II. Weiteres kasuistisches material und zusammenfassung. Arch Laryngol Rhin 13: 59

10. Kuhn FA (1996) Chronic frontal sinusitis: The endoscopic frontal recess approach. Op Tech Otolaryngol Head Neck Surg 7:222–229

11. Kuhn FA (1998) Lateral nasal wall and sinus surgical anatomy: Contemporary understanding. AAO-HNS, Renewal of certification study guide 171–181

12. Kuhn FA, Bolger WE, Tisdall RG (1991) The agger nasi cell in frontal recess obstruction: An anatomic, radiologic and clinical correlation. Oper Tech Otolaryngol Head Neck Surg 2:226–231

13. Kuhn FA, Citardi MJ (1997) Postoperative care following functional endoscopic sinus surgery. Otolaryngol Clin North Am 30:479–490

14. Lynch RC (1921) The technique of a radical frontal sinus operation, which has given me the best results. Laryngoscope 31:1–5
15. Merritt R, Bent JP, Kuhn FA (1996) The inter sinus septal cell. Am J Rhinol 10:299–302
16. Messerklinger W (1967) On the drainage of the normal frontal sinus of man. Acta Otolaryngol 63:176–181
17. Moriyama H, Yanagi K, Ohtori N, Asai K, Fukami M (1996) Healing process of sinus mucosa after endoscopic sinus surgery. Am J Rhinol 10:61–66
18. Mosher HP (1912) The applied anatomy and intranasal surgery of the ethmoid labyrinth. Trans Am Laryngol Assoc 34:25–39
19. Owen RG, Kuhn FA (1996) The supraorbital ethmoid cell in frontal recess obstruction. Otolaryngol Head Neck Surg 116:254–261
20. Reardon EJ (2002) Navigational risks associated with sinus surgery and the clinical effects of implementing a navigational system for sinus surgery. Laryngoscope 112: supplement 90
21. Reidel (1898) Schenke Inaug. Dissertation, Jena
22. Sillers MJ, Kuhn FA, Vickery CL (1995) Radiation exposure in paranasal sinus imaging. Otolaryngol Head Neck Surg 112:248–251
23. Van Alyea OE (1939) Ethmoid labyrinth: Anatomic study with consideration of the clinical significance of its structural characteristics. Arch Otolaryngol 29:881–901
24. Van Alyea OE (1946) Frontal sinus drainage. Ann Otol Rhinol Laryngol 55:267–277

Chapter 21

Revision Endoscopic Frontal Sinus Surgery

21

Alexander G. Chiu, David W. Kennedy

Core Messages

- Successful revision endoscopic frontal sinus surgery starts with proper patient selection and medical management of co-morbidities and environmental influences

- Pre-operative planning in at least two and preferably three CT planes is needed in order to plan the surgical approach

- Common anatomical causes for revision frontal surgery include a retained superior uncinate process, superior cap of the ethmoid bulla, agger nasi cells, lateralized middle turbinate remnants, frontal recess, and supraorbital ethmoid cells

- Surgical approach is most safely done from a posterior to anterior direction along the skull base, where the skull base can first be identified in the posterior ethmoid or sphenoid sinus

- All bony fragments must be removed from the frontal recess, and specialized through-cutting instruments should be used to spare frontal recess mucosa

- Nearly as important as a good technical surgery is meticulous long-term postoperative debridements and surveillance to insure frontal recess patency

Contents

Introduction

Many will agree that revision endoscopic frontal sinus surgery is one of the most difficult operations for the endoscopic surgeon. The fact that there exists an abundance of different technical operations to treat frontal sinus disease underscores the complexity and nature of its difficulty. Over the years, there has been a progression from external, obliterative procedures to endoscopic management of recurrent or persistent frontal sinus disease. Despite the change in techniques, the keys to successful revision frontal sinus

21

surgery have remained proper patient selection, meticulous technique, a thorough knowledge of the anatomy, and a significant commitment to follow-up care from both the patient and physician.

Patient Selection

When evaluating a patient for a revision endoscopic frontal procedure, it is important to review the patient's symptoms, associated co-morbidities, and radiographic studies. Before deciding on the necessity for any type of revision surgery, it is advisable to review the original CT scan, before any surgery was performed. This helps the surgeon to evaluate the indications for the original surgery and is particularly important for the frontal sinus, where the primary surgical indication may be headache. In general, the symptom of headaches correlate poorly with chronic rhinosinusitis, and it is important to establish the presence or absence of disease in the frontal sinus prior to the first operation. If this remains the primary symptom, a revision surgery on asymptomatic iatrogenic mucosal change may be avoided. This determination leads to the initial and most important decision to be made, whether or not the patient will benefit from a revision surgery.

As with other revision sinus surgeries, careful consideration should be given to the environmental and general host factors that predispose to recurrent disease. Underlying factors such as allergic rhinitis, underlying immune deficiencies, and smoking should be investigated and where possible, managed before any revision surgery is undertaken.

Frontal sinusitis following functional endoscopic sinus surgery (FESS) can represent:

- Persistent disease
- Recurrent disease
- Iatrogenic disease

Persistent disease may be the result of an incomplete initial surgery or underlying factors predisposing to chronic inflammation. In order to evaluate whether the initial surgery(s) was inadequate, the initial pre-

operative report should be reviewed along with an examination of the pre- and postsurgical CT scans. An initial operative report which does not mention the dissection of superior ethmoid cells, agger nasi, cells and/or frontal recess cells may mean that a proper frontal recess dissection was never performed. Reviewing postoperative CT scans is an appropriate next step, and is an objective aid in determining a cause for persistent disease.

Reviewing CT scans are best done in multiple planes. In-office consultation should result in a review of axial and coronal sections, at a maximum of 3-mm sections, through the paranasal sinuses. Many image guidance companies now offer workstations that allow for the review of CT scans in the sagittal plane, as well as the coronal and axial views.

The coronal view is excellent in determining the presence of the following:

- Remaining agger nasi
- Superior uncinate process
- Frontal recess
- Supraorbital ethmoid cells

Sagittal and axial views are important in determining the following:

- Anterior to posterior dimension of the frontal recess
- The identification of a supraorbital ethmoid cell
- Frontal recess
- Interseptal frontal sinus cell

The dimensions of the frontal recess, particularly in the antero-posterior diameter, should be reviewed. The presence of neo-osteogenesis may make it impossible to work with the normal fine through-cutting frontal recess instruments. The overall frontal sinus pneumatization should also be considered in deciding whether or not to proceed with a revision procedure. A poorly pneumatized frontal sinus, irrespective of the size of the frontal recess, may be less likely to remain patent.

Persistent Disease

The two most common local obstructive causes of persistent frontal recess obstruction are (1) a medially displaced uncinate process, and (2) obstruction from a remnant agger nasi cell (Table 21.1). In a series of 67 patients undergoing revision endoscopic frontal sinus surgery, 79% of patients had evidence of residual ethmoid bulla or agger nasi cells, and 49% had remnant uncinate processes [2]. A medially displaced uncinate process can result from disease within the terminal recess of the infundibulum, displacing the uncinate medially, where it can fuse to the middle turbinate. A frontal sinus drainage pathway that is medial to the displaced uncinate will be obstructed by this displacement.

The cap of a remnant agger nasi cell is a common finding in a dissection in which angled endoscopes were never used. A 45° or 70° endoscope is needed to visualize the top of the frontal sinus. When using a 30° or straight endoscope, true visualization of the frontal sinus is often unattainable. Entrance into an agger nasi or frontal recess cell can easily be mistaken for the frontal sinus, and the cap and offending frontal recess obstruction will remain.

Recurrent or Persistent Disease in the Presence of an Adequate Surgical Procedure

If it is determined that the initial surgery was adequate, it increases the chances of a patient having re-

Table 21.1. Common anatomical causes for revision frontal sinus surgery

Remnant superior uncinate process
Agger nasi cell
Remnant cap of ethmoid bulla
Frontal recess cells
Supraorbital ethmoid cells
Iatrogenic scarring or neo-osteogenesis
Polyps and/or mucocele formation

current or persistent frontal sinusitis as a result of either a general host or environmental problem. In these cases, revision surgery is not necessarily the answer to the problem, and treatment of the underlying condition should be more aggressively pursued, particularly in the symptomatic patient.

> ■ The most common sign of recurrent disease is mucosal thickening within the frontal recess and sinus

If a surgeon is able to pass a curved 4-mm suction past the polyps or swollen mucosa into the frontal sinus, then further surgical therapy is unlikely to be of additional benefit, unless residual osteitic bony partitions are present. If these are identified, they can frequently be removed in the office under local infiltrative anesthesia. Persistent frontal recess disease is often seen in patients with nasal polyposis, allergic fungal rhinosinusitis, and recurrent sinus infections. In these cases, appropriate medical therapy should be aggressively pursued. Oral and topical steroids, culture directed antibiotics and/or antifungals may be used to decrease the mucosal edema. In some cases, careful local infiltration with a small particle depot steroid into the thickened frontal recess mucosa may help to control the edema. However, given the known complications of this procedure, great care should be exercised to avoid any intravascular injection or injection under pressure. Environmental allergies should also be controlled, and an immune work-up may be warranted in a patient with recurrent, acute infections.

Iatrogenic Disease

While persistent disease may be due to incomplete initial surgery, and often is corrected with a meticulous revision procedure, iatrogenic problems represent some of the most difficult cases to treat. The incidence of frontal sinusitis following FESS is unknown. Published reports over the last decade quote a 2% to 11% rate of persistent frontal sinusitis symptoms with 1% to 5% of patients requiring revision surgery [5].

21

> ■ Iatrogenic disease is often the result of circumferential stripping of frontal recess mucosa

This can result in scarring and ultimately neo-osteogenesis. Neo-osteogenesis represents our most difficult challenge in revision frontal sinus surgery (Fig. 21.1). The inflamed and hardened bone is difficult to remove and often has to be drilled out to provide an adequate opening. Any procedure involving a drill creates the potential for a great amount of fibrin debris, neo-osteogenesis and stenosis, and requires more extensive postoperative debridements.

> ■ If not meticulously addressed in the postoperative period, sinuses in which the drill is used are more likely to re-stenose.

A second manifestation of iatrogenic disease is mucocele formation. Mucoceles may form years after in-

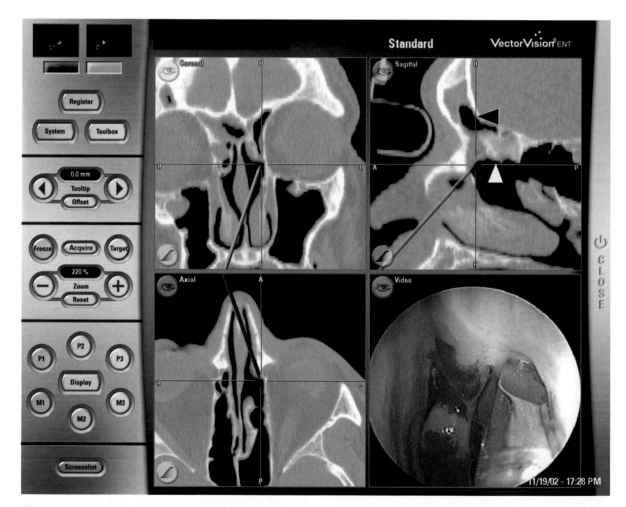

Fig. 21.1. Image-guided triplanar CT scan of the frontal recess in a patient undergoing revision endoscopic frontal sinus surgery. The coronal view shows the pointer at a left lateralized middle turbinate remnant. On the sagittal view, the *white arrow* points to extensive neo-osteogenesis along the posterior frontal recess. The *black arrow* shows a type 3 frontal recess cell

itial surgery, and can result in thinning or dehiscence of the anterior or posterior tables of the frontal sinus.

■ Mucoceles are proof that long-term follow-up is needed after any frontal sinus surgery, because the stenosis and obstruction that leads to the mucocele can be observed for years before it develops.

Neel et al. clearly demonstrated the necessity of long-term follow-up in their patients undergoing a modified Lynch procedure. Their failure rate with that procedure grew from 7% at a mean follow-up of 3.7 years to 30% at 7 years [4].

Pre-operative Planning

Once the decision has been made to perform a revision endoscopic procedure, it is imperative in the pre-operative period to review each patient's frontal sinus anatomy and determine the best procedure, taking into account anatomy, amount of disease, and underlying co-morbidities.

Anatomy

From a surgical standpoint, the frontal recess can be thought of as a box with four surrounding walls. Creating a wide frontal sinusotomy requires a step-wise approach to evaluate each wall of the box.

■ The best approach is to start with detailed pre-operative planning. Surgical navigation, using 1-mm axial sections reformatted into sagittal and coronal views, allows for three-dimensional analysis of the frontal recess. The surgeon should carefully scroll through the images in each of these planes until a three-dimensional concept of the regional anatomy, adjacent cells, and locations of the natural drainage pathway is established.

The anterior wall of the frontal recess is addressed by the dissection of the superior uncinate and agger na-

si cells. Posteriorly, the superior attachment of the ethmoid bulla and any supraorbital ethmoid cell must be opened to expose the box to its greatest anterior-posterior dimension. The anterior ethmoid artery is located along the skull base posterior to the frontal recess, typically where the dome of the ethmoid becomes horizontal. Most frequently, but not always, the anterior ethmoid artery lies posterior to the supraorbital ethmoid cell openings. Potential complications, related to a dehiscent anterior ethmoid artery, or an artery which travels in a bony mesentery below the skull base, can be evaluated prior to the operation and avoided during surgery (Fig. 21.2).

Along with the anterior ethmoid artery, the skull base should be evaluated prior to revision surgery. A fairly common complication following revision frontal surgery is a CSF leak or injury to the skull base. This is a more common occurrence in revision than primary frontal sinus surgery, given the distorted anatomy, possible dehiscence from prior surgeries, and more aggressive moves to eradicate disease and maximally enlarge the frontal recess. Adequate pre-operative planning may help to avoid these complications.

■ One of the most useful pieces of information is the distance from the nasofrontal beak to the olfactory cleft. This can be evaluated on the axial image and can give the surgeon a sense of how much room he or she has in the anterior-posterior dimension.

Choice of Procedure

Once the films have been reviewed, a decision should be made as to which procedure should be performed. Endoscopic frontal sinus surgery has been classified by Draf into three types, based on the extent of surgery.

A Draf I procedure is an anterior ethmoidectomy with drainage of the frontal recess without touching the frontal sinus outflow tract [6]. This is best reserved for primary cases of chronic sinusitis without polyposis and without evidence of frontal sinus disease.

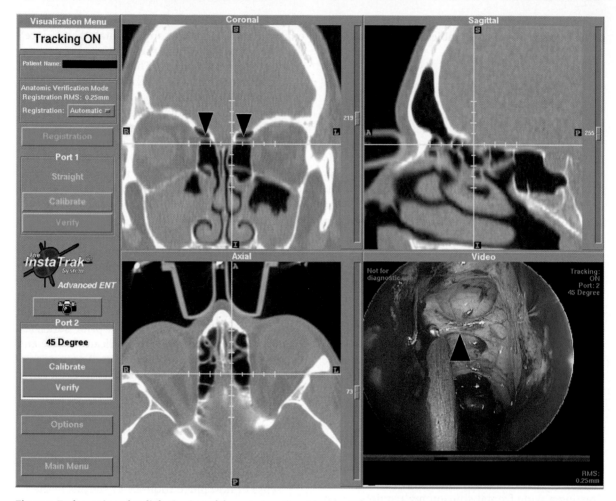

Fig. 21.2. Endoscopic and radiologic view of the anterior ethmoid artery (*black arrows*) as it courses below the skull base

A Draf IIA procedure involves the removal of ethmoid cells protruding into the frontal sinus, creating an opening between the middle turbinate medially and the lamina papyracea laterally. This incorporates the concept of "uncapping the egg" made popular by Stammberger. The key to this procedure is the delicate removal of bony partitions with preservation of the mucosa. When done properly, a Draf IIA is the adequate procedure for any frontal recess that is greater than 4 mm in the anterior-posterior dimension. As stated earlier, the majority of revision cases are secondary to remnant uncinate processes, agger nasi, and/or frontal recess cells. Clearance of these re-

maining obstructions can successfully result in a patent frontal sinusotomy without the use of a drill or external incision.

A Draf IIB involves the removal of the frontal sinus floor between the nasal septum medially and the lamina papyracea laterally. In order to allow for this, the anterior portion of the middle turbinate is resected where it lies medial to the frontal sinus. Opening the sinus in this fashion involves the use of angled through-cutting forceps and may require the use of an endoscopic drill. Although it is not usually performed as an initial procedure, a common indication for this procedure is the presence of a narrow anterior-posterior or medial-lateral dimension, osteitic middle turbinate and/or intersinus septal cell.

The frontal intersinus septal cell occurs in the septum between the two frontal sinuses. In a review of 300 CT scans, the intersinus septal cell was present in 101 or 34% of scans [3]. This cell may pneumatize only the lower intersinus septum or extend to the top of the frontal sinus. Utilizing the frontal sinus interseptal cell is another technique to widen the frontal recess. Removing the common wall that separates the cell from the frontal recess, and the floor of the sinus from the lamina papyracea to the middle turbinate, keeps the posterior and anterior mucosa of the frontal recess intact while enlarging the medial-lateral dimension.

A Draf III or trans-septal frontal sinusotomy involves the removal of the upper part of the nasal septum and the lower part of the frontal sinus septum, in addition to the Type IIB drainage of both frontal sinuses. Also known as a modified Lothrop procedure, this has been used an alternative to the frontal sinus obliteration in revision cases with significant neo-osteogenesis, narrow anterior-posterior dimension and/or significant polypoid thickening or debris.

Surgical Equipment

Once the decision has been made to perform a revision procedure, specialized instruments should be used to maximize sound surgical technique. Each of the following aid in achieving the principles for successful frontal sinus surgery, that is, sparing of frontal recess mucosa and accurate identification of frontal recess anatomy.

Surgical Navigation Systems

With the advent of surgical navigation in the late 1980's, endoscopic surgeons have been increasingly utilizing this technology for intraoperative localization and pre-operative planning. Fine-cut axial CT scans, often 1 mm in section, are reformatted into coronal and sagittal views and allow for greater understanding of anatomy that has been distorted by previous surgery, polypoid mucosa and/or anatomical variants.

Angled Endoscopes and Instruments

Angled instruments are essential in frontal sinus surgery; 45° and 70° endoscopes allow direct visualization of the frontal recess and anterior skull base.

Popularization of endoscopic techniques for frontal sinus surgery has brought about the development of specialized instruments. Powered instrument companies have devised angled drills, diamond and cutting, that may be attached to handheld microdebriders. The 70° diamond suction irrigation drill has, in particular, made a dramatic difference to this surgery. In particular, the drill reduces the amount of trauma and exposed bone during the approach, as well as decreasing the size of the septal perforation required [1]. There is a variety of 90° instruments designed to reach around the nasofrontal beak and into the frontal recess. Angled and malleable curettes have been devised to aid in the removal of the cap of obstructing ethmoid air cells. Revision procedures often become a methodical process of cut, remove, suction, and re-examine. These specialized instruments allow for preservation of mucosa and removal of fine bony fragments that if left behind, can serve as a nidus for scarring and infection.

After the patient has been properly selected, associated disease factors have been controlled, pre-operative planning has been performed, and adequate specialized equipment has been prepared, the surgeon is finally ready for surgery.

Revision Frontal Sinusotomy: General Principles of Surgical Technique (Table 21.2)

■ In revision surgical procedures, the anatomy is significantly distorted and landmarks such as the middle turbinate may be partially resected, making them unreliable for anatomic localization

Accurate identification of both the medial orbital wall and the skull base is essential if the risk of complications is to be minimized (Fig. 21.2).

Table 21.2. General principles of surgical technique

Accurate identification of medial orbital wall and skull base
First identify the skull base posteriorly in the sphenoid sinus, and then dissect from a posterior to anterior direction along the skull base
Use a 45° or 70° endoscope
Identify the anterior ethmoid artery as it crosses the ethmoid roof
Stay close to the medial orbital wall, keeping in mind that the opening of the frontal is often medial
Identify supraorbital ethmoid and frontal recess cell openings
Make sure all remnant osteitic bony fragments are removed from the frontal recess

■ As in all endoscopic surgical cases, it should be remembered that the skull base is usually most easily identified in the posterior ethmoid or sphenoid sinuses, where it is more horizontal and the cells are larger

Care always needs to be taken where the skull base slopes down medially towards the attachment of the middle turbinate in the region of the anterior ethmoid artery. The ethmoid roof is at its thinnest in this area, and may even be membranous in part, making it particularly vulnerable to injury. As this area is approached, it is important to stay close and parallel to the medial orbital wall, while keeping in the mind that the opening of the frontal sinus is most frequently medial, close to the attachment of the middle turbinate to the skull base.

As the dissection along the skull base is carried forwards, the anterior ethmoid artery typically lies in a superior extension of the anterior wall of the bulla ethmoidalis at, or somewhat below, the skull base and courses anteriorly as it travels medially. The openings of one, or more frequently two, supraorbital ethmoid cells often lie anterior to the vessel and extend laterally and superiorly (Fig. 21.3).

The opening to the frontal sinus is frequently not immediately evident. Very fine malleable probes have been developed which can be utilized to gently probe the openings and help determine which of these openings truly passes superiorly into the frontal sinus. Once the opening has been clearly identified, ad-

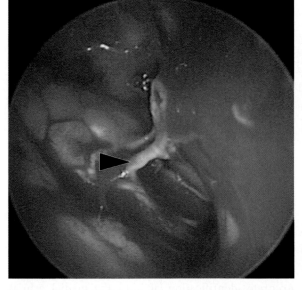

Fig. 21.3. View of the frontal sinus and supraorbital ethmoid cell from a 70° endoscope. The *arrow* points to the bony partition separating the two drainage pathways

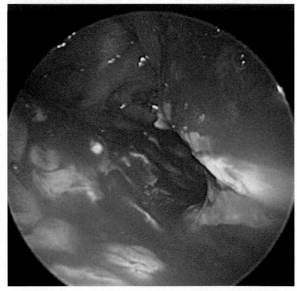

Fig. 21.4. Same patient as in Fig. 21.3, where the bony partition between the frontal sinus and supraorbital ethmoid cell has been removed to create one common drainage pathway

jacent bony partitions may be fractured with specialized frontal sinus instruments to open the frontal sinus. Bony fragments are then teased out, and redundant mucosa is trimmed with through-cutting instruments (Fig. 21.4). It is extremely important in revision surgery to not end the case until all bony partitions have been removed completely.

Postoperative Care

The actual surgery to open a frontal sinus is often the easy part in the management of frontal sinus disease. The postoperative period is where much of the difficulty lies.

> ■ Revision frontal sinusotomies must be carefully and diligently examined following surgery

A failure to actively debride the recess, ensure its patency, and suction contaminated blood and mucus from the sinus is a recipe for restenosis and failure. To do this in a setting of an awake, often anxious patient, with topical analgesia alone, makes this portion of the process very challenging, but can be aided by the careful application of topical cocaine solution to the site. Where local debridements are necessary, the region of the frontal recess can be infiltrated with 1% Xylocaine with 1:100,000 adrenaline using a fine bent needle and a small syringe.

The timing of the first postoperative debridement varies with the individual surgeon's preference. Some debride on postoperative day one, while others wait for an additional 3 to 7 days. It is advantageous to have a full set of frontal sinus instruments available in the clinic. This is coupled with angled suctions that are long and curved enough to reach into the frontal sinus. Debridements should be aimed at clearing away fibrin debris and any loose bony fragments, while keeping trauma to the surrounding mucosa to a minimum.

While the mechanical care of the frontal sinusotomy is important to prevent restenosis, medical management of the disease state is essential to long-term success. In a patient with significant polypoid edema, postoperative oral steroids can be used to keep the edema to a minimum. Intranasal steroids sprayed in

the Moffit or head-down position can help with delivery to the frontal recess. Postoperative antibiotics should also be given in an infectious setting, and antibiotics with good bone penetration should be used in patients with evidence of neo-osteogenesis.

This routine of mechanical debridement and postoperative medication should be continued on a weekly basis until the mucosa of the frontal recess is healed. Once the sinusotomy is secure, routine surveillance by nasal endoscopy should continue for the life of the patient.

Conclusion

Revision endoscopic frontal sinus surgery remains a great challenge to all who practice sinus surgery. The last decade has brought about a specialization of instruments and techniques aimed at treating frontal sinus disease endoscopically and avoiding frontal sinus obliteration. Surgical technique aside, the most important decisions are still made in the office. These entail assessing whether or not the patient is a good surgical candidate, the appropriate choice of endoscopic procedure given the individual patient's anatomy and disease process, and the institution of aggressive adjuvant medical therapy.

References

1. Chandra RK, Schlosser R, Kennedy DW (2004) Use of the 70-degree diamond burr in the management of complicated frontal sinus disease. Laryngoscope 114(2):188–192
2. Chiu AG, Vaughan WC (2004) Revision endoscopic frontal sinus surgery with surgical navigation. Otolaryngol Head Neck Surg 30:312–18
3. Merrit R, Bent JP, Kuhn FA (1996) The intersinus septal cell. Am J Rhinol 10:299–302
4. Neel HB, McDonald TJ, Facer GW (1987) Modified Lynch procedure for chronic frontal sinus diseases: Rationale, technique and long-term results. Laryngoscope 97:1274
5. Orlandi RR, Kennedy DW (2001) Revision endoscopic frontal sinus surgery. Otolaryngol Clin North Amer 34:77–90
6. Weber R, Draf W, Kratzsch B, et al (2001) Modern concepts of frontal sinus surgery. Laryngoscope 111:137–146

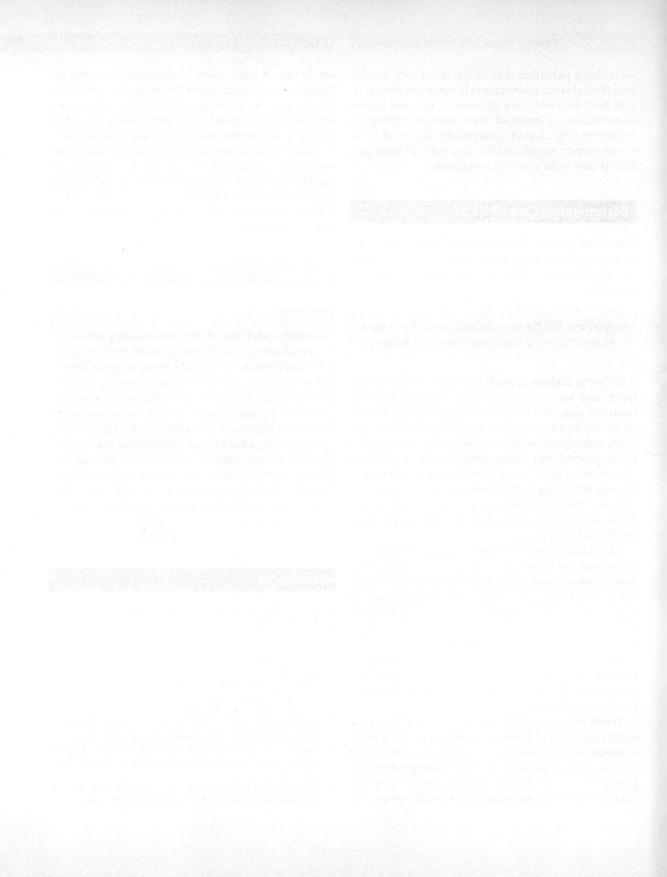

Chapter 22

Image-Guidance in Frontal Sinus Surgery

22

Ralph Metson, Feodor Ung

Core Messages

- The utilization of image-guidance systems continues to increase for sinus surgery, in general, and frontal sinus surgery in particular

- Image-guidance systems can assist surgeons with identification and enlargement of the frontal sinus ostium

- Image-guidance systems appear to be most beneficial for revision frontal sinus surgery in which normal anatomic landmarks are obscured

- Image-guidance systems have the potential to reduce complications from frontal sinus surgery

- Technology is no substitute for technique

Contents

Introduction

The ability of image-guidance systems to provide the surgeon with enhanced anatomic localization during frontal sinus surgery offers the potential for improved clinical outcome. Surgery of the frontal sinus is particularly well suited for surgical navigation systems because of the proximity of the sinus to the orbit and cranial cavities, which demands a high degree of precision and provides little room for misjudgments regarding anatomic relationships. The variable anatomical development of the frontal sinus and its anterior superior location within the nasal cavity increase the possibility of disorientation during surgery. The loss of surgical landmarks can be particularly problematic in patients with extensive disease or a history of previous surgery.

Image-guidance Systems

Commercially available image-guidance systems track the position of a surgical instrument relative to the patient's head using two different types of signals:

- Optical-based (infrared)
- Electromagnetic-based (radiofrequency)

This information is processed by a computer workstation, so the location of the instrument tip can be depicted on a three-dimensional video display of the patient's preoperative CT scan. Both electromagnetic and optical-based technologies have been found to be highly accurate, providing anatomical localization within 2 mm at the start of surgery [2, 6] and deteriorating by less than 1 mm at the conclusion of surgery [6].

■ **Equipment.** Electromagnetic-based systems use a radiofrequency transmitter mounted to a specialized headset, which is worn by the patient during the operative procedure. A radiofrequency receiver is incorporated into the hand-piece of a nonmagnetic instrument. Cables connect the transmitter and receiver to the central workstation, where the data are processed and displayed on a multiplanar video image of the patient's preoperative CT scan.

Optical-based image-guidance systems use an infrared camera array to determine instrument and head position (Fig. 22.1). The camera tracks the coordinate position of optical markers that are attached to a straight probe or surgical instrument. A separate set of optical markers is mounted to a reference headset worn by the patient during surgery to moni-

tor head movement (Fig. 22.2). These optical markers further differentiate optical-based systems into active or passive systems. Active optical-based systems track the position of infrared light-emitting diodes (LEDs), which are powered by cables or individual battery packs. Passive optical-based systems use an infrared emitter in the camera array, which illuminates highly reflective spheres (glions) attached to the surgical instrument and patient headset. This technology allows for the use of wireless instrumentation and eliminates the problem of multiple cables, which may become tangled and entwined. The camera tracks the infrared emissions reflected from the glions, and this spatial information is processed by an optical digitizer and displayed in multiplanar format on a video monitor (Fig. 22.3).

■ **Drawbacks.** Although both types of image-guidance systems are relatively easy to use, these tracking technologies are associated with different drawbacks. For those systems that use a radiofrequency signal for localization, metallic objects in the surgical field may cause signal distortion. Instrument tables, anesthesia equipment, and other sizable metallic devices need to be kept an appropriate distance from the surgical field.

Electromagnetic imaging protocols often require the patient to wear the same headset during both the preoperative CT scan and the operative procedure. Care must be taken not to allow objects, which could cause distortion, to push against the headset during the scan or procedure. The patient must bring the same headset worn during the CT scan to the hospital to wear during the surgery. The headsets are not interchangeable or reusable per recommendation of the manufacturer, although there is evidence to suggest headsets may indeed be reused or interchanged with little effect on accuracy [7]. The electromagnetic headset is typically secured at the ear canals and nasal bridge. This configuration necessitates intraoperative coverage of a portion of the medial orbit and frontal regions. For most sinus surgery this design is not of clinical importance; however, it does preclude use of this headset for procedures that involve external incisions when operating on the frontal sinus. To allow for an external approach to these areas, the headset would need to be secured in the upside-

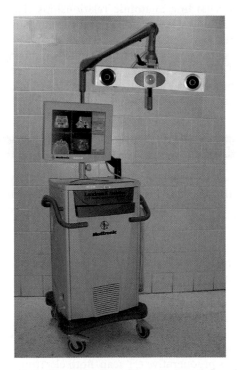

Fig. 22.1. Optical-based image-guidance system. Infrared camera is located within the horizontal bar above the video monitor

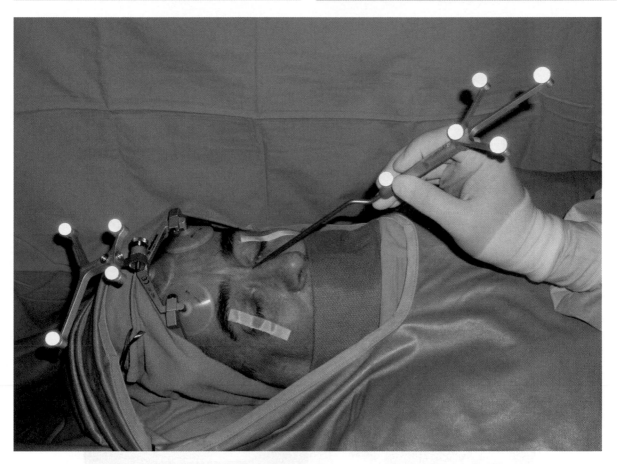

Fig. 22.2. Headset and hand-held probe used for the optical-based image-guidance system. The mirrored spheres reflect the infrared signal, enabling the camera to track the position of the patient's head and the probe tip

down position, resting on the upper lip instead of the nasion during the preoperative CT scan and operative procedure.

■ When using an optical-based system, it is necessary to maintain a clear line of sight between the infrared camera and the optical markers mounted on the surgical instrument and patient headset for the system to function properly.

The instrument must be held with LEDs or glions uncovered and pointed in the direction of the infrared camera. Furthermore, operating room personnel and equipment cannot be positioned between the patient headset and the camera lens, which is generally located six feet above the head of the table.

■ **Instrumentation.** Since the introduction of image-guidance technology in the mid-1990s, the number and variety of surgical instruments that may be used with surgical navigation systems has grown rapidly. From the initial straight pointers and suctions, a variety of instruments with multiple angles and configurations have been specifically developed to support frontal sinus surgery applications. Many of the optical systems now offer universal instru-

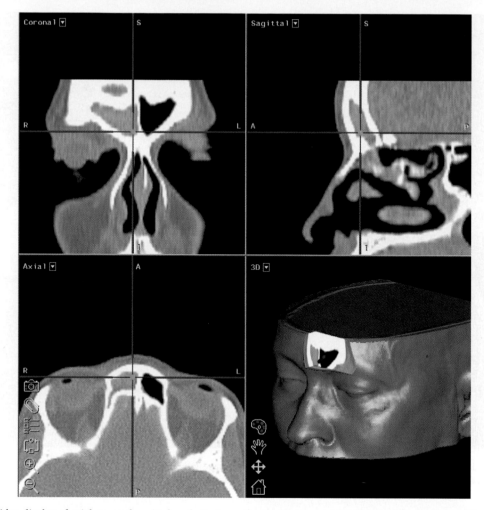

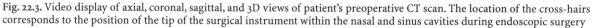

Fig. 22.3. Video display of axial, coronal, sagittal, and 3D views of patient's preoperative CT scan. The location of the cross-hairs corresponds to the position of the tip of the surgical instrument within the nasal and sinus cavities during endoscopic surgery

ment registration. With this process almost any rigid surgical instrument can be digitized during surgery and used for anatomical localization. Even microdebriders may be tracked with this technology. For external surgical approaches that would be obstructed by the presence of a headset, such as frontal sinus obliteration, skull reference arrays have been developed. These glion-equipped posts can be percutaneously affixed to the skull at an unobtrusive location and used to monitor patient head position.

Image-guidance for Endonasal Approaches to the Frontal Sinus

■ **Frontal Sinusotomy.** Image-guidance technology greatly facilitates preoperative understanding of intricate anatomy of the frontal sinus outflow tract. By depicting three-dimensional information in a multiplanar format, synchronized viewing of all three orthogonal planes is possible.

The advantages of using image-guidance technology in frontal sinusotomy are:

- The ability to rapidly and simultaneously scroll through all three planes promotes a better sense of the three-dimensional relationships of the frontal sinus in regard to important surrounding structures
- It is often possible to follow the entire course of the frontal drainage pathway and examine it for areas of pathology. In this way, surgical navigation systems are exceedingly helpful for preoperative planning
- Intraoperatively, image-guidance technology is used to help identify the frontal ostium in an atraumatic manner during frontal sinusotomy

In those patients with disease limited to the frontal recess, an anterior ethmoidectomy is performed and obstructing tissue removed from the recess with an angled Blakesley forceps. An image-guidance-equipped instrument such as a ball-tipped probe or curved suction cannula is then passed to confirm ostial location and patency (Fig. 22.4). The proximity to the adjacent skull base and orbit can also be assessed.

Surgical navigation systems can also assist in distinguishing the frontal sinus ostium from an adjacent supraorbital ethmoid cell. When a supraorbital ethmoid cell is present, its opening is typically found posterolateral to the more anteromedial location of the true frontal sinus ostium. However, within the narrow confines of the frontal recess, these two openings can be easily confused if image-guidance is not employed.

By providing anatomical localization and preventing surgical disorientation, image-guidance technology has been shown to increase surgeon confidence [3]. In a review of 800 sinus procedures done at a community hospital, Reardon [4] noted a significant increase in the number of frontal sinuses entered after the introduction of a surgical navigation system. The incidence of maxillary, ethmoid, and sphenoid sinus entry did not change with image-guidance application.

■ **Frontal Sinus Drillout.** Surgery on the frontal sinus remains a clinical challenge because of the high rate of ostial restenosis after frontal sinusotomy. In the past, patients who failed frontal sinusotomy proceeded to frontal sinus obliteration. More recently, the frontal sinus drillout procedure, also known as the Modified Lothrop or Draf 3 procedure, has been described.

Endoscopic frontal sinus drillout can be a technically demanding procedure because of the narrow anatomy of the frontal recess, the angled field of view at which the surgeon operates, and the paucity of landmarks from previous surgery. These factors increase the likelihood of surgical disorientation even for the experienced sinus surgeon. When an image-guidance system is utilized for drillout surgery, a calibrated curved probe can be used to assist in identification of the frontal ostium and to ensure that drilling is performed in the direction of the frontal sinus floor. Without an image-guidance system, initial drilling is "blind" until the frontal sinus is entered. Once the frontal sinus has been entered, bone removal continues under direct endoscopic visualization.

The advantages of using image-guidance in drillout surgery are:

- The surgical navigation system is used during bone removal to alert the surgeon to the proximity of the skull base, orbit, and anterior nasal skin (Fig. 22.5)
- At the conclusion of surgery, the image-guidance system is used to verify that all compartments of the frontal sinus, including supraorbital ethmoid cells, have been completely opened

Success rates for frontal drillout surgery with and without image-guidance are comparable, although there appears to be a trend toward a higher surgical success rate when surgical navigation systems are employed [8]. Even though image-guidance may not alter the overall long-term outcome of drillout surgery, the extent to which image-guidance systems enhances surgeon confidence, particularly when drilling in the vicinity of the orbit and skull base, cannot be overstated.

22

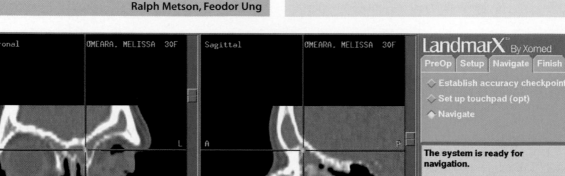

Fig. 22.4. Intraoperative view of image-guided frontal sinusotomy

Image-Guidance in External Approaches to the Frontal Sinus

■ **Frontal Sinus Obliteration.** When endoscopic approaches to the frontal sinus fail to control frontal sinusitis, frontal sinus obliteration must be considered. Although frontal sinus obliteration is highly successful, its rate of major intraoperative complications remains high, occurring in over 20% of patients [9]. These complications include dural exposure, dural injury with cerebrospinal fluid leak, and exposure of orbital fat [9].

■ Most complications during frontal sinus obliteration are due to misdirected osteotomies that extend beyond the confines of the frontal sinus and result in an the osteoplastic flap which is too large

Underestimation of the size of the frontal sinus can result in a bony flap that is too small, making complete removal of mucosa from the sinus interior difficult and increasing the risk of postoperative mucocele formation

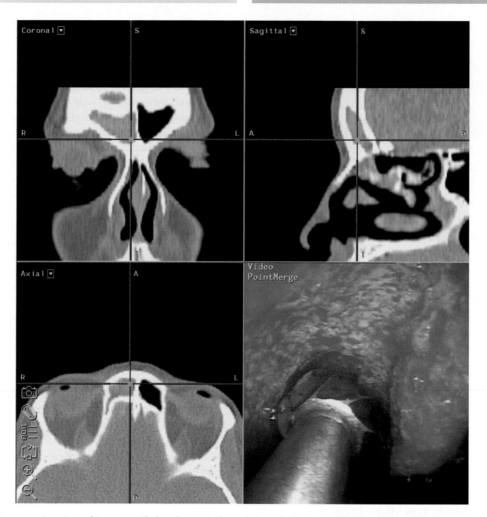

Fig. 22.5. Intraoperative view of image-guided endoscopic frontal sinus drillout (modified Lothrop or Draf 3 procedure)

To utilize image-guidance in frontal sinus obliteration, a skull reference array is anchored percutaneously near the vertex of the cranium at the start of surgery. This positioning affords unencumbered access to the frontal region throughout the procedure. Once the frontal bone is exposed through a coronal or mid-forehead incision, a hand-held probe is used to demarcate the perimeter of the frontal sinus. This information, in conjunction with the x-ray template, is used to direct bony cuts through the anterior table with a sagittal saw and expose the sinus interior (Fig. 22.6). Anatomic accuracy of the image-guidance system is verified once the frontal sinus has been opened. The mucosa is then stripped from the interior of the frontal sinus, and the entire surface is drilled with diamond burrs to obliterate mucosal remnants and promote neovascularization. Oxidized cellulose is used to seal the frontal sinus ostia, and the sinus is then filled with abdominal fat. A closed suction drain is placed and the incision is closed in layers.

Carrau et al. [5] were the first to report the use of image-guidance technology for the localization of the osteoplastic flap during frontal sinus obliteration surgery. Measuring the difference between the frontal sinus perimeter outlined by an image-guidance

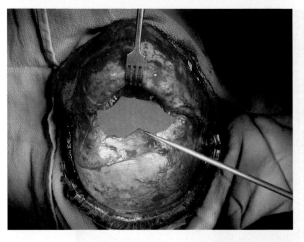

Fig. 22.6. Intraoperative view during image-guided frontal sinus obliteration surgery. The image-guidance probe is used to verify the proper location of the x-ray template and to direct bony cuts through the anterior table of the frontal sinus

probe and that obtained with a traditional radiographic template in six cases, the authors suggested that the surgical navigation system was more accurate. A later study [10] compared four frontal sinus mapping methods: 6-foot Caldwell radiography, sinus transillumination, sinus trephination with probing, and image-guidance technology. The authors concluded that image-guided mapping of the frontal sinus was the most accurate method of delineating the limits of the frontal sinus and least likely to overshoot the real sinus margins. Since successful frontal sinus obliteration surgery is predicated upon the precise localization of osseous anatomy, the utilization of a surgical navigation system may enhance the safety of this procedure. A recent study demonstrated a significant reduction in the rate of intraoperative complications during frontal sinus obliteration when this method of image-guided surgery was utilized [11].

■ **Endoscopic Frontal Sinus Obliteration.** The endoscopic approach to frontal sinus obliteration provides a minimally invasive alternative to traditional frontal sinus obliteration. This technique combines a supraorbital incision, similar to that used for frontal sinus trephination, with endoscopic instrumentation. Standard image-guidance headsets that do not conceal the medial canthal region may be employed.

A curvilinear incision is made along the inferior edge of the medial eyebrow and carried down through the subcutaneous tissue and periosteum. The location of the frontal sinus is then verified with the surgical navigation system and the medial floor of the sinus opened. This bony opening is enlarged to permit passage of both a nasal endoscope and surgical instruments. Using the 0° and 30° endoscopes, the frontal sinus mucosa is elevated and removed. The entire interior of the frontal sinus is then drilled with diamond burrs under endoscopic visualization to remove any mucosal remnants. The surgical navigation system is used to assist with orientation while drilling within the sinus. It is particularly helpful when exenterating frontal cells or removing septations within the frontal sinus. Once drilling is complete, the frontal sinus ostium is plugged with oxidized cellulose and the sinus is completely filled with abdominal fat. The incision is then closed in layers.

Thus far, the use of image-guidance technology in endoscopic frontal sinus obliteration has avoided complications associated with conventional frontal sinus obliteration such as dural exposure, dural tear with cerebrospinal fluid leak, and orbital entry. In addition, early results indicate that operative time, blood loss, and length of hospital stay were all significantly reduced for those undergoing endoscopic obliteration compared with conventional osteoplastic techniques [12]. However, these results should be interpreted with caution, as the long-term outcome of endoscopic frontal sinus obliteration has yet to be determined.

Conclusion

Image-guidance systems appear to be particularly well-suited to frontal sinus surgery. They can assist the surgeon with localization of the frontal sinus ostium during endonasal procedures and the sinus perimeter during external procedures. Navigation technology has the potential to improve the efficacy and safety of frontal sinus surgery; however, its use is no substitute for proper surgical training and technique.

References

1. Kennedy D, Shaman P, Han W, et al (1994) Complications of ethmoidectomy: A survey of the American Academy of Otolaryngology-Head and Neck Surgery. Otolaryngol Head Neck Surg 111:589–599
2. Metson R, Gliklich RE, Cosenza M (1998) A comparison of image-guidance systems for sinus surgery. Laryngoscope 108:1164–1170
3. Metson R, Cosenza MJ, Cunningham MJ, et al (2000) Physician experience with an optical image-guidance system for sinus surgery. Laryngoscope 110:972–976
4. Reardon EJ (2002) Navigational risks associated with sinus surgery and the clinical effects of implementing a navigational system for sinus surgery. Laryngoscope 112(suppl):1–19
5. Carrau RL, Snyderman CH, Curtin HB, et al (1994) Computer-assisted frontal sinusotomy. Otolaryngol Head Neck Surg 111:727–732
6. Metson R, Cosenza M, Gliklich RE, et al (1999) The role of image-guidance systems for head and neck surgery. Arch Otolaryngol Head Neck Surg 125:1100–1104
7. Javer AR, Kuhn FA (2000) Stereotactic computer-assisted navigational (SCAN) sinus surgery: Accuracy of an electromagnetic tracking system with the tissue debrider and when utilizing different headsets for the same patient. Am J Rhinol 14:361–365
8. Samaha M, Cosenza MJ, Metson R (2003) Endoscopic frontal sinus drillout in 100 patients. Arch Otolaryngol Head Neck Surg 129:854–858
9. Weber R, Draf W, Keerl R, et al (2000) Osteoplastic frontal sinus surgery with fat obliteration: technique and long term results using MRI in 82 operations. Laryngoscope 110(6):1037–1044
10. Ansari K, Seikaly H, Elford G (2003) Assessment of the accuracy and safety of the different methods used in mapping the frontal sinus. J Otolaryngol 32:254–258
11. Sindwani R, Metson R (2004) Impact of image-guidance on complications during osteoplastic frontal sinus surgery. Otolaryngol Head Neck Surg 131:150–155
12. Ung F, Sindwani R, Metson R (2004) Endoscopic frontal sinus obliteration: A new technique for the treatment of chronic frontal sinusitis. Annual Meeting of the American Academy of Otolaryngology-Head and Neck Surgery. New York, NY. September 19, 2004

Chapter 23

"Above and Below" FESS: Simple Trephine with Endoscopic Sinus Surgery

23

Ankit M. Patel, Winston C. Vaughan

Core Messages

■ In most cases of frontal sinus disease, endoscopic approaches are favored; however, in some situations where an endoscopic approach is insufficient, an "above and below" approach may be suitable, serving as an alternative to more invasive procedures

■ Situations where this may be considered include large or laterally-based frontal sinus cells, lesions of the frontal sinus lateral to the plane of the lamina papyracea, trauma, revision surgery, and complicated infection

■ Endoscopic frontal sinusotomy is performed first, followed by trephination

Contents

Background

Historically, frontal sinus disease was treated using external approaches, with the first written reports of frontal trephination dating back to the late 1800's. In 1921, Lynch reported on his experience and technique of external frontoethmoidectomy. In the 1950's and 1960's, Montgomery popularized the osteoplastic flap approach with obliteration of the frontal sinus.

In the late 1970's, Messerklinger and Wigand introduced endoscopic sinus surgery. Since that time, increased emphasis has been placed on atraumatic, mucosal-sparing endoscopic techniques that incorporate the natural drainage pathways of the paranasal sinuses–"functional" endoscopic sinus surgery (FESS). This led to improved healing, preservation of the mucociliary transport, and better results. In the mid 1980's, image-guided surgery was introduced.

Over the last two decades, there have also been tremendous advances in imaging. With these advances in imaging, knowledge of endonasal anatomy, instrumentation, and image-guided surgery, there has been an overwhelming move away from external approaches toward minimally invasive endoscopic approaches for frontal sinus surgery [1–6]. Functional endoscopic sinus surgery is now considered the first-line approach for frontal sinus disease. Table 23.1 summarizes the major approaches to the frontal sinus most often used.

However, there are cases when the endoscopic technique itself is insufficient. In these cases, an external approach with frontal sinus trephination (above), along with endoscopic sinus approach (below) can provide improved visualization and allow for

23

Table 23.1. Surgery for frontal sinus disease: from least aggressive to most aggressive treatment

Anterior ethmoidectomy
Frontal sinusotomy
Frontal sinus rescue procedure
"Above and below FESS" (trephine + endoscopic surgery)
Unilateral "frontal sinus drillout"
Endoscopic modified Lothrop, Transseptal frontal sinusotomy
External ethmoidectomy / Lynch approach
Osteoplastic flap without obliteration
Osteoplastic flap with obliteration

more precise surgery. This technique is especially useful for cases where endoscopic surgery is insufficient, but the osteoplastic flap approach is too aggressive. These situations may include cases where there are large or laterally-based frontal cells that cannot be approached safely endoscopically. A lesion in the frontal sinus that is lateral to the plane of the lamina papyracea on preoperative coronal CT scan may suggest the need for an "above and below" approach. Potential applications for this combined approach are listed in Table 23.2.

Table 23.2. Relative indications for "Above and Below" FESS

Electively, for visualization to facilitate endoscopic frontal sinusotomy
Inability to completely address disease endoscopically:
Laterally-based frontal sinus lesions
Type III or IV frontal cell, which cannot be addressed endoscopically
Large tumors or inflammatory lesions involving frontal sinus, including:
Osteoma
Inverted papilloma
Fibrous dysplasia
Trauma with distorted frontal recess or need to evaluate posterior frontal wall
Revision cases with extensive scarring or neo-osteogenesis
Distorted anatomy in the frontal recess
Pott's puffy tumor

Technique

Decongestant-soaked pledgets are placed in the nasal cavity. The image-guidance system, if being used, is calibrated and verified using known landmarks. Image-guided systems can also provide a guide for the initial brow incision and external entry site. If image-guidance is not being used, the position and size of the frontal sinus is confirmed on preoperative CT scan in relation to the supraorbital rim or with 6-foot Caldwell templates. Typically, incision and trephination location will be through the medial eyebrow at the supraorbital rim without shaving this region.

The endoscopic portion of the surgery is done first. A complete uncinectomy is performed. Superiorly, a complete uncinectomy will create additional space for endoscopic work as well as help to create a larger frontal sinus outflow drainage pathway. The superior uncinate process may attach to the middle turbinate, lamina papyracea, or skull base. Review of preoperative CT scan films will identify its attachment point.

Maxillary antrostomy is then performed to serve as a landmark. The ethmoid bulla may then be removed via the retrobullar recess. Superiorly, this is traced to the skull base. The lamina papyracea should be identified and preserved. The anterior ethmoid artery may often be identified at the skull base at this point as well. Preoperative review of coronal CT scans will reveal a medial dimpling of the lamina papyracea at the location of the anterior ethmoid artery. The artery may be dehiscent or coursing from medial to lateral at a position inferior to the skull base. In both these instances, the artery is at risk for injury.

If complete sphenoethmoidectomy is planned, it may be performed at this time, with removal of posterior ethmoid cells and sphenoidotomy. The skull base should be identified posteriorly, at the sphenoid face. It then is traced from posterior to anterior with removal of ethmoid cells along the skull base. If complete sphenoethmoidectomy is not necessary, then dissection may stop at the basal lamella, which is traced to the skull base.

Key landmarks should always be reconfirmed for frontal recess dissection.

These are:

- Lamina papyracea medially
- Skull base superiorly
- Anterior ethmoid artery superiorly and posteriorly, which marks the start of the frontal recess
- The middle turbinate and its attachment to the skull base
- The nasofrontal bone / beak

The agger nasi cell, which is present in a majority of patients, should be identified. Endoscopically, it will appear as a bulge of the lateral nasal wall at the junction of the lateral nasal wall and the middle turbinate. This must be removed downward (uncapping the egg) in its entirety. Next, the frontal recess is opened with mucosal preservation. Any frontal recess cells, supraorbital cells, and intersinus cells are opened endoscopically. Review of sagittal preoperative CT scans or image-guided scans is critical to maximize the diameter of the frontal sinus drainage pathway. The frontal recess can then be enlarged using a combination of curved mushroom punches, giraffe forceps, seekers and limited use of microdebriders. The mucosa of the frontal sinus should be preserved as much as possible to maintain the functional nature of FESS.

Once the endonasal frontal sinusotomy has been completed to its full extent, then the external approach is begun. Sometimes, due to tumor, trauma, previous surgery, or the patient's anatomy, endoscopic frontal sinusotomy cannot be completed endoscopically. In these cases, as much as possible of the previously described dissection is performed in a safe fashion. Trephination and endoscopic visualization through the trephine may also facilitate further dissection from below.

The external approach field is now prepped. If image guidance is being used, it is used to confirm the optimal eyebrow incision and frontal sinus entry point. Lidocaine with epinephrine is used to infiltrate the eyebrow incision. A 1–2-cm incision is carried through the medial eyebrow. The incision should be beveled to parallel the hair shafts of the eyebrow. No electrocautery should be used in the superficial dermis, to prevent injury to hair follicles. Bipolar cautery or pressure is less traumatic.

A self-retaining retractor is placed into the incision. The incision is carried down to bone. Deeper hemostasis is carefully achieved with bipolar cautery. Next, a 4-mm drill bit is used to perform the external trephine. The trephine may be enlarged using Kerrison rongeurs. Angled endoscopes (adult or pediatric) are used to visualize the frontal sinus through the trephine. The remaining pathology of the frontal sinus may then be addressed via the trephine, with the trephine enlarged (max: 6–8 mm) to accommodate both endoscope as well as instrumentation.

If the frontal sinus outflow tract is still not seen endonasally, the frontal sinus can be irrigated through the trephine. The endoscope is used within the middle meatus to visualize the draining irrigation fluid (this can be colored with methylene blue). This will facilitate further dissection. The endoscope is now placed back through the trephine, and angled instruments from within the nose are used to complete frontal sinusotomy. If necessary, a stent may be placed upon completion of the above-and-below procedure from below and visualized from above. The external incision is closed in layers using absorbable suture for deep tissues and permanent 5-0 sutures for the skin.

Illustrative Case

This patient has a laterally-based frontal sinus mucocele with left forehead pain, and has failed medical treatment. There is a large obstructing type III frontal cell. Because of the large size of the frontal cell, the patient was counseled regarding the possible need for trephination in conjunction with FESS. Intraoperatively, the lateral wall of the type III frontal cell could not be sufficiently opened endoscopically from below. "Above and below" FESS with the addition of a simple trephine was performed, to remove more of the lateral border of the type III frontal cell and drain the mucocele. Figures 23.1–21.9 illustrate the anatomy and technique.

23

Fig. 23.1.
A laterally-based muco-
cele, symptomatic and
persistent despite medi-
cal management. A large,
obstructing type III
frontal cell is present

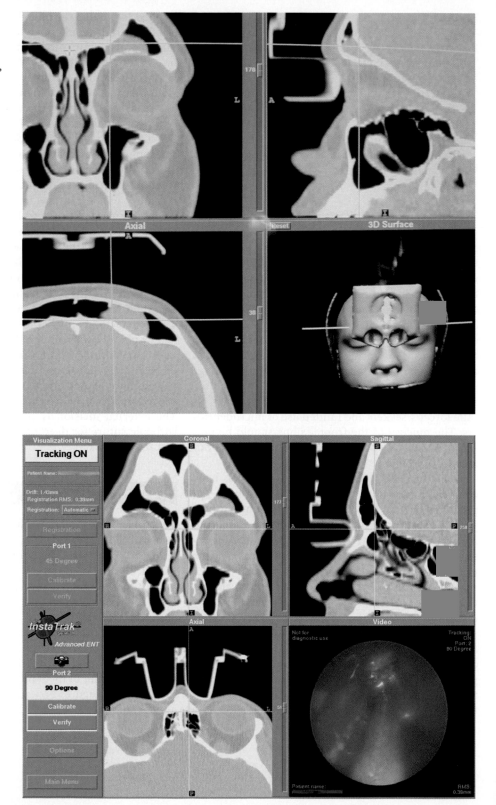

Fig. 23.2.
Endoscopic approach,
at the base of the type
III frontal cell, above
agger nasi and at the
'beak'

Fig. 23.3.
Cross-hairs depict dissection of the type III frontal cell medially

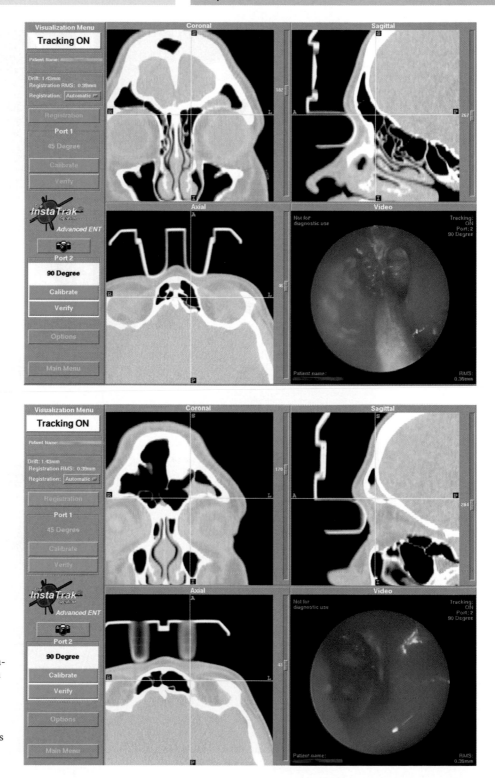

Fig. 23.4.
Laterally-based mucocele, endoscopic view. Endonasal instrumentation is insufficient to take down the lateral septation sufficiently and drain the mucocele. At this point, trephination is needed to help facilitate more complete surgery

23

Fig. 23.5.
External approach. Image-guidance is used to confirm incision site and entry point of trephination through the medial eyebrow

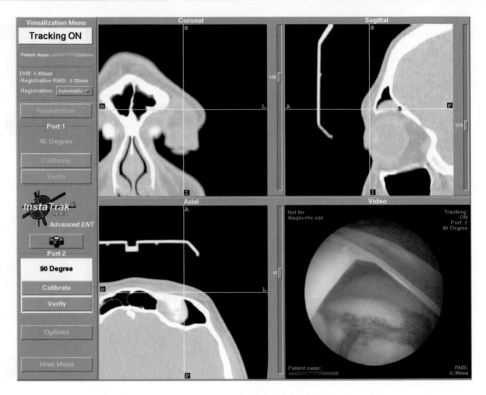

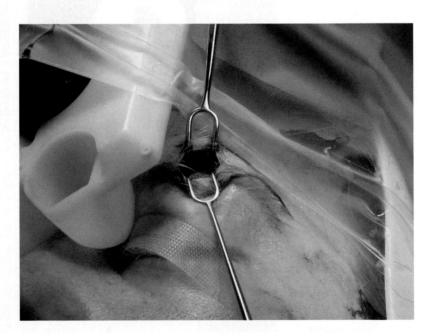

Fig. 23.6.
Trephination incision. Alcohol-prepped image-guidance headset is in place. This may be retracted and put back into position as needed

Fig. 23.7.
Reverse 70° endoscope through trephine site. Curved (90°) giraffe forceps used endonasally under endoscopic visualization from above

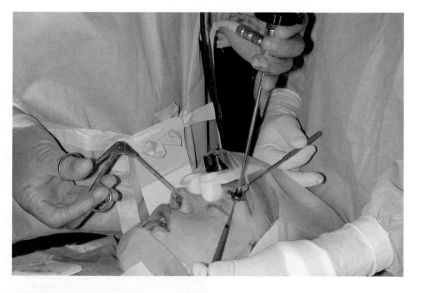

Fig. 23.8.
Angled endoscope through trephine looking down into recess from above. Angled image-guidance suction from below, guided by endoscope from above

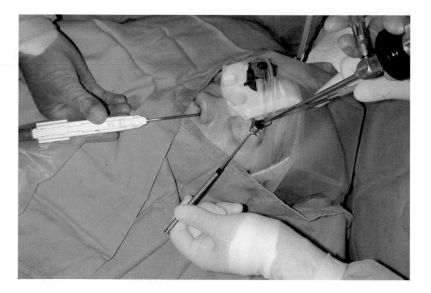

Fig. 23.9.
Additional instrumentation for
frontal sinus trephination

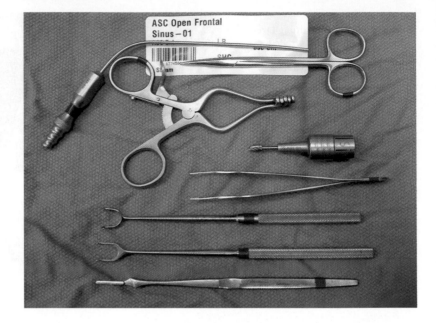

Conclusion

While endoscopic approaches are preferred for management of disease of the frontal sinus, in some situations, transnasal techniques alone will not allow sufficient access to the frontal sinus. One alternative in these cases to more aggressive open approaches is the "above and below" approach utilizing a small trephination to assist the dissection. This technique allows access to lesions located cephalad and laterally in the frontal sinus, and may also be beneficial in the setting of trauma, revision surgery, and complicated acute sinusitis. This simple technique is well-tolerated by patients and may be easily incorporated into the rhinologist's practice.

References

1. Benoit CM, Duncavage JA (2001) Combined external and endoscopic frontal sinusotomy with stent placement: A retrospective review. Laryngoscope 111 (7):1246–1249
2. Bent JP 3rd et al (1997) Combined endoscopic intranasal and external frontal sinusotomy. Am J Rhinol 11 (5): 348–354
3. Chiu AG, Vaughan WC (2004) Revision endoscopic frontal sinus surgery with surgical navigation. Otolaryngol Head Neck Surg 130(3):312–318
4. El-Silimy O (1996) Combined endonasal and percutaneous endoscopic approach to Pott's puffy tumour. Rhinology 34 (2):119–122
5. Gallagher RM, Gross CW (1999) The role of mini-trephination in the management of frontal sinusitis. Am J Rhinol 13 (4):289–293
6. Gerber ME, Myer CM 3rd, Prenger EC (1993) Transcutaneous frontal sinus trephination with endoscopic visualization of the nasofrontal communication. Am J Otolaryngol 14 (1):55–59

Chapter 24

Endonasal Frontal Sinus Drainage Type I–III According to Draf

24

Wolfgang Draf

Core Messages

■ The *Endonasal Type I–III Drainages* allow the surgeon to adapt the frontal sinus surgery to the underlying pathology

■ From type I–III upwards, surgery is increasingly invasive

■ The type III median drainage (Draf 1991) is identical to the endoscopic modified Lothrop procedure (Gross 1995)

■ The concept of endonasal drainage of the frontal sinus implicates preservation of bony boundaries of frontal sinus outlet, in contrast to the classic external frontoorbital procedure [11, 14, 21, 29]. This means less danger of shrinking and reclosure with development of mucocele. It is a surgical strategy, not just a technique. The frontoorbital external operation should not be used anymore for treatment of inflammatory diseases

■ When the type III drainage is technically not possible (anterior-posterior diameter of the frontal sinus less than 0.8 cm) or has failed, osteoplastic frontal sinus obliteration must be considered

Contents

24

Introduction

Endonasal surgery of the paranasal sinuses began, apart from a couple of earlier reports, some hundred years ago [5, 6, 12, 30, 31]. Only a few skilled surgeons have been able to perform endonasal ethmoidectomy and adequate drainage of the frontal sinus using just a headlight and the naked eye, whereas others created serious complications such as CSF leak, meningitis, brain abscess, and encephalitis ending in the preantibiotic era mostly with the death of the patient. This is why for decades, until the 1970s, endonasal sinus surgery was not accepted in most leading institutions.

The renaissance of endonasal surgery was due to several advances:

- New optical aids such as the microscope and endoscope
- Improved understanding of the physiology and pathophysiology of nasal and paranasal sinus mucosa
- Patients no longer accepting the sometimes serious sequelae of external operations in addition to an unsatisfactory outcome
- Remarkable progress in anesthesiology providing the endonasal surgeon with an almost bloodless field

Between 1980 and 1984, an endonasal surgical concept with different degrees of frontal sinus opening was worked out and intensively tested before being published [2].

With increasing experience and referrals of difficult frontal sinus cases, it became obvious that not all problems can be solved via an endonasal route. Therefore the osteoplastic obliterative frontal sinus operation [34] was included in the concept, in order to deal with all different kinds of frontal sinus problems. In difficult revision cases, the endonasal operation sometimes has to be combined with the osteoplastic, mostly obliterative procedure [2].

Operative Technique, Indications

For the endonasal frontal sinus, an operation using some type of general anesthesia is required. In addition, topical decongestion helps to provide a dry field.

Surgery on the frontal recess is usually preceded at least by an anterior, more often than not by a complete ethmoidectomy. Exceptions are those cases where a complete ethmoidectomy has already been performed. It is important to remove agger nasi cells and to visualize the attachment of the middle turbinate medially, the lamina papyracea laterally, and the anterior skull base with the anterior ethmoidal artery superiorly.

Type I: Simple Drainage (Fig. 24.1A)

The type I drainage is established by ethmoidectomy including the cell septa in the region of the frontal recess. The inferior part of Killian's infundibulum and its mucosa is not touched. This approach is indicated when there is only minor pathology in the frontal sinus and the patient does not suffer from 'prognostic risk factors" like aspirin intolerance and asthma, which are associated with poor quality of mucosa and possible problems in outcome (Table 24.1). In the majority of cases the frontal sinus heals because of the improved drainage via the ethmoid cavity.

Type II a/b: Extended Drainage (Fig. 24.1B–D)

Extended drainage is achieved after ethmoidectomy by resecting the floor of the frontal sinus between the lamina papyracea and the middle turbinate (type II a) or the nasal septum (type II b) anterior to the ventral margin of the olfactory fossa.

In the classification of May and Schaitkin [22] type IIa corresponds with NFA II (nasofrontal approach) and type IIb with NFA III. Hosemann et al. [7, 8, 9] showed in a detailed anatomical study that the maximum diameter of a neo-ostium of the frontal sinus (type IIa), which could be gained using a spoon or a curette, was 11 mm with an average of

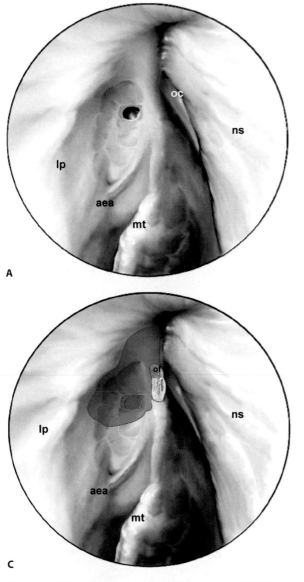

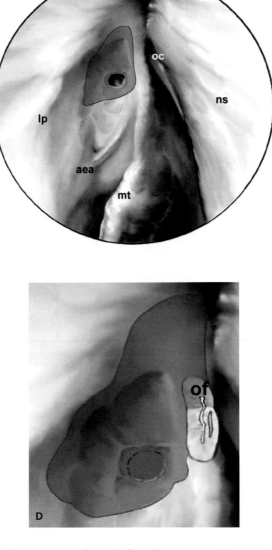

Fig. 24.1A–F. Endonasal frontal sinus drainage 2. (A) Type I drainage (Simple drainage, right side). aea, anterior ethmoidal artery; lp, lamina papyracea; mt, middle turbinate; ns, nasal septum; oc, olfactory cleft. (B) Type II a drainage (enlarged drainage, a, right side). Opening of frontal sinus between lamina papyracea and middle turbinate. Mostly possible without drill. (C) Type IIb drainage (enlarged drainage, b, right side). Drainage of the frontal sinus between lamina papyracea and nasal septum. Usually medially drill necessary. (D) Type IIb drainage Detail with identification of the first olfactory fiber (detail of 1c; of, olfactory fiber). (E) Type III drainage (median drainage) with "Frontal T" (red) and first olfactory fiber on both sides (View from left inferior). (F) Type III drainage (median drainage) sagittal view: removal of the frontal sinus floor in front of the olfactory cleft

Fig. 24.1E,F

24

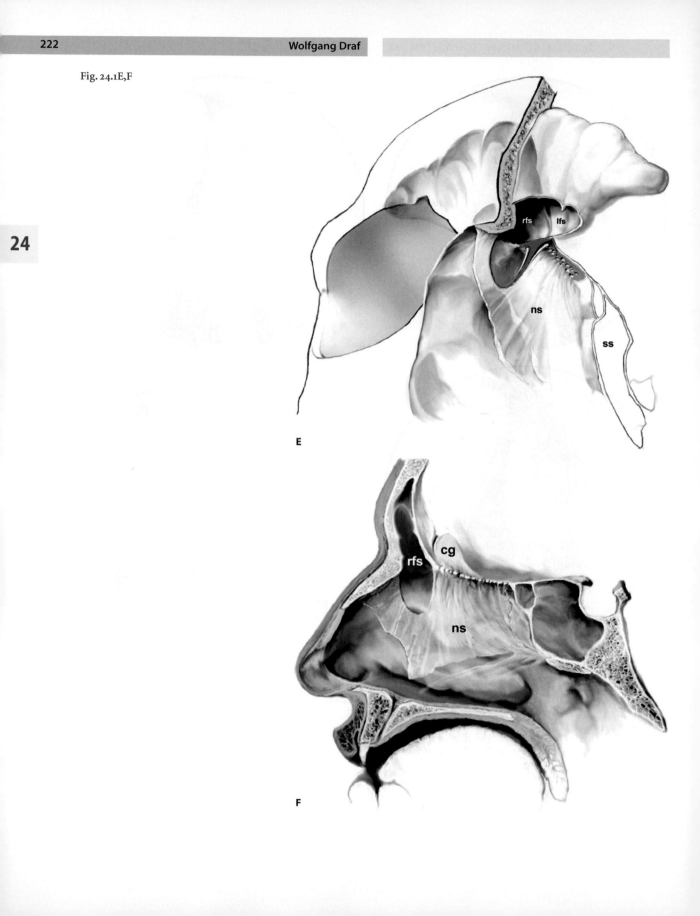

E

F

Table 24.1. Indications for endonasal frontal sinus drainage Type I–III

(A)	*Indications type I drainage*	
	Acute sinusitis	– failure of conservative surgery
		– orbital and endocranial complications
	Chronic sinusitis	– first time surgery
		– no risk factors (aspirin intolerance, asthma, triad)
		– revision after incomplete ethmoidectomy
(B)	*Indications type IIa drainage*	– serious complications of acute sinusitis
		– medial muco- pyocele
		– tumor surgery (benign tumors)
		– good quality mucosa
	Indications type IIb drainage	– all indications of type IIa, if the resulting IIa is smaller than 5×7 mm. For type II b drill necessary
(C)	*Indications type III drainage*	– difficult revision surgery
		– primarily in patients with prognostic risk factors and severe polyposis particularly patients with triad mucoviscidosis
		– mucoviscidosis
		– Kartagener's syndrome
		– ciliary immotility syndrome
		– benign and malignant tumors(see text)

5.6 mm. They also presented an excellent critical evaluation and results [9].

If one needs to achieve a larger drainage opening like type II-b, a drill is used because of the increasing thickness of the bone medially towards the nasal septum. During drilling with the diamond burr, bone dust fogs the endoscope, demanding repeated cleaning. At this point the microscope is useful, allowing one to work with two hands, while an assistant holds a simple self-retracting speculum according to Cholewa (1888) [1]. The endoscopic four–hand technique, introduced by May [21], is also a useful alternative, allowing the surgeon to work with two hands while an assistant holds the endoscope.

In revision cases after incomplete ethmoidectomy, it is recommended that a wide approach to the ethmoid sinuses is created using a microscope and drill or punch when possible. Punches and through-cutting instruments [23] help preserve the mucosa, whereas the drill is more destructive in this respect. The wide approach to the ethmoid is obtained by exposing the lacrimal bone and reducing it, as well as parts of the agger nasi and part of the frontal process of the maxilla, until the lamina papyracea is clearly seen through the microscope. This facilitates better visualization of the frontal recess to allow further work on the frontal sinus floor, but also makes the postoperative treatment less painful. As soon the frontal recess is identified using the middle turbinate and where identifiable, the anterior ethmoidal artery as landmarks, the frontal infundibulum is exposed and the anterior ethmoidal cells are resected. During surgery, repeated considerations of the pre-operative CT scans will establish the presence of so-called frontal cells [17] (Fig. 24.2, see also Chapter 2) which can develop far into the frontal sinus, giving the surgeon the erroneous impression that the frontal sinus has been properly opened. Sagittal CT slices and navigation may be helpful in difficult situations. When frontal cells are present, a procedure called "uncapping the egg" by Stammberger [33] uses a 45° telescope and results in a type IIa drainage.

An alternative when the middle turbinate has been retracted laterally after previous surgery and is obstructing the frontal sinus drainage is the so-called "frontal sinus rescue procedure" [16] (see Chapter 26). The decision should be left to the patient as to whether or not he desires a more conservative procedure like this, which has a relatively higher frequency of recurrence and need for re-operation.

If, after a type IIa drainage has been performed, further widening to produce a type IIb is required, the diamond burr is introduced into the clearly visible gap in the infundibulum and drawn across the

24

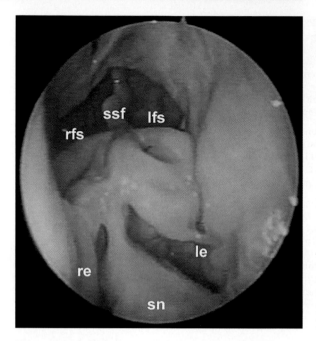

Fig. 24.2. Type III drainage 1 year postoperatively. ssf, septum sinuum frontalium; rfs, right frontal sinus; lfs, left frontal sinus; sn, septum nasale; re, right ethmoid; le, left ethmoid

Type III: Endonasal Median Drainage
(Fig. 24.1E,F)

Endonasal median drainage or type III: The extended IIb opening is enlarged by resecting portions of the superior nasal septum in the neighborhood of the frontal sinus floor. The diameter of this opening should be about 1.5 cm. This is followed by resection of the frontal sinus septum or septa, if more than one are present. Starting on one side of the patient, one crosses the midline until the contralateral lamina papyracea is reached.

To achieve the maximum possible opening of the frontal sinus, it is very helpful to *identify the first olfactory fibers* on both sides: the middle turbinate is exposed and is resected in very small pieces from an anterior to posterior direction, along its origin at the skull base. After about 5 mm one will see the first olfactory fiber coming out of a small bony hole, slightly medial to the origin of the middle turbinate. The same is done on the contralateral side. Finally the so-called *"Frontal T"* [3] (Fig. 24.1E) results. Its long crus is represented by the posterior border of the perpendicular ethmoid lamina resection, and the shorter wings on both sides are provided by the posterior margins of the frontal sinus floor resection.

After that, the ethmoidectomy on the left side is performed exactly as it was on the right.

To perform the type III drainage in the technically most efficient way, it is helpful to interchange the use of the endoscope and microscope. Alternatively, this procedure can be done with the endoscope alone, though it is more time-consuming. Curved drills of different angles used with the shaver motor are helpful [41]. They allow a more superior reach into the frontal sinus and resection of the interfrontal sinus septum or septa, if more than one are present. They also allow removal of superiorly located frontal cells when present, and thus they help achieve a more complete operation. These measures help to create excellent landmarks for the anterior border of the olfactory fossa on both sides, which allow for an easier and safer complete resection of the frontal sinus floor as far posteriorly as the location of the first olfactory fiber.

Finally, a rubber finger stall is placed into each frontal sinus, and two more are placed in the ethmoid

bone in a medial direction. Care is taken to ensure that the frontal sinus opening is bordered by bone on all sides and that mucosa is preserved at least on one part of the circumference. To also safely create medially the widest possible opening of the frontal sinus floor, one should identify the first ipsilateral olfactory fiber (for details see type III drainage, Fig 2B,C). At the end a rubber finger stall can be introduced into the frontal sinus for about 5 days.

The indications for one or the other Type II drainage in general are listed in Table 24.1B. If the surgeon feels that the type IIa drainage is too small in regard to the underlying pathology, it is better to perform the type II b drainage procedure.

Some authors [11, 27, 39] advocated the use of soft, flexible silicone stents in cases of a frontal sinus neo-ostium less than 5 mm in diameter, since more rigid silicone tubes have not given satisfying results [24, 29]. So far the techniques using soft silicone drainage devices showed promising results although long term observation is still lacking.

Fig. 24.3.
Frontal sinus view from above after coronal osteoplastic revision. Several frontal cells of different sizes narrow the drainage into the nose. (fc, frontal cell)

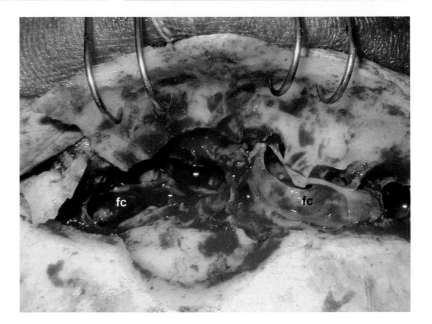

cavity and the inferior nasal meatus bilaterally. This packing is left for 7 days (!) under prophylactic antibiotic treatment. The rubber finger stalls do not stick to the surrounding tissue and are therefore easily and painlessly removed. The packing allows re-epithelialization of a major portion of the surgical cavity, which simplifies the postoperative treatment.

In difficult revision cases, one can begin the type III drainage primarily from two starting points, either from the lateral side as already described or from medially. The *primary lateral approach* is recommended if the previous ethmoidal work was incomplete and the middle turbinate is still present as a landmark. One should adopt the primary medial approach, if the ethmoid has been cleared and/or if the middle turbinate is absent.

The *medial approach* begins with the partial resection of the perpendicular plate of the nasal septum, followed by identification of the first olfactory fiber on each side as already described.

The endonasal median drainage is identical with the NFA IV [21] and the "modified Lothrop procedure" [4]. Lothrop [18, 19] himself warned against using the endonasal route, judging it as too dangerous during his time; he performed the median drainage via an external approach. Halle [6] in 1906 created a large drainage from the frontal sinus directly to the nose using the endonasal approach, and using only a headlight and the naked eye.

The principle difference between the endonasal median frontal sinus drainage and the classic external Jansen, Lothrop, Ritter, Lynch, and Howarth operations is that the bony borders around the frontal sinus drainage are preserved. This makes it more stable in the long term and reduces the likelihood of reclosure by scarring, which may lead to recurrent frontal sinusitis or a mucocele, not to mention the avoidance of external scar.

The endonasal median drainage (type III) is indicated (Table 24.1C) after one or several previous sinus operations have not resolved the frontal sinus problem, including an external frontoethmoidectomy. It is also justified as a primary procedure in patients with severe polyposis and other prognostic "risk factors" affecting outcome, such as aspirin intolerance, asthma, Samter's triad (aspirin hypersensitivity, asthma, and allergy), Kartagener's syndrome, mucoviscidosis, and ciliary dyskinesia syndrome (Table 24.1C). Its use in patients with severe polyposis without these risk factors is undetermined and needs to be evaluated. It seems that patients with generalized polyposis but who still show air on coro-

Table 24.2. Indications for the osteoplastic flap procedure

1. Correctly performed Type III drainage failed

2. Patients after many endonasal and various external frontal sinus operations, so-called problem frontal sinus, sometimes in combination with complete endonasal ethmoidectomy

3. Type III drainage technically not possible (anterior-posterior diameter less than 8 mm)

4. Laterally located muco-pyocele

5. Major destruction of posterior wall

6. Inflammatory complications after trauma (e.g. alloplastic material, without or with obliteration)

7. Aesthetic correction of pneumatosinus dilatans frontalis (mostly without obliteration)

8. Major benign tumors (e.g. osteoma) without or with obliteration

nal CT ("halo sign") in the periphery of the sinuses along the skull base have a comparatively better prognosis than those without, and can be managed by a more conservative technique. The procedure is also useful for removal of benign tumors in the frontal and ethmoid sinuses, as long as the main portion of the tumor in the frontal sinus is medial to a vertical line through the lamina papyracea. In addition, the use of the type III drainage makes the removal of malignant tumors which are just reaching the frontal sinus safer.

Results of Endonasal Frontal Sinus Surgery

Judging the *results* of endonasal frontal sinus surgery requires a postoperative follow-up of ten or more years [14, 25, 26]. The failure rate of Neel et al. [14] with a modified Lynch procedure grew from 7% at a mean follow-up of 3.7 years to 30% at 7 years.

Kikawada et al. [16] presented a retrospective review of 22 consecutive cases of extended frontal sinus surgery (Draf type III) in patients with obstructive frontal sinusitis caused by postoperative scarring, with a follow-up time of at least 12 months after surgery. Of the 16 patients who underwent the type III procedure, in 14 (88%) the patency of the newly created frontal sinus drainage and an aerated sinus were confirmed. Of 12 sides in nine patients who underwent Draf type II procedure, 5 sides (42%) were also confirmed as cured. In the opinion of the authors, the median drainage operation (type III) on the frontal sinus showed excellent long-term results compared with the type II procedure.

Weber et al. [36, 40] carried out two studies in 1995 and 1996. In the first retrospective study, patients who underwent endonasal frontal sinus drainage (471 type I drainages, 125 type II drainages, and 52 type III drainages) between 1979 and 1992 were evaluated. From these groups, random patients were examined: 42 patients with type I drainage, 43 with type II drainage, and 47 with type III drainage were included in the study. In each patient, the indication for surgery was chronic polypoid rhinosinusitis, except in five patients with type III drainage, in whom an orbital complication presented associated with acute sinusitis. The follow-up period was between 1 year and 12 years with a median of 5 years. The subjective estimation of operative results by the patients is shown in Figure 24.4a–c. Applying subjective and objective criteria to evaluate the success of endonasal frontal sinus drainage (Grade 1 = endoscopically normal mucosa, independent of the subjective complaints; Grade 2 = subjectively free of symptoms, but with endoscopically visible inflammatory mucosal changes; Grade 3 = no subjective improvement and pathologic mucosa = failure), it was possible to achieve a success rate of 85.7% with type I drainage, 83.8% with Type II drainage, and 91.5% with type III drainage. This means that, despite the choice of prognostically unfavorable cases, type III drainages appeared to show the best results, though this was not statistically significant among the three groups.

In the second study [39], endoscopic and CT examinations were systematically carried out (Figs. 24.5, 24.6). After 12–98 months follow-up of patients with type II drainage, 58% of 83 frontal sinuses were ventilated and normal. A ventilated frontal sinus with hyperplastic mucosa was seen in 12%. Scar tissue occlusion with total opacification on CT was evident in 14%. In 16%, total opacification was due to recurrent polyposis. Seventy-nine percent of the patients were free of symptoms or had only minor problems.

Twelve to 89 months following type III drainage, 59% of 81 frontal sinuses were ventilated and normal.

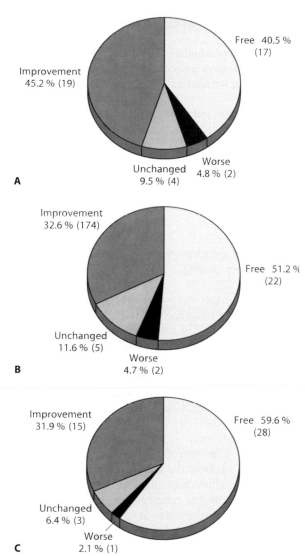

A

B

C

Fig. 24.4A–C. Subjective judgment of results of frontal sinus surgery 1 to 12 years after surgery. (A) Type I drainage. (B) Type II drainage. (C) Type III drainage

A ventilated frontal sinus with hyperplastic mucosa was seen in 17%. Scar tissue occlusion with total opacification on CT was obvious in 7% and, in 16%, there was total opacification due to recurrent polyposis. Ninety-five percent of the patients were free of symptoms or had only minor problems. Already this

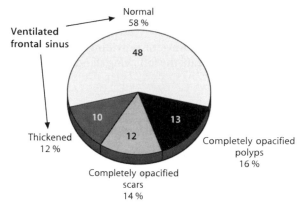

Fig. 24.5. Synopsis of CT and endoscopy 12 to 98 months following Type II drainage 41.

first series of re-evaluation of long-term results demonstrates the value of the endonasal frontal sinus surgery.

In a retrospective study Mertens et al. [22] compared the results of 236 patients operated on between 1985 and 1993 using different techniques. After follow-up of 3–10 years only 8% of patients needed revision. The lowest revision rate was seen after endonasal technique according Draf's classification (5.9%) compared to the osteoplastic techniques according to Jansen-Ritter (Lynch) and Riedel (10.6%).

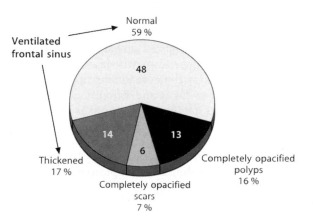

Fig. 24.6. Synopsis of CT and endoscopy 12 to 98 months following Type III drainage 41.

24

Postoperative Care

There are different ways of providing *postoperative care*. Within the years the following standards proved to be efficient:

Packing

Rubber finger stalls (Rhinotamp; Vostra Aachen) filled with sponge have stood the test of time. They provide safe hemostasis, are a stimulator of re-epithelialization of bare bone, are cost-effective and painless to remove. In cases of type I-type IIb drainage, the packing is left between 2–5 days maximum without antibiotic prophylaxis. It is of utmost importance to fix the rubber finger stalls with threads at the nasal dorsum to avoid aspiration. The more stable the middle turbinate at the end of operation is, the shorter the time of uncomfortable packing can be. The risk of adhesions and synechiae is low because this type of packing suppresses the development of granulations

After a type III drainage, we leave the packing in place for 7 days postoperatively as recommended by Toffel [35].

Leaving rubber finger stalls for one week carries the following advantages [40]:

1. The fibrinoid phase of wound healing is somehow overcome. Reclosure of the large drainage by scars is remarkably reduced, since bare bone is re-epithelialized almost completely.
2. Sedation and general anesthesia are not necessary for packing removal. Rubber finger packs do not bind to the wound. Removal of the tamponade does not lead to renewed tissue trauma. The patients are prepared preoperatively for a somewhat uncomfortable postoperative time. This is by far compensated by the optimal wound healing and easy postoperative care with less crusting.

Postoperative Therapy

The question of whether postoperative intensive mechanical cleansing is necessary or the wound cavity is self-cleaning without external measures is very controversial.

In an obstructed nose or sinus, when the patient has complaints that can be explained with occlusion of the sinus ostial region by crusts, mechanical cleaning must be done. However, since each cleaning leads to injury, freshly granulating tissue, and partial removal of new epithelium, a rather controlled and conservative approach to instrument cleaning seems appropriate.

The patients are given the following instructions to ensure proper healing:

1. Irrigate the nasal cavities with saline solution at least once a day, sometimes more frequently.
2. Use one of the corticosteroid sprays 1–3 times/day.
3. The recommendation is made to use peanut oil 1 hour after the use of corticosteroid spray, for general care of the mucosa.

In patients with extreme crusting, the physician should inquire about the use of medications because as a side effect, they cause mucosal desiccation. These include psychotropic medications or beta-blockers. Spectacular improvement is possible once these medications are changed.

General Postoperative Medication

1. *Antibiotics*: They are indicated in the postoperative period for 1–2 weeks in cases of acute or purulent sinusitis. In type III drainage, we recommend prophylactic antibiotic use, as long as the tamponade is in place.

2. *Antiallergic medical therapy:* This is recommended for 6 weeks postoperatively if allergy is diagnosed by history or specific tests. The presence of a large number of eosinophils in the inflamed tissue may provide additional guidance in the decision-making process. In less severe cases we prescribe day antihistamines. In severe allergy patients (e.g. Samter's triad), the combination of antihistamines with low-dose corticosteroid medication for 6 weeks is helpful to prevent early recurrence of polyps.

Failures

Postoperative Frontal Sinusitis after Type I and Type II Drainage

Sometimes after ethmoidectomy and type I as well as type II drainage, the patients may develop more problems in the frontal sinus than before surgery. Postoperative sinus CT will provide information if frontal sinusitis has developed.

The pathogenesis of recurrent frontal sinusitis after surgery can involve various mechanisms. Either remnant ethmoidal cells developed recurrent sinusitis or mechanical irritations of the mucosa in the frontal recess can result in a severe scar around Killian's infundibulum. Both pathologies may result in blockage of the frontal sinus drainage.

This can be avoided by performing at least a complete anterior ethmoidectomy and using extremely atraumatic handling of the frontal recess mucosa. For treatment we recommend the following procedures: a type IIa drainage if a type I procedure was performed previously, a type IIb drainage if a type IIa procedure was performed previously, and a type III drainage after a previous type IIb.

Reclosure after Type III Drainage

Several technical details can lead to this problem:

a) The "chimney" between the anterior ethmoid and the frontal sinus has not been opened well. It is important that after the anterior ethmoidal artery is identified, the surgeon proceeds along the skull base medial to the lamina papyracea to enter into the frontal sinus.
b) The anterior-posterior opening of the frontal sinus floor, particularly in the midline, is too small. The identification of the first olfactory fiber bilaterally and the creation of the "Frontal T" are very helpful to avoid this problem.
c) The resection of the septum/a sinuum frontalium has been missed or was not performed to a satisfying degree. The new curved drills between 15° and 60° angle are ideal for this purpose.
d) The resection of the superior nasal septum was too small. The diameter of resection must be 1.5 cm just in front of the "Frontal T" and below the frontal sinus floor.
e) The packing between the ethmoid and the frontal sinus was not left long enough. 7 days proved to be the best time frame for using rubber finger packings.

Complications

In principle, the complication rate of endonasal frontal sinus drainage procedures is low and similar to the frequency of complications of endonasal pansinus operations.

An evaluation of complications with special respect to endonasal frontal sinus surgery was not performed. The operation can be classified as very safe, even with identification of the first olfactory fibers, when optical aids such as microscope and/or endoscope are used and the techniques described are followed.

We have analyzed the complications of our endonasal micro-endoscopic pansinus operations in two studies [37, 38].

The significant complications were:

1. Injury to the periorbit in 14% of cases. This had no further consequences except in one patient, who developed periorbital hematoma. No cases of blindness or other orbital lesions like muscle injury with double vision or lacrimal drainage obstruction occurred.
2. Dural injury occurred in 2.3% of cases. The subsequent course was uneventful and free of complications after immediate plastic closure of the defect with preserved fascia and fibrin glue. Persistent CSF leakage or meningitis was not observed.
3. A postoperative disturbance of the sense of smell was confirmed by a smell test in only one patient.

General Guidelines for Surgical Therapy of Frontal Sinus Inflammatory Diseases not Responding to Conservative Measures

How to treat frontal sinusitis, which has not responded to conservative measures nor has been operated before?

Depending on the individual situation, in most of the cases, the endonasal type I or type II drainage will be sufficient, whereas in severe polyposis with Samter's triad or other risk factors, a primary type III operation may be indicated.

What to do in cases of chronic postoperative frontal sinusitis after one or even several previous operations, otherwise referred to as "iatrogenic" sinusitis [12, 27, 33]?

The term "iatrogenic sinusitis" suggests that previous surgeons have made a mistake. Since many other factors may have contributed to an unsatisfactory surgi-

cal outcome, such as a particular anatomic variant, it seems more appropriate to use the term "*postoperative sinusitis*"(see also above) indicative that such a patient has already undergone surgery, an important fact in further decision-making.

In many patients one can prove with CT that the ethmoidectomy was incomplete. Inflamed residual anterior ethmoid cells often cause symptoms of chronic frontal sinusitis, whereas the more posteriorly located, well-drained parts of the sinus system are aerated. In this situation completion of the ethmoidectomy in combination with a type IIa/b procedure is indicated. In cases of Samter's triad and other prognostic risk factors, the type III drainage procedure is the best choice. If the patient had numerous prior operations and wishes to have only one more "final" sinus surgery, the surgeon has to choose between the type III drainage and the osteoplastic flap procedure with obliteration. If the frontal sinus is large enough and has an anterior-posterior diameter of at least 0.8 mm, the type III drainage may be attempted. If the frontal sinus has a smaller diameter, the frontal sinus fat obliteration is the safer technique, although more extensive.

How "radical" the extent of primary surgery should be in patients with extensive polyposis of the frontal sinus?

In this situation, particularly in the presence of aspirin hypersensitivity or/and asthma, experience has shown that the primary type III drainage is most likely to be successful. In cases of recurrence and severe frontal sinus symptoms, the osteoplastic operation is indicated.

Should patients with so-called spontaneous or postoperative mucoceles of the frontal sinus, be operated endonasally or via an external approach?

As long as the endonasal route using a type II or type III drainage procedures provides a sufficient opening and not a bottleneck situation, the *endonasal marsu-*

pialization is reliable and the least traumatic measure. However, if the medial border of the mucocele is laterally to a vertical line through the lamina papyracea, the endonasal approach is rarely possible. This is also the case if, usually after several previous operations, multiple mucoceles are diagnosed. In this situation the frontal sinus obliteration is usually indicated. The final decision is made on the basis of a multiplanar sinus CT, often in combination with MR, since MR gives the best diagnostic information of a mucopyocele. A previous Jansen-Ritter, Howarth, or Lynch operation is not a contraindication to endonasal drainage.

Is a Pott's puffy tumor always an indication for an external procedure?

If the anterior-posterior diameter of the frontal sinus is 0.8 mm or greater, the likelihood of a successful type III drainage is high enough to be tried. Long-term postoperative antibiotic therapy is mandatory.

However, these general guidelines cannot replace personal experience!

Conclusion

The endonasal frontal sinus type I–III drainage procedures provide suitable surgical options for the treatment of frontal sinus disease. In cases where the endonasal approach is not possible or is unsuccessful, the osteoplastic flap procedure with or without obliteration may provide a solution. The chance of complete reepitheliazation of eventually bare bone is very likely with the endonasal frontal sinus operations, since they respect the outer osseous borders of the newly created frontal sinus drainage and minimize the danger of frontal sinus outlet shrinking, thus preventing mucocele formation. This concept has revolutionized frontal sinus surgery, so that the classic external frontoorbital frontal sinus operations according to Jansen-Ritter or Lynch or Howarth are considered obsolete for the treatment of chronic inflammatory diseases of the frontal sinus.

References

1. Cholewa ER (1888) Cited after Tange RA, Pirsig W Het neusspeculum. Door de eeuwen heen. Universiteitsmuseum van de Universiteit van Utrecht. Glaxo BV
2. Draf W (1991) Endonasal micro-endoscopic frontal sinus surgery. The Fulda concept. Op Tech Otolaryngol Head Neck Surg 2:234–240
3. Draf W, unpublished data
4. Gross WE, Gross CW, Becker D, Moore D, Phillips D (1995) Modified transnasal endoscopic Lothrop procedure as an alternative to frontal sinus obliteration. Otolaryngol Head Neck Surg 113:427–434
5. Halle M (1915) Die intranasalen Operationen bei eitrigen Erkrankungen der Nebenhoehlen der Nase. Arch Laryngol Rhinol 29:73–112
6. Halle M (1906) Externe und interne Operation der Nebenhoehleneiterungen. Berl klin Wschr 43:1369–1372, 1404–1407
7. Hosemann W, Gross R, Goede U, Kuehnel T (2001) Clinical anatomy of the nasal process of the frontal bone (spina nasalis interna). Otolaryngol Head Neck Surg 125:60–65
8. Hosemann W, Kuehnel T, Held P, Wagner W, Felderhoff A (1997) Endonasal frontal sinusotomy in surgical management of chronic sinusitis: A critical evaluation. Am J Rhin 11:1–9
9. Hosemann WG, Weber RK, Keerl RE, Lund VJ (2000) Minimally invasive endonasal sinus surgery. Thieme, Stuttgart, pp 54–59
10. Howarth WG (1921) Operations on the frontal sinus. J Laryngol Otol 36:417–421
11. Hoyt III WH (1993) Endoscopic stenting of nasofrontal communication in frontal sinus disease. ENT Journal 72:596–597
12. Ingals EF (1905) New operation and instruments for draining the frontal sinus. Ann Otol Rhinol Laryngol 14:513–519
13. Jansen A (1894) Zur Eroeffnung der Nebenhoehlen der Nase bei chronischer Eiterung. Arch Laryng Rhinol(Berl) 135–157
14. Kennedy DW, Senior BA (1997) Endoscopic sinus surgery. A review. Otolaryngol Clin North Am 30:313–329
15. Kikawada T, Fujigaki M, Kikura M, Matsumoto M Kikawada K (1999) Extended endoscopic frontal sinus surgery to interrupted nasofrontal communication caused by scarring of the anterior ethmoid. Arch Otolaryngol Head Neck Surg 125:92–96
16. Kuhn FA, Javer AR, Nagpal K, Citardi MJ (2000) The frontal sinus rescue procedure: early experience and three-year follow-up. Am J Rhinol 14:211–216
17. Lang J (1989) Clinical anatomy of the nose nasal cavity and paranasal sinuses. Thieme, Stuttgart, pp 58–59
18. Lothrop HA (1914) Frontal sinus suppuration. Ann Surg 59:937–957
19. Lothrop HA (1899) The anatomy and surgery of the frontal sinus and anterior ethmoidal cells. Ann Surg 29:175–215
20. Lynch RC (1921) The technique of a radical frontal sinus operation which has given me the best results. Laryngoscope 31:1–5

24

21. May M, Schaitkin B (1995) Frontal sinus surgery: endonasal drainage instead of an external osteoplastic approach. Op Tech Otolaryngol Head Neck Surg 6:184–192
22. Mertens J, Eggers S, Maune S (2000) Langzeitergebnisse nach Stirnhoehlenoperationen: Vergleich extranasaler und endonasaler Operationstechniken. Laryngorhinootol 79:396–399
23. Moriyama H, Fukami M, Yanagi K, Ohtori N, Kaneta K (1994) Endoscopic endonasal treatment of ostium of the frontal sinus and the results of endoscopic surgery. Am J Rhinol 8:67–70
24. Neel HB III, Whitaker JH, Lake CF (1976) Thin rubber sheeting in frontal sinus surgery: Animal and clinical studies. Laryngoscope 86:524–536
25. Neel HB, McDonald TJ, Facer GW (1987) Modified Lynch procedure for chronic frontal sinus diseases: Rationale, technique, and long term results. Laryngoscope 97:1274
26. Orlandi RR, Kennedy DW (2001) Revision endoscopic frontal sinus surgery. Otolaryngol Clin North Am 34:77–90
27. Rains III BM (2001) Frontal sinus stenting. Otolaryngol Clini North Am 34:101–110
28. Ritter G (1906) Eine neue Methode zur Erhaltung der vorderen Stirnhoehlenwand bei Radikaloperationen chronischer Stirnhoehleneiterungen. Dtsch Med Wochenschr 32:1294–1296
29. Schaefer SD (1990) Close LG Endoscopic management of frontal sinus disease. Laryngoscope 100:155–160
30. Schaeffer M (1890) Zur Diagnose und Therapie der Erkrankungen der Nebenhoehlen der Nase mit Ausnahme des Sinus maxillaris. Dtsch Med Wschr 19:905–907
31. Spiess G (1899) Die endonasale Chirurgie des Sinus frontalis. Arch Laryngol 9:285–291
32. Stammberger H (1991) Functional endoscopic sinus surgery, the Messerklinger technique. BC Decker, Philadelphia
33. Stammberger H (2000) F.E.S.S., "uncapping the egg". The endoscopic approach to frontal recess and sinuses. Storz Company Prints
34. Tato JM, Bergaglio OE (1949) Surgery of frontal sinus. Fat grafts: A new technique. Otolaryngologica 3:1
35. Toffel PH (1995) Secure endoscopic sinus surgery with middle meatal stenting. Oper Tech Otolaryngol Head Neck Surg 6:157–162
36. Weber R, Draf W, Keerl R, Schick B, Saha A (1997) Micro-endoscopic pansinusoperation in chronic sinusitis. Results and complications. Am J Otolaryngol 18:247–253
37. Weber R, Draf W (1992) Die endonasale mikro-endoskopische Pansinusoperation bei chronischer Sinusitis. II. Ergebnisse und Komplikationen. Otorhinolaryngologia Nova 2:63–69
38. Weber R, Draf W (1992a) Komplikationen der endonasalen mikro-endoskopischen Siebbeinoperation. HNO 40:170–175
39. Weber R, Hosemann W, Draf W, Keerl R, Schick B, Schinzel S (1997) Endonasal frontal sinus surgery with long-term stenting of the nasofrontal duct. Laryngorhinootologie 76:728–734
40. Weber R, Keerl R, Huppmann A, Draf W, Saha A (2000) Wound healing after endonasal sinus surgery in time-lapse video: a new way of continuous in vivo observation and documentation in rhinology. In: Stamm A, Draf W (ed) Micro-endoscopic surgery of the paranasal sinuses and skull base. Springer, Berlin, Chapter 26 pp 329–345
41. Wormald PJ, Ananda A, Nair S (2003) Modified endoscopic Lothrop as a salvage for the failed osteoplastic flap with obliteration. Laryngoscope 11:1988–1992

Chapter 25

Endoscopic Modified Lothrop Procedure

Stilianos E. Kountakis

Core Messages

- The endoscopic modified Lothrop procedure is recommended as a surgical option when open osteoplastic flap frontal surgery is contemplated

- The success of the modified Lothrop procedure depends on the underlying mucosal pathology and its effective management

- The modified Lothrop procedure is the preferred approach for benign tumors of the frontal sinus such as inverted papilloma, since it allows for direct endoscopic postoperative surveillance for tumor recurrence

- In order to perform the modified Lothrop procedure, the total anterior-posterior dimension at the cephalad margin of the frontal recess between the nasal bones at the root of the nose and the anterior skull base should be at least 1.5 cm. This dimension includes the anterior-posterior thickness of the nasal beak and the distance from the beak to the anterior skull base

- While performing the modified Lothrop procedure, avoid drilling on the posterior margin of the frontal recess and posterior frontal sinus wall to prevent injury to the skull base with cerebrospinal fluid rhinorrhea and postoperative circumferential stenosis of the frontal opening

- Absolute contraindications in performing the endoscopic modified Lothrop procedure include inadequate surgical training and the lack of proper instrumentation

Contents

Introduction

Frontal sinus surgery has remained a frustrating and dangerous endeavor for many surgeons despite continued advances in instrumentation and surgical techniques.

Partly to blame is the relatively inaccessible location of the frontal recess, posterior and cephalad to the anterior insertion of the middle turbinate, hiding away from the surgeon's direct line of vision. Moreover, multiple anterior ethmoid cells may occupy the frontal recess during the embryologic development of the frontal sinus, as early forming ethmoid sinusoids invade and pneumatize the frontal bone to form the frontal sinus [13]. The variable size and location of these air cells contribute to the numerous patterns of the frontal sinus outflow pathway that is actually a potential space amongst the surface of these frontal recess cells, leading to the internal frontal sinus ostium. The remote location and anatomic complexity of the frontal recess along with its close proximity to the lamina papyracea and anterior skull base, led Lothrop [14] to state that an intranasal approach for frontal sinus drainage was too dangerous to perform. Instead, he described an external approach, which consisted of external ethmoidectomy to enlarge the nasofrontal drainage pathway. This included removal of the frontal sinus floors that were connected through a large nasal septectomy, and bilateral removal of the lacrimal bone and portion of the lamina papyracea that caused medial orbital fat collapse, with later stenosis of the newly created nasofrontal outflow communication.

The development of the external osteoplastic flap procedure [10] with or without frontal sinus obliteration in the 1940s–1960s eliminated the need for a nasofrontal communication and quickly became the standard of care. However, failure rates averaged 10% in early reports [2, 10] and more recently, Weber et al. [18] reported frontal mucoceles seen by magnetic resonance imaging in 9.4% of the patients approximately 2 years after osteoplastic frontal sinus obliteration.

The introduction of the nasal endoscope and endoscopic sinus surgery techniques allowed for better visualization of the frontal recess during surgery and provided an alternative to the open techniques for the surgical treatment of frontal sinus disease. Furthermore, endoscopic frontal surgery precisely addresses the exact location of chronic frontal sinus disease, which involves obstruction of the frontal sinus outflow pathway, in comparison to the open mucosal destructive procedures. Despite all endoscopic technique and instrumentation advances, the frontal sinus continues to remain challenging for many otolaryngologists, with the extent of surgery performed in the frontal recess being constantly debated in the literature. Excessive mucosal damage during endoscopic surgery can lead to scarring with obstruction of frontal drainage, and resection of the middle turbinate can lead to lateralization of the turbinate and obstruction of the frontal recess, as reported by Kuhn et al. [12]. As endoscopic advances continued, the Lothrop procedure was revisited as an alternative to the open destructive techniques. Draf in 1991 described removal of the frontal sinus floor bilaterally using endoscopic and microscopic techniques, and classified the extent of surgery in the frontal recess [5]. Close et al. in 1994 reported their results with 11 patients, and soon thereafter a series of reports established the legitimacy of the procedure with successful long-term surgical outcomes [4] (Table 25.1).

Table 25.1. Chronological advances leading to the endoscopic modified Lothrop procedure

1914	Lothrop procedure
1960s	Open osteoplastic flap frontal surgery becomes standard of care
1970s	Linear tomography and improved preoperative anatomic evaluation
1980s	Computed tomography
	Popularizing of endoscopic sinus surgery
1990s	Powered instrumentation
	Computer image-guided endoscopic surgery
1991	Extended frontal sinusotomy by Draf
1994	Endoscopic resection of the intranasal frontal sinus floor by Close
1995	Endoscopic modified Lothrop procedure by Gross

In the process, the procedure was renamed to accurately reflect the location and extent of surgery. The endoscopic modified Lothrop procedure offers several distinct advantages over open techniques and is slowly displacing the osteoplastic flap approach as the procedure of choice in persistent frontal disease after failure of medical therapy and more conservative endoscopic surgery.

The advantages of the endoscopic modified Lothrop procedure are:

- No external incision with improved cosmesis
- Decreased morbidity
- No hospital stay necessary
- No drains
- No abdominal wound and possible associated complications
- Avoidance of supra-orbital and supra-trochlear nerve injury
- Reduced blood loss
- No burying of mucosa
- Less pain
- Lower total cost
- Can still convert to open approaches if necessary
- Allows for endoscopic postoperative evaluation for persistent or recurrent disease

Indications and Patient Selection

The success of the modified Lothrop procedure depends on the anatomy of the frontal recess and the underlying mucosal pathology. Sinus surgery in patients with chronic rhinosinusitis in general is indicated when maximum medical therapy fails to control the symptoms of the disease. Initial surgical intervention in primary cases should avoid overly excessive manipulation in the frontal recess unless absolutely necessary. More extensive frontal surgery is performed in revision cases when scarring or persistent disease in the frontal recess and internal frontal ostium interferes with frontal sinus drainage. The endoscopic modified Lothrop procedure is recommended as a surgical option when open osteoplastic flap surgery is contemplated [6–9, 11, 16]. Table 25.2 lists all frontal sinus procedures available for the otolaryngologist as part of a protocol in the surgical management of frontal sinus disease. Patients with underlying mucosal disease such as hyperplastic rhinosinusitis with nasal polyposis, sarcoidosis, Wegener's granulomatosis, and Samter's triad require aggressive postoperative care to control mucosal inflammation and prevent re-stenosis of the nasofrontal drainage pathway with symptom recurrence. One of the advantages of the endoscopic modified Lothrop procedure is that once performed, it does not prevent a surgeon from resorting to open osteoplastic flap techniques if the modified Lothrop procedure fails and frontal sinus obstruction recurs.

Table 25.2. Frontal sinus procedure protocol

Endoscopic uncinectomy and anterior ethmoidectomy without surgery in the frontal recess
Frontal recess surgery
Minitrephination of the frontal sinus as an aid in endoscopic sinus surgery
Surgical manipulation of the internal frontal sinus ostium
Unilateral resection of frontal sinus floor (Draf II procedure)
Endoscopic modified Lothrop
Osteoplastic flap surgery

The anatomy of the frontal sinus and the cephalad margin of the frontal recess at the level of the internal frontal ostium are critical in the selection of patients for the endoscopic modified Lothrop procedure.

As Part of the Preoperative Evaluation, the Surgeon Should Do the Following

- Carefully review the anatomy on high-resolution computer tomography (CT) to identify the number, size, and location of air cells present in the frontal recess.

- Measure and calculate distances on the CT. The total anterior-posterior dimension at the cephalad margin of the frontal recess between the nasal bones at the root of the nose and the anterior skull base should be at least 1.5 cm (Fig. 25.1).

- The anterior-posterior thickness of the nasal beak (Fig. 25.2) should not exceed 1 cm.

The number of air cells in the frontal recess is important, since it indicates the number of sinus cell walls that should be removed in order to reach the internal frontal sinus ostium. The measurements and distances on CT determine whether the patient is a candidate for the modified Lothrop procedure. The total anterior-posterior dimension at the cephalad margin of the frontal recess (1.5 cm) includes the anterior-posterior thickness of the nasal beak and the distance from the beak to the anterior skull base (Fig. 25.1). Thick nasal beaks narrow the space between the nasal beak and the anterior skull base, making introduction of instruments into the frontal sinus very difficult, and increase the chances for skull base injury with cerebrospinal fluid (CSF) rhinorrhea.

As experience with the technique has grown, the procedure has been used successfully not only for chronic frontal sinus obstruction but also for resection of osteomas and benign tumors such as inverted papillomas. The advantages of using the modified Lothrop technique to remove frontal sinus inverted papillomas include the ability to directly inspect the sinus postoperatively for recurrence of the tumor.

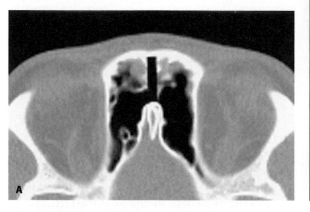

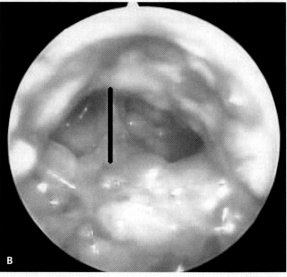

Fig. 25.1A,B. The total anterior-posterior dimension at the cephalad margin of the frontal recess, between the nasal bones at the root of the nose and the anterior skull base (solid black line) should be at least 1.5 cm. A Axial sinus CT through the cephalad margin of the frontal recess. B Endoscopic picture 3 weeks after the modified Lothrop procedure

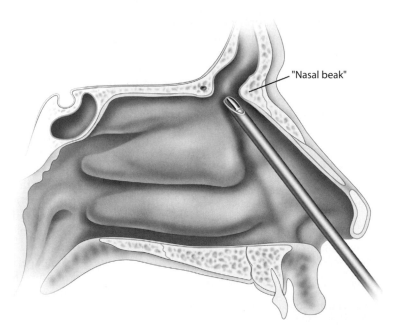

Fig. 25.2. Nasal beak

Indications and Contraindications for the Endoscopic Modified Lothrop Procedure Are as Follows

■ Indications
  - Persistent chronic frontal sinusitis with failure of appropriate medical therapy and after unsuccessful primary endoscopic frontal sinusotomy
  - Frontal sinus mucoceles
  - Inverted papilloma
  - Osteoma
  - Trauma
  - Last-resort procedure prior to osteoplastic frontal sinus obliteration

■ Contraindications
  - Hypoplastic frontal sinus and frontal recess
  - Lack of experience by the surgeon
  - Lack of proper instrumentation
  - Sinus disease located in a supra-orbital ethmoid air cell and not in the frontal sinus

Surgical Technique

The endoscopic modified Lothrop procedure requires general anesthesia, and best results are obtained when the surgical field is dry with minimal bleeding. The nasal cavities are first decongested using topical oxymetazoline, and then the septum and the lateral nasal wall at the anterior insertion of the middle turbinate are injected with up to 10 ml of 1% lidocaine and 1:100,000 epinephrine solution. The extent and type of local decongestant applied depends on the medical condition of each individual patient. The patient's CT is reviewed, rigid nasal endoscopy is performed, and the side with the most approachable frontal recess is chosen to start the procedure. The middle turbinate or remnant is medialized, and the superior attachment of the uncinate process remnant is resected using a microdebrider. In the most common configuration, the uncinate process attaches to the lamina papyracea forming the recessus terminalis (Fig. 25.3). The frontal ostium is identified posterior and medial to the recessus terminalis.

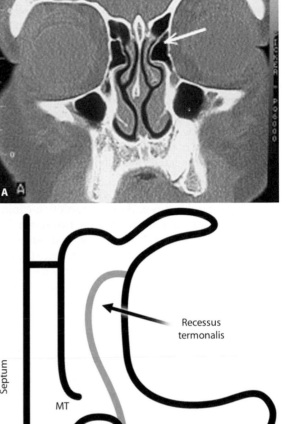

Fig. 25.3A,B. Recess terminalis: formed when the uncinate process attaches to the lamina papyracea superiorly

is. Computer image guidance may be used to help with the identification of the internal frontal sinus ostium. Drilling is initiated in an anterior direction through the anterior insertion of the middle turbinate to enlarge the frontal sinus ostium until the level of the nasal bone is reached. Similarly, drilling is performed in a lateral direction until the level of the plane of the lamina papyracea is reached. Care is taken not to remove the mucosa over the lateral wall of the frontal recess at the plane of the lamina papyracea to preserve the ciliated epithelium responsible for transporting secretions out of the frontal sinus. Care is also taken to prevent mucosal injury at the posterior margin of the frontal sinus and ostium to prevent circumferential mucosal injury with possible postoperative ostial stenosis (Fig. 25.4) and to avoid injury to the skull base with possible CSF rhinorrhea.

Once the level of the nasal bones is reached anteriorly, drilling is directed medially until the plane of the nasal septum is reached. In the process, part of the nasal beak is removed (Fig. 25.2). To avoid going through the nasal bones and causing soft tissue injury over the nasal root at the glabella, two fingertips are placed over the nasal root to feel and sense the closeness of the drill to the nasal bones. Once the nasal septum is reached, a partial septectomy necessary for the creation of a large common nasofrontal drainage pathway is performed. The center of the surgical septal perforation is located right under the floors of the frontal sinuses (Fig. 25.5). The size of the septectomy should be approximately 2 cm. Smaller septal perforations accumulate crusting despite aggressive nasal saline irrigation and thus cause inflammation and delayed healing. Drilling then is continued though the nasal beak, removing the frontal sinus floor on the opposite side and continued until the opposite lamina papyracea is reached (Fig. 25.6).

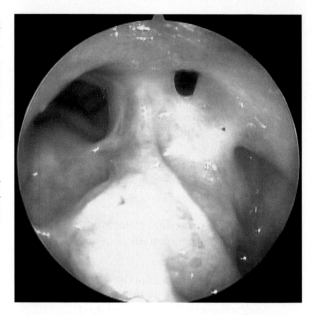

Fig. 25.4. Unilateral frontal stenosis after circumferential scar formation

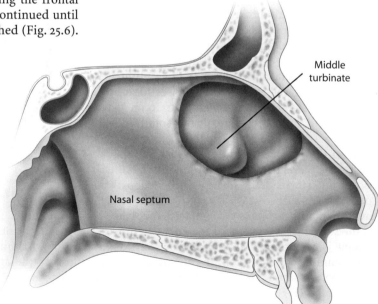

Middle turbinate

Nasal septum

Fig. 25.5.
Partial nasal septectomy

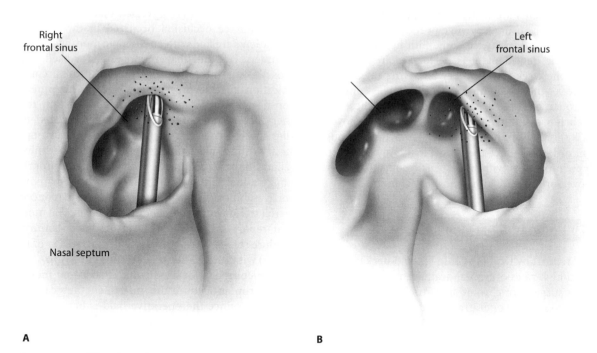

A   B

Fig. 25.6A,B. Drilling through the nasal beak to remove the opposite frontal sinus floor and complete the modified Lothrop procedure. A Drilling through the midline. B Completion of the toward the opposite frontal sinus modified Lothrop procedure

In the process, the posterior wall of the frontal sinus is protected to prevent injury to the skull base and to avoid circumferential mucosal scarring with stenosis. There is no need to remove the frontal sinus septum all the way posteriorly to the skull base. Drilling in this area may lead to violation of an anteriorly displaced skull base. With successful surgery, the common frontal sinus cavities can be easily inspected using a nasal endoscope (Fig. 25.7).

Postoperative Care

Aggressive medical management to remove crusting and control mucosal disease is necessary for successful outcomes. All patients are placed on postoperative antibiotics for 10 days, with high-dose mucolytics and intranasal steroid sprays. Patients with hyperplastic sinusitis and nasal polyposis, and patients with asthma with or without aspirin sensitivity may benefit from short-term tapering doses of systemic

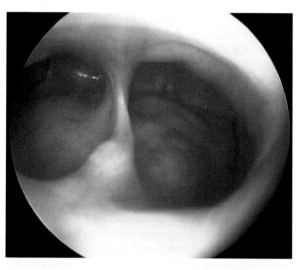

Fig. 25.7. Endoscopic view of the common frontal sinus cavities two years after the endoscopic modified Lothrop procedure

25

steroids. Patients are instructed to perform nasal saline irrigations using a syringe or mechanized irrigation devices at least twice daily until healing ensues. Endoscopic debridement is performed in the office setting one week after surgery and is repeated every two weeks thereafter until crusting in the common nasofrontal pathway is not an issue. During these visits, debris present in the open frontal sinus is removed. This is very important in cases of allergic fungal sinusitis in order to reduce the fungal load. Any persistent polyps in patients with hyperplastic sinusitis may be removed or injected with depository steroids.

Results and Complications

Initial reports by Draf [5], Close [4], and Becker [1] indicated high rates of frontal drainage pathway patency after surgery for chronic sinusitis, but it was quickly realized that the operative site after the endoscopic modified Lothrop procedure requires at least 12 to 18 months after surgery for stabilization. Casiano [3] reported that 12 of 21 patients (57%) had patent common frontal opening by flexible fiber optic examination with a mean follow-up of 6.5 months. Gross et al. [9] found a 95% frontal drainage patency rate with a mean follow-up of 12 months, but as experience with the procedure accumulated and patients were followed for longer periods of time, the overall patency success rate was reduced. When 44 patients were followed for an average of 40 months after endoscopic modified Lothrop procedure, nine (20%) required revision modified Lothrop surgery and eight of 44 (18%) patients eventually required osteoplastic flap with frontal sinus obliteration, with an overall frontal drainage patency rate of 82% [16]. This number is more realistic when patients are followed long-term, especially if one considers that as we gain more experience with the procedure, endoscopic modified Lothrop surgery is more often performed in patients with more aggressive mucosal disease, and this probably contributes to the long-term failure rate of this surgery. In their report however, Gross and colleagues reported that surgical outcomes were not influenced by comorbidities such as hyperplastic sinusitis with nasal polyposis and aspirin-sensitive asthma [7]. Close follow-up and management of early polyps prevented frontal sinus obstruction in these patients.

A literature review [15] revealed that in one study, frontal drainage occlusion occurred in three of 24 (12.5) patients treated with endoscopic modified Lothrop surgery [17] and that one investigator used free mucosal grafts to epithelialize the nasofrontal communication and thus prevent stenosis [19]. Instrumentation advances also may have played a role in the higher success rates recently reported compared to earlier studies. Powered microdebriders can now operate at drilling speeds of 12,000 revolutions per minute, and finesse drill-bits are available with appropriate angulation and decreased size, allowing for more maneuverability in the frontal recess with reduced mucosal trauma and postoperative stenosis. The most recent report on the endoscopic modified Lothrop procedure shows a 93% primary patency rate (77 of 83 patients) with mean follow-up of 22 months [19].

Major complications with the endoscopic modified Lothrop procedure are infrequent but can be devastating, since the operative field is between the orbits and just anterior to a very thin skull base. Lack of proper surgical training and instrumentation should preclude attempts to perform this procedure. Skull base violations with CSF leaks and pneumocephalus has been reported even in the most experience hands [16], but none of the studies have reported more than one patient having skull base violation per study. Serious eye injury has not been reported in any of the studies. Minor complications are more frequent, with one study reporting up to 9% of the patients having easily controlled epistaxis [16].

Conclusion

The endoscopic modified Lothrop procedure appears to be an effective alternative to osteoplastic flap frontal surgery. With continued instrumentation improvement, proper training, and patient selection, the endoscopic modified Lothrop procedure is a welcome addition to the rhinologist's armamentarium. In selected cases such as inverted papilloma of the frontal sinus, it has become the procedure of choice since it allows for endoscopic frontal sinus inspection and postoperative surveillance.

References

1. Becker DG, Moore D, Lindsey WH, Gross WE, Gross CW Modified transnasal endoscopic Lothrop procedure: Further considerations. Laryngoscope 1995 105(11):1161–1166
2. Bosley WR (1972) Osteoplastic obliteration of the frontal sinuses. A review of 100 patients. Laryngoscope 82:1463–1476
3. Casiano RR, Livingston JA (1998) Endoscopic Lothrop procedure: The University of Miami experience. Am J Rhinol 12:335–339
4. Close LG, Lee NK, Leach LJ, Manning SC (1994) Endoscopic resection of the intranasal frontal sinus floor. Ann Otol Rhinol Laryngol 103:952–958
5. Draf W (1991) Endonasal micro-endoscopic frontal sinus surgery, the Fulda concept. Oper Tech Otolaryngol Head Neck Surg 2:234–240
6. Gross CW (1999) Surgical treatments for symptomatic chronic frontal sinusitis. Arch Otolaryngol Head Neck Surg 126:101–102
7. Gross CW, Schlosser RJ (2001) The modified Lothrop procedure: Lessons learned. Laryngoscope 111:1302–1305
8. Gross CW, Zachmann GC, Becker DG et al (1997) Follow-up of University of Virginia experience with the modified Lothrop procedure. Am J Rhinol 11:49–54
9. Gross WE, Gross CW, Becker D et al (1995) Modified transnasal endoscopic Lothrop procedure as an alternative to frontal sinus obliteration. Otolaryngol Head Neck Surg 113:427–434
10. Hardy JM, Montgomery WW (1976) Osteoplastic frontal sinusotomy: An analysis of 250 operations. Ann Otol Rhinol Laryngol 85:253–232
11. Kountakis SE, Gross CW (2003) Long-term results of the Lothrop operation. Curr Opin Otolaryngol Head Neck Surg 11:37–40
12. Kuhn FA, Javer AR, Nagpal K, Citardi MJ (2000) The frontal sinus rescue procedure: Early experience and three-year follow-up. Am J Rhinol 14:211–216
13. Libersa C, Laude M, Libersa JC (1981) The pneumatization of the accessory cavities of the nasal fossae during growth. Anat Clin 2:265–273
14. Lothrop HA (1914) Frontal sinus suppuration. Ann Surg 59:937–957
15. Metson R, Gliklich RE (1998) Clinical outcome of endoscopic surgery for frontal sinusitis. Arch Otolaryngol Head Neck Surg 124:478–479
16. Schlosser RJ, Zachmann G, Harrison S et al (2002) The endoscopic modified Lothrop: Long-term follow-up on 44 patients. Am J Rhinol 16:103–108
17. Stennert E (2001) Rhino-frontal sinuseptotomy (RFS): A combined intra-extra nasal approach for the surgical treatment of severely disease frontal sinuses. Laryngoscope 111:1237–1245
18. Weber R, Draf W, Kratzsch B et al (2001) Modern concepts of frontal sinus surgery. Laryngoscope 111:137–146
19. Wormald PJ (2003) Salvage frontal sinus surgery: The endoscopic modified Lothrop procedure. Laryngoscope 113:276–83

Chapter 26

Frontal Sinus Rescue

26

Martin J. Citardi, Pete S. Batra, Frederick A. Kuhn

Core Messages

■ The frontal sinus rescue procedure, more formally known as the revision endoscopic frontal sinusotomy with mucoperiosteal flap advancement, is a technique for the management of frontal sinus obstruction after middle turbinate resection.

■ In this procedure, the frontal stenosis is removed, and a small mucoperiosteal flap is advanced over the denuded region of the frontal neo-ostium.

■ In this way, normal frontal mucociliary clearance is restored to the frontal sinus that had been obstructed by previous middle turbinate resection.

■ The procedure offers several distinct advantages in the setting of frontal recess stenosis related to previous middle turbinate resection, including preservation of lateral frontal recess mucosa and less trauma to the frontal recess than alternative procedures such as the Modified Lothrop.

Contents

Introduction

Since the late 1980's, endoscopic frontal sinusotomy has emerged as the preferred technique for the surgical management of chronic frontal sinusitis that is refractory to routine medical treatment [9]. During endoscopic frontal sinusotomy, the partitions of the cells that pneumatize the frontal recess are carefully identified and removed under endoscopic visualization. Throughout the procedure, mucosa is preserved, and the boundaries of the frontal recess are not disturbed. Thus, after endoscopic frontal sinusotomy, the frontal recess should be a widely patent, mucosa-lined structure with rigid walls.

If a frontal recess boundary is not fixed, then it may collapse into the frontal recess and cause secondary frontal recess/ostium stenosis. Today, this most commonly occurs after resection of the middle turbinate (which forms the medial boundary of the frontal recess). Because the middle turbinate remnant that remains after middle turbinate resection is often destabilized, it may fall laterally and compromise frontal recess patency. Simply stated, standard endoscopic frontal sinusotomy is often inadequate for the surgical treatment of chronic frontal sinusitis after middle turbinate resection, since the technique cannot compensate for frontal recess stenosis due to collapse of the middle turbinate. Revision endoscopic frontal sinusotomy with mucoperiosteal flap advancement, termed the frontal sinus rescue procedure (FSR), has been developed as a modification of the standard endoscopic frontal sinusotomy technique [5, 10].

The important principles of FSR are:

- FSR is not the creation of a simple hole to drain an obstructed frontal sinus
- In FSR, bony and soft tissue obstruction caused by the destabilized middle turbinate remnant is removed, and then a mucosal flap is advanced across the denuded bone at the medial aspect of the frontal ostium
- Critical lateral frontal recess mucosa is preserved; thus mucociliary clearance is restored, since the normal drainage pattern is down the lateral aspect of the frontal recess
- Of course, the entire FSR procedure is performed under endoscopic visualization.

Historical Perspective

In 1921, Lynch described the external frontoethmoidectomy procedure for management of frontal sinus disease [12]. It soon became apparent that frontal recess stenosis was the most important cause of failure of frontoethmoidectomy, and the failure rates were unacceptably high. In attempting to minimize this problem, in 1935, Sewall developed a medially-based mucoperiosteal flap, which he used to reline the frontal opening [16]. In 1936, McNaught reported a variation on Sewall's strategy when he introduced a laterally-based mucoperiosteal flap, which was also used to reline the frontal opening [13]. In 1952, Boyden described his experience in 57 operations in which he had successfully employed the Sewall procedure [2]. The success of the mucoperiosteal flap for frontal sinus surgery has also been corroborated by the work of Ogura [14] and Baron [1].

In the 1996–1997, Kuhn developed the FSR, and initial experiences were reported later [5, 10]. FSR builds upon the concepts outlined by Sewall, McNaught, Boyden, and others who were able to use mucoperiosteal flaps to cover denuded areas of a sur-

gically-enlarged frontal neo-ostium. Thus, the importance of avoiding exposed bone in the frontal recess has been recognized for many decades. Similarly, the ability of a mucoperiosteal flap to minimize secondary stenosis is not a new idea.

Technique

Most FSR procedures are performed with intraoperative surgical navigation [3, 4]. Review of the preoperative high-resolution sinus CT at the computer workstation greatly facilitates the comprehension of complex three-dimensional frontal recess anatomy, and this knowledge can be directly applied through intraoperative surgical navigation. Of course, the surgeon may rely upon CT scan images on a standard x-ray view box; but this approach may be more difficult.

The procedure may be performed under general anesthesia or local anesthesia with intravenous sedation. Achieving adequate levels of anesthesia with local blocks may be problematic; therefore, almost all patients require general anesthesia.

At the beginning of the surgery, detailed endoscopic examination of the nasal cavity with particular attention to the frontal recess region must be performed. Topical 0.05% oxymetazoline provides significant mucosal decongestion with relatively long duration. Intraoperative surgical navigation may be invaluable during the initial diagnostic nasal endoscopy. Often gentle palpation may help to delineate critical anatomic features. The relationship of the middle turbinate remnant to the medial orbital wall must be established (Fig. 26.1A). In addition, the relative position of the skull base, including the cribriform plate, should be determined. Because the frontal recess is far anterior along the skull base, the 30°, 45°, and 70° telescopes must be used to provide adequate visualization. A 0-degree telescope will not provide an adequate view of the area. After this initial examination is complete, the middle turbinate stub and adjacent medial orbital wall should be infiltrated with 1% lidocaine with 1:100,000 epinephrine, which is used for its vasoconstrictive effect. Over-infiltration of local anesthetic will tend to distort the soft-tissue anatomy, and suboptimal infiltration will be associated with greater mucosal oozing.

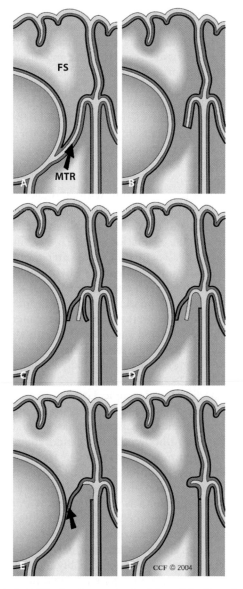

Fig. 26.1A–F. The fundamental principles of the frontal sinus rescue procedure. A The middle turbinate remnant (MTR) has scarred across the outflow tract frontal sinus (FS). B The lateral attachment/adhesion of the middle turbinate remnant has been released. C Mucosa from the medial and lateral aspects of the middle turbinate remnant has been partially elevated. D The mucosa from the medial aspect of the middle turbinate remnant has been removed and discarded. E The bony middle turbinate remnant has been resected, and the remaining mucosa from its lateral aspect has been preserved. This mucosa, indicated by the *arrow*, forms the mucoperiosteal flap. F The mucosal flap has been advanced across the former middle turbinate attachment point.

The initial step is a parasagittal incision along the most anterior aspect of the middle turbinate stub (Fig. 26.1B). A sickle knife may be passed above the 30°, 45°, or 70° telescope to achieve this objective. Alternatively, a frontal recess curette may be used to create a controlled tear, but this approach often induces unacceptable collateral tissue damage. Small, through-cutting giraffe forceps, which have just been introduced recently, provide a direct means to create this incision. The parasagittal incision releases the scar band that has pulled the middle turbinate laterally across the frontal recess outflow track. At this point, the middle turbinate stub should be apparent. This bony remnant may be directly attached to the skull base, or it may simply be encased in thickened, scarred mucosa. The mucosa along the medial and lateral aspects of the bony middle turbinate remnant is then gently elevated from the underlying bone (Fig. 26.1C). The medial mucosa as well as a very small area of adjacent mucosa along the nasal roof (frontal sinus floor) is removed and discarded (Fig. 26.1D). The lateral mucosal flap is preserved; this mucosa is the mucoperiosteal flap for which FSR is formally named. After elevation, the mucoperiosteal flap mucosa is gently pushed superiorly so as to avoid inadvertent trauma and damage. Next, the bony middle turbinate stub must be removed (Fig. 26.1E). If it is merely a free fragment, then a noncutting giraffe forceps may be used to grasp and take it from the operative field. If the bony middle turbinate stub is attached to the skull base, then it must be freed of that attachment and removed. Today, the through-cutting frontal giraffe forceps are ideally suited for this function. Alternatively, a frontal recess curette may be used to fracture the middle turbinate stub. Finally, the mucoperiosteal flap, which had been displaced superiorly, is repositioned over the former middle turbinate site (Fig. 26.1F). The raw surface of the underside of the flap faces the denuded bone of the middle turbinate removal site; these two surfaces are likely to stick together throughout the healing process.

In most instances, a frontal recess stent should not be used, since the stent may displace the delicate flap and thus undo what the procedure aims to accomplish. Of course, in certain instances, a soft, low-caliber frontal recess stent will be appropriate.

It must be emphasized that the mucosa of the lateral frontal recess is not disturbed. The natural mu-

26

cociliary clearance process for the frontal sinus is along the lateral frontal recess; preservation of this mucosa helps to achieve restoration of frontal sinus function.

After FSR, thorough and comprehensive postoperative care must be performed [8]. Serial nasal endoscopy provides a simple means for monitoring the frontal neo-ostium as well as a platform for early intervention for the release of early fibrinous adhesions. Gentle debridement under endoscopic visualization is necessary. Acute suppurative exacerbations of chronic rhinosinusitis may be cultured and appropriate culture-directed antibiotics should be instituted. All patients should perform irrigations with isotonic or hypertonic saline solution. Some patients will also receive systemic corticosteroids for a few weeks. (Full discussion of the strategy for postoperative care is beyond the scope of this chapter.)

The steps for FSR are schematically illustrated in Fig. 26.1.

Indications

- FSR was designed for the surgical treatment of chronic frontal sinusitis due to frontal recess obstruction after middle turbinate resection.

FSR compensates for the destabilized middle turbinate and secondary bony frontal ostium stenosis, while standard endoscopic frontal sinusotomy inadequately addresses these issues.

Concomitant issues may include frontal sinus/recess osteitis/osteoneogenesis, frontal bone osteomyelitis, and mucocele with or without bony erosion. Since acute infection is associated with greater bleeding which may obscure visualization, FSR may not be feasible for the surgical management of acute frontal sinusitis requiring surgical drainage; however, consideration for FSR in this scenario may be appropriate. In addition, FSR may play a significant role in the surgical management of allergic fungal sinusitis involving the frontal sinus after middle turbinate resection, since FSR creates a patent functional tract that permits long-term endoscopic monitoring and debridement.

In the situation of frontal sinusitis after middle turbinate resection, the central problem is obstruction of the frontal sinus outflow tract by residual bony and soft tissue scar. Both the modified endoscopic Lothrop procedure and frontal sinus obliteration have been presented as alternatives for surgical management of refractory frontal sinusitis, due to frontal recess/ostium stenosis after middle turbinate amputation. It must be emphasized that both of these procedures carry significant morbidity, and the long-term prognosis after these procedures is often suboptimal.

Frontal sinus obliteration with autologous fat [6] may be complicated by perioperative morbidity, chronic pain, and delayed mucocele formation [15]. Furthermore, the evaluation of the frontal sinus in a patient with persistent symptoms after fat obliteration is typically impossible, since MRI signal characteristics of the fat graft are inconsistent and mixed, even in the asymptomatic patient [11]. Frontal sinus obliteration focuses on the frontal sinus contents, but the real issue in frontal sinusitis is the frontal recess. As a result, frontal sinus obliteration is a misdirected procedure that destroys a potentially healthy frontal sinus.

The modified endoscopic Lothrop procedure, a technique for the resection of frontal sinus floor under endoscopic visualization, has gained some popularity [7]. Although this is an endoscopic procedure, it is not minimally invasive. The frontal drillout inevitably causes significant frontal recess trauma, including destruction of mucosa, which leads to soft tissue and bony stenosis. The long-term impact of this procedure is unknown. Because frontal recess mucosa is inevitably disrupted by the modified endoscopic Lothrop procedure, normal frontal mucociliary clearance is often irreversibly altered. Thus, even a frontal sinus with a patent frontal neo-ostium after drillout may not clear its mucus appropriately.

FSR should be considered in the context of frontal sinus obliteration and modified endoscopic Lothrop procedure. FSR re-establishes normal frontal sinus/recess mucociliary clearance, while these other procedures tend to disrupt this physiology. In particular, frontal sinus obliteration destroys the frontal sinus, and the modified endoscopic Lothrop procedure destroys the frontal recess. FSR seeks to preserve these structures and promote normal sinus function.

FSR Outcomes

The published surgical results demonstrate that FSR achieves frontal recess patency and function. In a preliminary report, relief from frontal recess scar and frontal ostium stenosis was achieved in 14 of 16 sides (87.5%) in 12 patients with average follow-up of 8.5 months [5]. In an update of the initial publication, Kuhn noted frontal recess patency (confirmed by nasal endoscopy) and complete resolution of symptoms in 29 of 32 operative sides in 24 patients [10]. It should be noted that 18 sides were successfully treated with FSR on the first attempt, seven sides required a revision FSR procedure, and four sides required two revision FSR procedures. Mean follow-up was 9.6 months, and one patient had long-term patency at 37 months.

Representative endoscopic images of the healed frontal recess after FSR are shown in Figures 26.2 and 26.3.

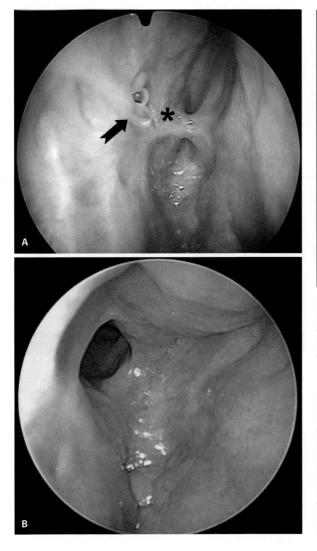

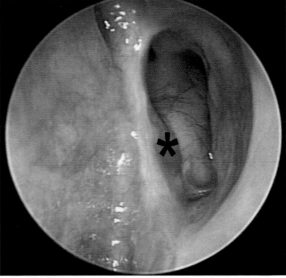

Fig. 26.3. The FSR mucoperiosteal flap heals across the former insertion point for the destabilized middle turbinate stub. This endoscopic image of the left frontal recess shows a patent left frontal neo-ostium, 7 years after revision FSR. The flap (indicated by *) has healed well, and the mucosa is quite healthy

Fig. 26.2. A After middle turbinate resection, the remnant middle turbinate may scar the frontal recess, leading to formal frontal recess/ostium stenosis. In this endoscopic view of the right frontal recess, the frontal ostium (*arrow*) is stenotic, and middle turbinate remnant (indicated by *) is simply encased in scar. Purulent secretions drain slowly from the narrowed frontal ostium. **B** This endoscopic image of the right frontal recess was obtained 8 years after FSR. The frontal neo-ostium is clearly patent and functional. The preoperative view of this frontal recess is shown in **A**

Advantages

FSR offers several distinct advantages:

- Because the lateral frontal recess mucosa is not disturbed by the procedure, mucociliary clearance is restored.
- FSR compensates for both bony and soft tissue stenosis induced by middle turbinate resection.
- FSR builds upon established techniques for endoscopic frontal sinusotomy, and FSR incorporates mucoperiosteal flaps that were first used as means to re-line surgically created frontal neo-ostia created via an external ethmoidectomy.
- FSR mucoperiosteal flap minimizes the tendency for granulation tissue and stenosis.
- FSR is truly minimally invasive; in contrast, the alternative procedure of frontal sinus obliteration is quite extensive with significant morbidity.
- FSR is also a truly functional procedure; in contrast, the alternative procedure of modified endoscopic Lothrop causes significant frontal recess trauma that may ultimately compromise the final surgical result.
- Because FSR is not destructive to the frontal recess, surgical revision under endoscopic visualization is reasonably easy to pursue.

Disadvantages

The potential disadvantages of FSR must be considered as well:

- The mucoperiosteal flap, which is the key feature of FSR, is extremely delicate. If the flap is disrupted, the procedure cannot be completed.
- FSR is a difficult technique. The entire procedure is performed with curved frontal recess instruments under the visualization provided by the angled telescopes.

- Endoscopic frontal recess instrumentation is required; in particular, fine through-cutting giraffe forceps greatly facilitate the procedure.
- The cribriform plate is just behind the site of the surgical manipulations. Hence, FSR carries the risk of skull-based injury with concomitant cerebrospinal fluid leak.
- In some instances, revision FSR will be required.

Conclusion

Frontal sinusitis after middle turbinate resection is a serious surgical challenge, for which standard endoscopic frontal sinusotomy is poorly suited. The frontal sinus rescue procedure, more formally known as revision endoscopic frontal sinusotomy with mucoperiosteal flap advancement, is uniquely designed for the correction of frontal stenosis due to middle turbinate resection. In this procedure, the bone and soft-tissue stenosis is removed, and the surgically enlarged frontal neo-ostium is relined with a small mucoperiosteal flap. Mucosa of the lateral frontal recess is preserved. In this way, frontal sinus rescue procedure may restore appropriate mucociliary clearance to a frontal sinus obstructed due to previous middle turbinate resection.

References

1. Baron SH, Dedo HH, Henry CR (1973) The mucoperiosteal flap in frontal sinus surgery (The Sewall-Boyden-McNaught operation). Laryngoscope 83:1266–1280
2. Boyden GL (1952) Surgical treatment of chronic frontal sinusitis. Ann Otol Rhinol Laryngol 61:558–566
3. Citardi MJ (2001) Computer-aided frontal sinus surgery. Otolaryngol Clin North Am 34:111–122
4. Citardi MJ (2002) Computer-aided otorhinolaryngology-head and neck surgery. Marcel Dekker, New York
5. Citardi MJ, Javer AR, Kuhn FA (2001) Revision endoscopic frontal sinusotomy with mucoperiosteal flap advancement: The frontal sinus rescue procedure. Otolaryngol Clin North Am 34:123–132

26

6. Goodale RL, Montgomery WW (1958) Experience with osteoplastic anterior wall approach to frontal sinuses. Arch Otolaryngol 68:271–283

7. Gross WE, Gross CW, Becker DG, et al (1996) Modified transnasal endoscopic Lothrop procedure as an alternative to frontal sinus obliteration. Otolaryngol Head Neck Surg 113:427–434

8. Kuhn FA, Citardi MJ (1997) Advances in postoperative care following functional endoscopic sinus surgery. Otolaryngol Clin North Am 30:479–490

9. Kuhn FA, Javer AR (2001) Primary endoscopic management of the frontal sinus. Otolaryngol Clin North Am 34:59–75

10. Kuhn FA, Javer AR, Nagpal K, Citardi MJ (2000) The frontal sinus rescue procedure: Early experience and three-year follow-up. Am J Rhinol 14:211–216

11. Loevner LA, Yousem DM, Lanza DC, et al (1995) MR evaluation of frontal sinus osteoplastic flaps with autogenous fat grafts. Am J Neuroradiol 16:1721–1726

12. Lynch RC (1921) The technique of radical frontal sinus operation that has given me the best results. Laryngoscope 31:1–5

13. McNaught RC (1936) A refinement of the external frontoethmosphenoid operation: A new nasofrontal pedicle flap. Arch Otolaryngol 23:544–549

14. Ogura JH, Watson RK, Jurema AA (1960) Frontal sinus surgery: The use of a mucoperiosteal flap for reconstruction of a nasofrontal duct. Laryngoscope 70:1229–1243

15. Sessions RB, Alford BR, Stratton C, et al (1972) Current concepts of frontal sinus surgery: An appraisal of the osteoplastic flap fat obliteration operation. Laryngoscope 82:918–930

16. Sewall EC (1935) The operative technique of nasal sinus disease. Ann Otol Rhinol Laryngol 44:307–316

Chapter 27

Endoscopic Trans-septal Frontal Sinusotomy

27

Pete S. Batra, Donald C. Lanza

Core Messages

- Middle turbinate resection contributes to refractory frontal sinus disease after primary sinus surgery

- The trans-septal frontal sinusotomy technique (TSFS) utilizes the relationship of the nasal septum to the midline floor of the frontal sinus

- Safe completion of the TSFS procedure requires that the frontal sinus floor has an anterior-posterior diameter of at least 1.2 cm

- When performing the TSFS procedure, all efforts are made to preserve sinus mucosa, especially in the frontal recess

Contents

Introduction

The successful surgical management of chronic frontal sinus disease remains a significant challenge for otolaryngologists. From an anatomic standpoint, the drainage pathway of the frontal sinus is hidden from direct view by a complex and variable pneumatization pattern of anterior ethmoid and frontal cells. The close proximity to critical structures, including the lamina papyracea, anterior cranial fossa, and anterior ethmoid artery, adds to the dilemma of effective surgical treatment of these patients. The recent advances in endoscopic sinus surgery and image guidance have afforded direct visualization and easier access to the frontal recess and have made surgery feasible for chronic frontal sinusitis [4, 9, 14, 16, 18, 20].

Despite these advances, frontal sinus disease remains refractory in a subset of patients. This is typically related to neo-osteogenesis resulting in complete or near-complete stenosis of the nasofrontal pathway. A common contributing factor to the frontal recess stenosis is resection of the middle turbinate [19]. The destabilized middle turbinate remnant with excoriated mucosa on its lateral surface lateralizes across the floor of the frontal sinus and compromises the frontal recess patency (Fig. 27.1) [19]. Standard endoscopic techniques are generally inadequate for treatment of chronic frontal disease in these patients. In the past, they required external approaches such as frontal sinus obliteration or cranialization. These open techniques have the potential for significant morbidity. In 250 consecutive osteoplastic procedures, Hardy and Montgomery reported an operative complication rate of 19% and intraoperative cerebrospinal fluid (CSF) leak rate of 2.8% [7]. These difficult patients can now be successfully treated

27

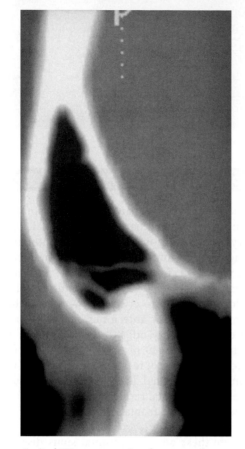

Fig. 27.1. Sagittal CT reconstruction demonstrating narrow anterior-posterior dimensions of the frontal sinus

with extended endoscopic approaches to the frontal sinus.

The novel technique of endoscopic trans-septal frontal sinusotomy (TSFS) augments management of refractory frontal sinus disease in this setting. TSFS is a unique endoscopic surgical approach that utilizes the relationship of the nasal septum to the midline floor of the frontal sinus. Like the Draf III or modified Lothrop procedure, the trans-septal approach provides good access to the midline floor of the frontal sinus and permits but does not require intersinus septum removal [5, 6]. TSFS can be utilized even in circumstances where the severity of the stenosis prohibits cannulation of the frontal recess as a primary landmark.

Translocation of the nasal septum, especially in cases of a narrow nasal vault, allows for:

- Improved visualization
- Improved instrumentation
- Minimizing the size of the planned septal perforation

In addition, TSFS also has several theoretical advantages over frontal sinus obliteration including:

- Decreased morbidity
- Improved cosmesis
- Ease of endoscopic and radiographic surveillance postoperatively

Historical Perspective

An external approach to restore the communication between the nose and the frontal sinus began with the Lynch Howarth fronto-ethmoidectomy [13]. In 1914, Lothrop described a combined intranasal ethmoidectomy and external Lynch type approach to create a common nasofrontal communication by resecting the floor of the frontal sinus, the intersinus septum, and the superior nasal septum [12]. Early attempts at intranasal approaches were largely abandoned due to the inadequate visualization of the frontal recess and frequent treatment failures [3, 17].

In 1991, Draf described a median drainage approach to the frontal sinus utilizing a combined microscopic and endoscopic technique [5]. By using the operating microscope, the lateral bony walls were preserved, thus preventing medial collapse of the orbital soft tissues with subsequent obstruction of the frontal recess. In 1995, Gross et al. described an extended endoscopic approach to create a similar common frontal opening [6]. In this procedure the frontal recess is cannulated and a posteriorly guarded drill is used to resect the frontal sinus floor from both sides. However, the success of this technique depends on the ability to cannulate the frontal recess, which is not always possible in cases of frontal recess stenosis. TSFS builds on the concepts from these previous techniques and allows for entry into the medial frontal sinus floor where the bone is thinnest, especially in cases of extensive neo-osteogenesis that preclude identification and cannulation of the frontal recess.

Preoperative Planning

Symptomatic patients with complete or near-complete opacification of the frontal sinus(es) on CT imaging are candidates for TSFS. They are considered refractory to maximal medical therapy. Each patient is given a comprehensive explanation of the advantages and disadvantages of the different surgical approaches available to manage the frontal sinus disease. Consent is also obtained for an external approach when it was unclear whether the frontal sinus would be amenable to TSFS.

A detailed CT review is performed prior to considering surgical intervention. Coronal and axial CT scans or triplanar views on an image-guidance station are evaluated to determine the pattern of frontal sinus pneumatization, the nature of agger nasi pneumatization, presence of intersinus septal cells, frontal cells, and/or supra-orbital ethmoid cells, and frontal sinus mucocele formation. "Y-shaped" nasal septal attachment to the floor of the frontal sinus is sought. Imaging is also evaluated for the presence of pneumatized crista galli, the integrity of the skull base in the area of the proposed dissection, and the relationship of the middle turbinate to the frontal sinus.

The width and depth of the frontal sinus floor is estimated in either direct coronal or reconstructed sagittal planes on CT images.

- An anterior-posterior diameter of at least 1.2 cm was considered requisite to safe endonasal drilling
- A diameter less than this is considered a relative contraindication and limitation to successfully performing the TSFS given the currently available technology (Fig. 27.1).

Anatomic Considerations

The anterior-most aspect of the middle turbinate can be a helpful landmark in determining the position of the frontal sinus relative to the cribriform plate when consideration is given to performing a drillout procedure. Classic teaching holds that the anterior insertion of the middle turbinate lies adjacent to the cribriform plate. In a radiographic study evaluating 35 coronal CT scans, only 13 of 35 (37%) patients had the superior insertion of the middle turbinate within the anterior 2 mm of the cribriform plate. In 22 of 35 (63%), the insertion of the middle turbinate was anterior to the cribriform plate with 47% of these inserting into the ascending process of the maxilla. Additionally, six of 35 patients (17%) had a superior insertion into the floor of the frontal sinus. Recognizing these variations in the middle turbinate insertion can help the surgeon avoid inadvertent skull base injury. "Y-shaped" nasal septal attachment to the floor of the frontal sinus was noted in three patients. This unique configuration allows for entry into the frontal sinus through the superior nasal septum [1].

Operative Technique

All surgery is performed under general anesthesia. The patient is positioned, prepped and draped as for routine endoscopic sinus surgery. Although this technique was first applied without a computer-aided technique, it is now typically performed using image guidance. This helps confirm critical anatomic landmarks throughout a technically challenging procedure. At the outset of the procedure, the image guidance is properly registered and verified. Oxymetazoline is instilled in each nasal cavity. Injections with 1% lidocaine with 1:200,000 epinephrine are performed bilaterally on the septum, lateral nasal wall (agger nasi region), and middle turbinate remnant. A bilateral greater palatine foramen block is also performed with the same agent. Because most of these patients have undergone previous endoscopic sinus surgery, the adjacent paranasal sinus disease, if present, is addressed first since superiorly created bleeding with TSFS can result in significant difficulty in performing the remainder procedures.

The septum may be endoscopically mobilized to one side for surgical access if necessary. The technique for endoscopic septoplasty has been described [8]. A hemi-transfixion incision is made with an ophthalmic crescent knife (Alcon Labs, Ft. Worth, TX) at the mucocutaneous junction on the appropriate side of the septum. Bilateral inferior and unilateral (left) anterior tunnels are created by sub-perichondral dissection. The quadrilateral cartilage is separated at the bony-cartilaginous junction, and the anterior septum is mobilized from the maxillary crest. Resection of any deviated portions of septal cartilage and bone further improves surgical exposure. A high septal perforation is then created.

Alternately, if space permits a septoplasty may be avoided and a 1.5–2 cm iatrogenic septal perforation is created just across from the leading edge of the middle turbinate/agger nasi region below the skull base. This permits further exposure, ventilation, future endoscopic inspection, and sinus debridement through the nasal cavity. The incisions for the perforation are created utilizing an ophthalmic crescent knife. Through-cutting endoscopic forceps or a soft-tissue shaver is helpful in completing the perforation. Exposed areas of bone or cartilage are minimized throughout the procedure.

The floor of the frontal sinus is identified by intraoperative surgical navigation or, alternately, by using surgical landmarks that are helpful in gauging the position of the frontal sinus relative to the cribriform plate. The midline position of floor of the frontal sinus is typically localized posterior-superior to the most anterior-superior aspects of the septal bony-cartilaginous junction. This location is approximated adjacent to the most anterior remnant or root of the middle turbinate and the agger nasi (ascending process of the maxilla). This is considerably more anterior than the position of the naturally occurring frontal recess area. In patients with a Y-shaped septum at the floor of the frontal sinus, the midline floor of the frontal sinus has an appearance similar to that of the anterior wall of the sphenoid sinus that has been described during trans-septal sphenoid surgery. It appears as the "prow of a ship", albeit in a much narrower region (Fig. 27.2).

After careful inspection of the roof of the nasal vault, the frontal sinus is entered. The evolution of surgical instrumentation has permitted the use of angled drills with concurrent suction/irrigation (Fig. 27.3). Larger burrs can give a critical advantage while drilling around corners anteriorly, but may also pose a hazard by permitting inadvertent drilling the posterior table of the frontal sinus. Concurrent saline irrigation is essential to avoiding inadvertent

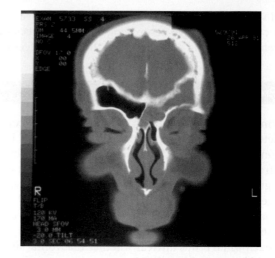

Fig. 27.2. Coronal CT scan demonstrating the "Y-shaped" bony attachment of the nasal septum to the floor of the frontal sinus. Note presence of mucocele in the left frontal sinus

heat injury to bone and surrounding tissue. If straight drills are used without concurrent suction irrigation, irrigation can be applied through a 5 FR ureteral catheter with the help of an assistant and is positioned through the contralateral nares into the operative field. Alternatively, depending upon the thickness of the floor of the sinus, curetting may be sufficient to enter the frontal sinus (Fig. 27.4A).

After successful entry into the lumen of the frontal sinus, the opening can be enlarged further by drilling anteriorly and laterally. Depending on the extent of the disease, dissection can be carried laterally to include the frontal recess. Note that the frontal recess is located posteriorly, and drilling directly across from one frontal recess to the other is not advised. This straight path of drilling will traverse the olfactory fossa and anterior cranial vault and place the patient at risk for CSF leak or even intracranial injury. All efforts are made to preserve the mucosa throughout the procedure, especially in the frontal recess. By reducing mucosal injury, bone exposure is minimized and risk of delayed stenosis is reduced. When drilling anteriorly, care must be taken to preserve the integrity of the radix. The inferior aspect of the intersinus septum may be resected in order to provide a common outlet for both right and left frontal sinuses at the midline. In this fashion, a "neo-ostium" is created as illustrated in Figures 27.4B and 27.5.

Fig. 27.3.
Sagittal illustration demonstrates drilling of the frontal sinus floor through a superiorly-created septal perforation (dotted line). Anterior dotted line represents the hemi-transfixion incision for the septoplasty

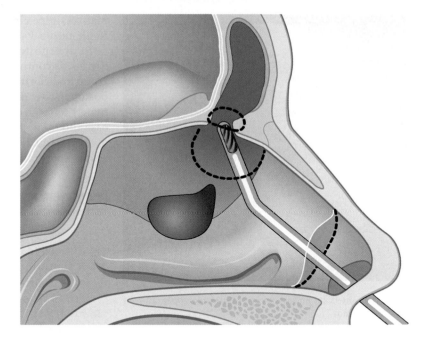

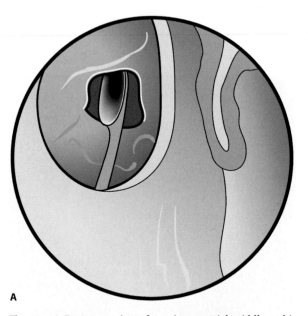

A

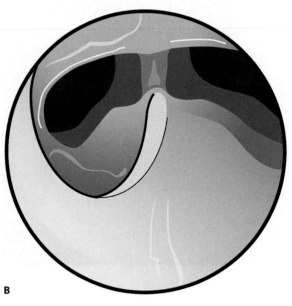

B

Fig. 27.4. A Demonstration of previous partial middle turbinate resection and lateralization in left nasal cavity and entry into the frontal sinus utilizing a frontal sinus curette in right nasal cavity. **B** C-shaped "neo-ostium" created via TSFS. Note that the more lateral aspects including the frontal recess are more posterior than the midline opening

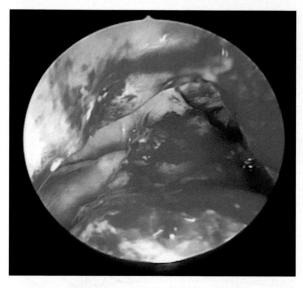

27

Fig. 27.5. Immediate endoscopic postoperative appearance of the "neo-ostium"

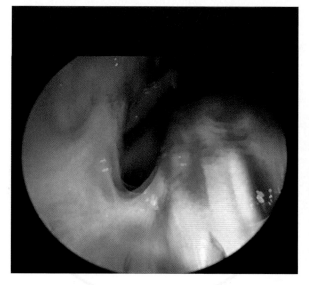

Fig. 27.6. Endoscopic appearance of healed "neo-ostium" at 6 weeks

If septal dislocation was performed earlier, it is now corrected and the hemi-transfixion incision is closed with interrupted 4–0 chromic suture. The septal flaps are re-approximated using a running trans-septal

mattress-type closure with 4–0 plain gut suture on a Keith needle. Packing is not typically required.

In the postoperative period, maximal medical therapy is continued and meticulous debridement of blood and fibrin clots is initiated. It is performed on postoperative day 1, and then weekly for approximately 6 weeks depending on the severity of the disease and the appearance of the postoperative surgical bed [10]. Figure 27.6 demonstrates the healed endoscopic appearance of the "neo-ostium" at 6 weeks.

Indications

- Chronic frontal sinusitis after failed endoscopic sinus surgery, especially in the setting of "neo-osteogenesis" or middle turbinate resection
- Frontal sinus mucocele formation (Fig. 27.7)
- Inverted papilloma (Fig. 27.8)
- Sinonasal malignancies
- Fibro-osseous lesions
- Trauma

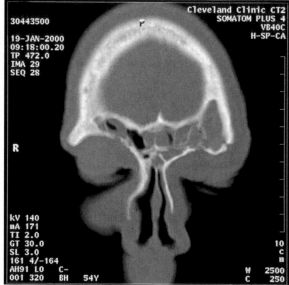

Fig. 27.7. Coronal CT scan shows a complex, multi-septate frontal mucocele

Fig. 27.8.
Coronal T1- weighted MRI with gadolinium demonstrates an extensive
frontal sinus inverted papilloma

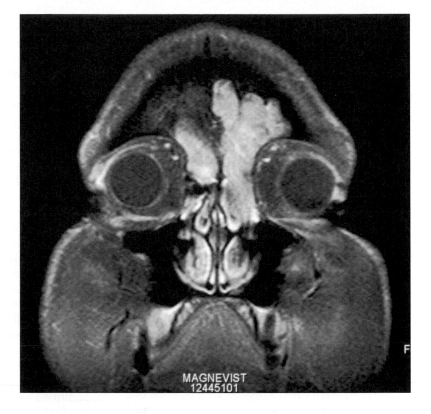

Advantages

- Functional restoration of frontal sinus drain-
  age
- Utilizes inherent anatomic landmarks to facili-
  tate surgery
- Allows for mucosal preservation
- Allows for endoscopic and radiographic
  surveillance postoperatively
- Improved cosmesis through avoidance of
  facial incisions
- Decreased morbidity compared to open
  approaches
- May resort to open approaches if required

Disadvantages

- Requirement of endoscopic expertise
- Need for specialized surgical instrumentation,
  including image guidance
- Risk of inadvertent skull base injury and CSF
  leak
- Possible bone loss at radix
- Drill-related heat injury to nasal sill
- Septal perforation with potential for chronic
  crusting

27

Outcomes

Retrospective analysis was performed to determine the incidence of drillout procedures in management of complex frontal sinus disease in a tertiary academic-based rhinology practice (Cleveland Clinic Foundation). From May 1999 to April 2004, 207 endoscopic frontal sinus procedures were performed in 186 patients. In this group, 161 patients (86.6%) were addressed with endoscopic frontal sinusotomy. Twenty-five patients (13.4%) required 30 drill-out procedures for management of frontal sinus disease. The breakdown of the procedures was as follows: TSFS, six patients; Draf III, 17; Draf II, five; and Draf IB, two. The indications for the procedure included mucocele (11 cases), frontal sinusitis (two cases), invasive fungal sinusitis (two cases), mucosal melanoma (two cases), inverted papilloma (two cases), CSF leak (one case) and fibrous dysplasia (one case). Since the TSFS procedure was only required on six occasions over a 5-year period, one must be cognizant that it is not a common procedure and is reserved for specific anatomy and circumstances.

Of the six patients undergoing TSFS, three patients (50%) were cured symptomatically, while two (33%) were improved and one (17%) was unchanged after the surgical intervention. Endoscopically, frontal patency was noted in five cases (83%). Two of these patients were noted to have partial stenosis of the "neo-ostium"; no patients required stenting to maintain patency. One patient (17%) had complete stenosis though CT demonstrated aeration of the frontal sinus. One intraoperative CSF leak was encountered in a patient with a history of severe maxillofacial trauma secondary to a motor vehicle accident. CT imaging demonstrated a multi-septate mucocele with posterior table erosion. The CSF was encountered upon entering the frontal sinus and was not attributed to technical issues such as drill injury. It was recognized and repaired intraoperatively utilizing fat, cartilage, and floor-of-nose mucosa without any long-term sequelae. The average follow-up was 16 months with a range from 3 to 37 months [2].

■ Lanza et al. reviewed 29 patients undergoing TSFS between 1995 and 1999. The male:female ratio was 21:8. All 29 patients were deemed candidates for frontal sinus obliteration or cranialization. The main indication for TSFS was chronic frontal sinusitis in the setting of previously failed endoscopic surgery. Other indications for surgery were mucocele formation and nasofacial trauma. Twenty-four patients (83%) were available for telephone interview postoperatively. The mean follow-up period was 45 months (range 9–69 months). In this group, 18 of 24 (75%) reported at least 50% improvement of symptomatology, while 14 of 24 (58%) reported 80% or greater improvement of their symptoms. Four (16.6%) patients underwent further frontal sinus surgery with three having frontal sinus obliteration [11, 15].

■ Complications included two CSF leaks, one unplanned anterior inferior septal perforation, and one patient with chronic crusting at the planned perforation in these cases. One leak was attributable to surgical trauma with a drill in a patient with narrow anterior posterior dimensions, and the second occurred during debridement of scarred mucosa in a patient with history of severe trauma. Both CSF leaks were identified and repaired intra-operatively without further sequelae. Both patients with septal difficulties had prior septoplasty.

Conclusions

Endoscopic TSFS represents a novel surgical advance in the management of patients with recalcitrant frontal sinus disease, especially in the setting of new bone formation. The approach utilizes the unique relationship of the nasal septum to the midline floor of the sinus. From an anatomic standpoint, it is best suited for patients with adequate anterior-posterior dimensions of the midline floor of the frontal sinus and a Y-shaped dorsal nasal septum. Given the potential pitfalls of the technique, cumulative endoscopic experience, appropriate surgical instrumentation, and image guidance are requisite to performing successful TSFS.

References

1. Agarwal RP, Loevner L, Becker DG et al (2000) The relationship of the middle turbinate and nasal septum to the frontal sinus floor: A radiographic study. Abstract presented at the annual AAO-HNS meeting, San Antonio, TX. September 1998
2. Batra PS, Lanza DC (2004) Surgical outcomes for drillout procedures for management of complex frontal pathology. Manuscript in preparation
3. Becker D, Moore D, Lindsey W et al (1995) Modified transnasal endoscopic Lothrop procedure: Further considerations. Laryngoscope 105:1161–1166
4. Citardi MJ (2002) Image-guided functional endoscopic sinus surgery. In Citardi MJ (ed) Computer-aided otorhinolaryngology–Head and neck surgery. Marcel Dekker, Inc., New York, pp 201–222
5. Draf W (1991) Endonasal micro-endoscopic frontal sinus surgery: The Fulda concept. Op Tech Otolaryngol Head Neck Surg 2:234–240
6. Gross W, Gross C, Becker D et al (1995) Modified transnasal endoscopic Lothrop procedure as alternative to frontal sinus obliteration. Otolaryngol Head Neck Surg 113: 427–434
7. Hardy JM, Montgomery WM (1976) Osteoplastic frontal sinusitis: An analysis of 250 operations. Ann Otol Rhinol Laryngol 85:523–532
8. PH, McLaughlin RB, Lanza DC et al (1999) Endoscopic septoplasty: Indications, technique, and complications. Otolaryngol Head Neck Surg 120:678–682
9. Kennedy DW (1985) Functional endoscopic sinus surgery: Technique. Arch Otolaryngol 111:643–649
10. Kennedy D, Josephson J, Zinreich J et al (1989) Endoscopic sinus surgery for mucocoeles: A viable alternative. Laryngoscope 99:885–895
11. Lanza DC, McLaughlin RB, Hwang PH (2001) The five-year experience with endoscopic trans-septal frontal sinusotomy. Otolaryngol Clin North Am 34:139–152
12. Lothrop HA (1914) Frontal sinus suppuration. Ann Surg 59:937–957
13. Lynch RC (1921) The technique of a radical frontal sinus operation which has given me the best results. Laryngoscope 31:1–5
14. May M (1991) Frontal sinus surgery: Endonasal endoscopic osteoplasty rather than external osteoplasty. Operative techniques. Otolaryngol Head Neck Surg 2:247–256
15. McLaughlin RB, Hwang PH, Lanza DC (1999) Endoscopic trans-septal frontal sinusotomy: The rationale and results of an alternative technique. Am J Rhinol 13:279–187
16. Olson G, Citardi MJ (2000) Image-guided functional endoscopic sinus surgery. Otolaryngol Head Neck Surg 123: 188–194
17. Schaefer S, Close L (1990) Endoscopic management of frontal sinus disease. Laryngoscope 100:155–160
18. Stammberger H (1986) Endoscopic endonasal surgery–Concepts in treatment of recurring rhinosinusitis. Part II. Surgical technique. Otolaryngol Head Neck Surg 94:147–156.
19. Swanson PB, Lanza DC, Vining EM et al (1995) The effect of middle turbinate resection upon the frontal sinus. Am J Rhinol 9:191–197
20. Wigand ME (1981) Transnasal ethmoidectomy under endoscopical control. Rhinol 19:7–10

Chapter 28

Frontal Sinus Stenting

28

Seth J. Kanowitz, Joseph B. Jacobs, Richard A. Lebowitz

Core Messages

- ■ Postoperative stenting of the frontal sinus outflow tract has been demonstrated to improve long-term patency rates

- ■ Soft (Silicone) sheets or stents are superior to rigid stents

- ■ A minimum six-week period of stenting is generally recommended

- ■ Routine care after stent placement includes appropriate antibiotic therapy, nasal irrigation, gentle debridement, and topical nasal steroid spray

Contents

Introduction

The concept of frontal sinus stenting to minimize postoperative stenosis and improve mucosalization of the frontal sinus outflow tract (FSOT) following frontal sinus surgery has been reported in the literature for nearly 100 years. The external fronto-ethmoidectomy, as originally described by Lynch, involved postoperative stenting of the nasofrontal communication. Technological advances in sinus endoscopes, surgical instruments, high-resolution computed tomographic (CT) scanning, and image guidance have allowed for improved visualization and intranasal surgical access to the nasofrontal region. However, despite these advances, postoperative stenosis of the FSOT with recurrent frontal sinus disease remains a significant problem (Fig. 28.1).

Factors such as polyposis, osteitic bone, and lateralization of the middle turbinate/middle turbinate remnant may lead to FSOT stenosis, regardless of the

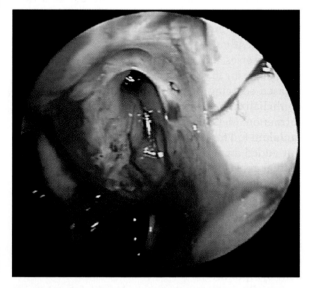

Fig. 28.1. Endoscopic view of stenotic right frontal sinus neo-ostium

28

surgical approach and the adequacy of the frontal sinusotomy. Failure rates of nearly 30% have been reported in the literature – and because of this propensity for postoperative stenosis of the FSOT, stenting remains an important component in the surgical management of chronic frontal sinusitis.

Stenting Materials

The concept of frontal sinus stenting dates back to 1905 when Ingals reported the use of a gold tube, placed endonasally, to help stent the surgical bed until the nasofrontal duct was mucosalized [11]. In 1921, in the initial description of the fronto-ethmoidectomy procedure that now bears his name, Lynch placed a firm rubber tube in the nasofrontal duct to help maintain patency [14]. The stent remained in place for five days postoperatively. Lynch initially reported a 100% success rate in 15 patients treated with this technique and followed for a period of 2.5 years. Unfortunately, the long-term failure rate for this procedure was found to be approximately 30% [16, 17].

In the 1940's and 50's, Goodale, Harris, and Scharfe described their experiences with the use of tantalum for frontal sinus stenting [5, 6, 8, 20]. Originally discovered by Eckenberg in 1902, tantalum is an inert basic element. Goodale described the use of a thin sheet of tantalum sutured to the orbital periosteum, while Harris and Scharfe both employed tantalum tubes extending from the frontal sinus into the nose. In their series, the authors reported success rates that were superior to the classic Lynch operation with decreased scarring of the nasofrontal duct, improved epithelialization, and decreased granulation tissue formation. Metson employed similar techniques and tantalum foil for drainage of frontal sinus mucoceles, but added an acrylic tube for mucoceles with intracranial extension [13]. In 1972, Barton described similar results in 34 patients implanted with a 6 or 8 millimeter (mm) Dacron Woven Arterial Graft sutured into the frontal sinus floor and extending downward into the middle meatus [2]. None of the implants were removed during the 17-year study period, and all of the patients were relieved of their frontal headache symptoms.

Initially, most surgeons used rigid frontal sinus stents. However, in animal and clinical trials published in 1976, Neel demonstrated the superiority of thin, pliable Silastic sheeting [16, 17]. He reported a 29% failure rate with rubber tubing and a 17% failure rate with thin Silastic sheeting, in patients followed for an average of 13.5 years postoperatively. In his canine model, Neel demonstrated significant fibrosis and osteoblastic activity, with little or no epithelialization, in frontal ostia that had been stented with firm rubber stents. In contrast, a normal mucosal lining was observed on histological specimens in ducts stented with thin Silastic sheeting. The difference was felt to be due to local ischemia, impaired drainage, and infection around the rigid tubes.

Schaefer and Close employed Silastic tubing for small endoscopic frontal sinusotomies (4 to 6 mm) in four of 36 patients treated [19]. However, a 50% stenosis rate resulted, which was attributed to a failure to maintain a postoperative communication between an air passage and the mucosa, thus resulting in massively hypertrophied mucosa and obstruction of the frontal sinus ostium. More recently, numerous authors have described the use of a variety of Silicone tubes, as well as rolled Silicone sheeting, placed either externally or endoscopically, to help maintain patency of the nasofrontal duct. [1, 3, 4, 7, 9, 10, 12, 15, 18, 21, 22].

Indications for Stenting

There are no standard, accepted indications for postoperative stenting of the FSOT. Routine stenting is not advocated, and the decision to place a frontal sinus stent is based on the surgeon's assessment of the patient's risk for stenosis of the FSOT. A number of conditions need to be considered as risk factors for FSOT stenosis, and thus, as potential indications for stenting.

Hosemann demonstrated a doubling (16% vs. 33%) of the rate of FSOT stenosis when the intraoperative diameter of the neo-ostium was less than 5 mm [9]. Therefore, a FSOT diameter of less than 5 mm is often considered an indication for stenting. Other indications include extensive demucosalization, particularly with circumferential exposure of bone, at the level of the frontal sinus ostium; osteitic bone (as determined by pre-operative CT) in the FSOT; extensive polyposis [as is often seen in patients with allergic

Fig. 28.2.
Intraoperative image guidance with probe in stenotic left frontal sinus outflow tract

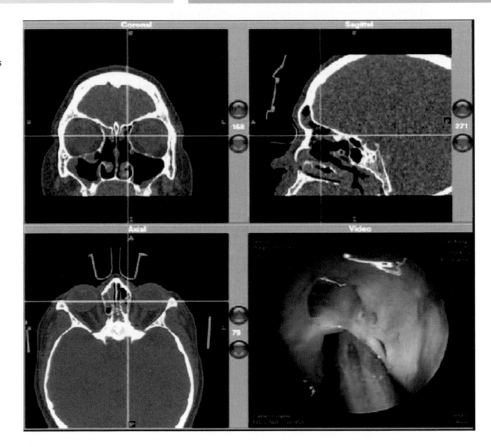

fungal sinusitis (AFS)]; flail middle turbinate, particularly in cases of partial middle turbinate resection; and revision frontal sinus surgery with pre-operative scarring or lateralization of the middle turbinate (Fig. 28.2).

Indications for FSOT Stenting

- Frontal sinus neo-ostium diameter less than 5 mm
- Extensive or circumferential exposure of bone in the FSOT
- Polyposis/AFS
- Flail/lateralized middle turbinate
- Revision frontal sinus surgery

External Versus Endoscopic Approach

The initial works of Lynch, Goodale, Harris, and Scharfe predated the availability of fiberoptic nasal endoscopes and endoscopic sinus instrumentation. Therefore, the techniques of those authors involved an external approach to the frontal sinus and placement of the stent. As the surgical management of frontal sinus disease shifts from external to endoscopic approaches, the techniques of frontal sinus stenting have changed as well.

However, some authors still report the use of an external approach for the placement of a frontal sinus stent. Barton employed a modified Lynch external frontal sinusotomy for the placement of a Dacron graft with a reported 100% success rate for relief of frontal headache symptoms [2]. Neel also employed a modified Lynch external approach (Neel-Lake) for

28

the placement of thin Silastic sheeting to stent the frontal ostium. In 13 patients (14 ducts), there was one (7%) short-term failure at four months, which was treated with frontal sinus obliteration. After an additional seven years of observation, the overall failure rate was 20% (three ostia), with both long-term failures being successfully treated with revision frontal sinusotomy [16, 17]. Using a similar external approach in 18 patients who failed a previous transnasal widening of the nasofrontal communication, Yamasoba placed a Silicone T-tube in the frontal sinus outflow tract [22]. Complete epithelialization of the nasofrontal communication, and resolution of symptoms was reported in all patients after tube removal. Two patients subsequently suffered closure of the FSOT. More recently, Amble placed thin silicone rubber sheeting to reconstruct the nasofrontal communication after a modified external Lynch procedure in which the frontal process of the superior maxilla was preserved [1]. Of the 164 patients studied, 96% achieved resolution of their symptoms.

In 1990, Schaefer and Close first reported their experience with endoscopic placement of thin Silastic tubing as a frontal sinus stent, resulting in a 50% failure rate in the four patients studied [19] (Fig. 28.3). Employing three different kinds of stents (Rains self-retaining silicone tube, U-shaped silicone tube, and

H-shaped silicone tube) and various Draf endoscopic frontal sinus drainage procedures in 12 patients, Weber reported complete resolution or significant improvement in 10 patients' frontal sinus symptoms, and moderate improvement in two patients. However, while clinically significant stenosis of the FSOT did not occur, stenting could not prevent the recurrence of endoscopically or radiographically visible polypoid mucosal disease [21]. Hoyt reported similar results in 21 patients (32 stents) who had vented tubular plastic stents placed endoscopically [10]. Freeman placed a bi-flanged Silicone tube (Freeman frontal sinus stent) endoscopically in 55 sinuses and externally in nine sinuses with follow-up of 12–45 months [4]. Six sinuses eventually required fat obliteration, four due to restensosis secondary to lateralization of the middle turbinate with scarring, and two due to the development of frontal sinus polyps. Rains also employed a soft Silicone tube with a tapered collapsible bulb placed endoscopically in 67 patients. With a total of 102 stents placed, and follow-up of 8–48 months, a failure rate of 6% was reported. Allergic fungal sinusitis was present in all cases requiring revision [18].

Ultimately, the success of all nonobliterative frontal sinus surgery, whether external or endoscopic, is judged by the long-term *functional* patency of the FSOT. In many instances the FSOT may not be visibly patent, but can be endoscopically probed in asymptomatic patients [12].

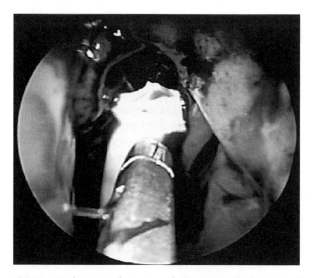

Fig. 28.3. Endoscopic placement of silastic stent in left frontal sinus outflow tract

To Pre-operatively Assess the Need for FSOT Stenting

- Carefully review the sinus anatomy on CT to determine the potential surgical diameter of the frontal sinus neo-ostium, as limited by the frontal beak, anterior skull base, medial orbit, and cribiform plate.

- Evaluate the pre-operative CT for radiographic evidence of AFS, and/or osteitis of the bone of the FSOT.

- Perform a thorough nasal endoscopic examination with particular attention to polyposis in the frontal recess, scarring from prior surgery, and previous partial middle turbinectomy.

Duration of Stenting

Currently no prospective controlled studies or definitive standards for the duration of frontal sinus stenting exist in the literature. Stenting duration ranges from as little as five days to as long as 17 years; however, most recommendations fall somewhere in-between [2,14].

Neel demonstrated, histologically, that re-epithelialization of the nasofrontal communication of canines stented with thin Silicone rubber is complete within approximately eight weeks. Based upon this work, Neel removed Silastic sheeting stents in his patients beginning after a minimum of six weeks (mean six months). This resulted in a failure rate of 20% with a seven-year follow-up period [16].

Employing a six-week duration of stenting using 4 mm Silastic tubing, Schaefer encountered a 50% failure rate. However, this technique was only utilized in four patients, and failure was attributed to the extent of frontal sinus disease, lateral extent of the disease, and the difficulty in placing the catheter within the frontal sinus [19]. Benoit employed the Rains frontal sinus stent for an average of five weeks with a FSOT patency rate of 79% at 12 months follow-up [3]. Rains reported a 96% patency rate at 48 months follow-up, with the same stent and the same average duration of stenting (five weeks; range 6–130 days) [18]. Hoyt removed the plastic tubing stenting material at eight weeks with a failure rate of 9.5% in 21 patients, but follow-up was unspecified and limited [10]. Similarly, Amble removed the Silicone rubber sheeting between six and eight weeks postoperatively in most patients, with an 18% revision rate at an average of 47 months follow-up.

Citing improved patency with a longer duration of stenting, Weber recommended removal of the Rains frontal sinus stent, U-shaped Silicone tube, and H-shaped Silicone tube at six months. In the 15 sinuses available for evaluation at an average of 19.4 months after surgery, no relevant restenosis of the FSOT was appreciated with this longer period of stenting [21]. Freeman also described a period of stenting lasting between six and 12 months for patients' stented to *correct* FSOT stenosis, while a period of four weeks was employed for those used to *prevent* postoperative stenosis [4]. Whenever stent removal is deemed appropriate, all authors report successful removal of the stenting material in the office using endoscopes and endoscopic sinus instrumentation.

Postoperative Stent Management

Most authors agree that regular debridement and irrigation of the nasal cavity and stent, regardless of material and placement technique, are necessary to maintain stent patency, minimize scarring and adhesions, and improve long-term results. Even during the early days of frontal sinus stenting, Goodale and Harris routinely probed and cleaned the tantalum tubes with a curved suction [5, 6, 8].

Nasal irrigation usually begins within the first few postoperative days and is maintained for at least the duration of stenting. Amble employed a regimen of nasal irrigation two to three times daily, twice daily placement of petroleum jelly into the nasal cavity, broad-spectrum antibiotics for 10 to 21 days, and the application of a heating pad for 30 min two to three times daily [1]. Routine postoperative endoscopic removal of blood clots, debris, dried secretions, and granulation tissue from within the nasal cavity and within the stent itself is performed in the office as needed.

The use of topical and/or oral steroids has been recommended to reduce postoperative inflammation and scar formation. Weber advocated saline nasal irrigation and a six-month course of topical inhaled nasal steroids [21]. Rains initiated inhaled topical nasal steroids at two to three weeks after surgery, with oral steroids prescribed when marked polypoid disease is present [18].

Appropriate antibiotic therapy is also recommended, but not for the entire duration of longer stenting periods. However, if an episode of acute frontal sinusitis occurs it should be treated accordingly with antibiotics. If purulent drainage persists despite appropriate medical therapy, the stent may act as a foreign body and consideration should be given to removing it.

Conclusion

Frontal sinus stenting has demonstrated the ability to improve FSOT patency in specific cases; however, failure rates of approximately 30% still persist. Long-term patency is improved with the use of soft Silicone sheets or stents as opposed to rigid stenting material. While duration of stenting varies widely in the literature, an average of approximately six weeks is generally accepted. Routine endoscopic debridement, nasal irrigation, appropriate antibiotic therapy, and topical nasal spray are important to help maintain stent patency. Acute episodes of frontal sinusitis during stenting should be treated appropriately, and if purulent discharge persists, consideration should be given to removing the stent.

References

1. Amble FR, Kern EB, Neel B, et al (1996) Nasofrontal duct reconstruction with silicone rubber sheeting for inflammatory frontal sinus disease: Analysis of 164 cases. Laryngoscope 106:809–815
2. Barton RT (1972) Dacron prosthesis in frontal sinus surgery. Laryngoscope 82:1795–1802
3. Benoit CM, Duncavage JA (2001) Combined external and endoscopic frontal sinusotomy with stent placement: A retrospective review. Laryngoscope 111:1246–1249
4. Freeman SB, Blom ED (2000) Frontal sinus stents. Laryngoscope 110:1179–1182
5. Goodale RL (1954) Ten years' experience in the use of tantalum in frontal sinus surgery. Laryngoscope 64:65–72
6. Goodale RL (1945) The use of tantalum in radical frontal sinus surgery. Ann Otol Rhinol Laryngol 45:757–762
7. Har El G, Lucente FE (1995) Endoscopic intranasal frontal sinusotomy. Laryngoscope 105:440–443
8. Harris HE (1948) The use of tantalum tubes in frontal sinus surgery. Cleve Clin Q 15:129–133
9. Hosemann W, Kuhnel TH, Held P, et al (1997) Endonasal frontal sinusotomy in surgical management of chronic sinusitis: A critical evaluation. Am J Rhinol 11:1–19
10. Hoyt WH (1993) Endoscopic stenting of nasofrontal communication in frontal sinus disease. Ear Nose Throat J 72:596–597
11. Ingals EE (1905) New operation and instruments for draining the frontal sinus. Tr Am Layng Rhin Otol Soc 11:183–189
12. Jacobs JB (1997) 100 years of frontal sinus surgery. Laryngoscope 107:1–36
13. Kaplan S, Schwartz A, Metson BF (1950) Mucocele of the frontal and ethmoid sinuses. Arch Otolaryngol 51:172–187
14. Lynch RC (1921) The technique of radical frontal sinus surgery operation which has given me the best results. Laryngoscope 31:1–5
15. Mirza S, Johnson AP (2000) A simple and effective frontal sinus stent. J Laryngol Otol 114:955–956
16. Neel HB, McDonald TJ, Facer GW (1987) Modified Lynch procedure for chronic frontal sinus diseases: Rationale, technique, and long-term results. Laryngoscope 97:1274–1279
17. Neel HB, Whicker JH, Lake CF (1976) Thin rubber sheeting in frontal sinus surgery: Animal and clinical studies. Laryngoscope 86:524–536
18. Rains BM (2001) Frontal sinus stenting. Otolaryngol Clin North Am 34:101–110
19. Schaefer SD, Close LG (1990) Endoscopic management of frontal sinus disease. Laryngoscope 100:155–160
20. Scharfe ED (1953) The use of tantalum in otolaryngology. Arch Otolaryngol 58:133–140
21. Weber R, Mai R, Hosemann W, et al (2000) The success of 6-month stenting in endonasal frontal sinus surgery. Ear Nose Throat J 79:930–932, 934, 937–938, 940–941
22. Yamasoba T, Kikuchi S, Higo R (1994) Transient positioning of a silicone T tube in frontal sinus surgery. Otolaryngol Head Neck Surg 111:776–780

28

Chapter 29

Complications of Frontal Sinus Surgery

29

Scott M. Graham

Core Messages

■ Safe and successful frontal surgery requires careful planning

■ Careful preoperative review of CT scans may reveal anatomic variations of importance for safe frontal sinus surgery

■ If intraoperative bleeding compromises adequate visualization, the surgery should be stopped

■ If a CSF leak is discovered intraoperatively, it should almost always be repaired at the same surgical setting

■ If an orbital hematoma occurs, while an ophthalmology consultation should be obtained, practical management in most cases falls to the otolaryngologist

■ Powered instrumentation provides efficient dissection but can also contribute to potentially devastating complications

■ Coronal incisions for osteoplastic flap surgery require a strategy to preserve the frontal branch of the facial nerve

Contents

Every surgeon and every patient must consider the potential for complications in making decisions about forthcoming frontal sinus surgery. An often quoted figure is that the risk of serious complications of sinus surgery is approximately half of one percent [1]. This figure is for sinus surgery in general and while discrete figures are not available for isolated frontal sinus surgery, the risk is unlikely to be lower. Challenging intranasal access to the frontal sinus, as well as close proximity to the brain and orbit, make frontal sinus surgeries among the most difficult to perform. Appropriate informed consent requires a full and frank discussion of potential complications as well as alternative treatments. The possibility of "surgical failure" or failure of the operation to successfully correct the patient's symptoms and the potential for revision surgery need also to be addressed. Surgical "success" and "failure" rates are covered in the appropriate chapters and will not be further discussed here. The impact of image-guided surgery on

29

complication rates is as yet unclear. While a conceptually attractive argument can be made for increased safety of frontal sinus surgery using image guidance, complications still occur with its use [2], and its principal legacy thus far seems to be an increase in the number of sinuses opened.

Safe and successful frontal sinus surgery requires careful planning and a deliberate effort to positively influence as many surgical variables as possible. First and foremost in minimizing surgical variables is the CT scan. The CT scan should be appropriately timed after intensive medical treatment and contain finely cut coronal images. Limited cut CT scans, while useful in resolving diagnostic issues, play no part in surgical planning. Axial cuts provide useful information in assessing frontal sinus wall integrity, and sagittal reconstructions provide invaluable information for endoscopic approaches to the frontal sinus. Image-guided surgery is an unquestioned advance in dealing with the complex anatomy of the frontal recess. While this is no substitute for surgical judgment and experience, it is of particular benefit in revision cases.

All of our surgical efforts and planning are aimed at reducing intraoperative bleeding with consequent increased visualization and by implication, enhanced surgical safety. These efforts include reduction of inflammation by the use of antibiotics and, in selected cases, corticosteroids. Patients are instructed to avoid the use of any substances which may effect the bleeding time. Intraoperative use is made of topical vasoconstricting solutions as well as hemostatic injections at selected sites. Head of bed elevation and judicious control of blood pressure are employed. In the event that bleeding of sufficient severity to preclude adequate surgical endoscopic visualization persists, the surgery should be stopped. Intraoperative blood loss is, of course, recorded in the anesthetic record and, from a medico-legal point of view, an operative complication in the face of significant bleeding becomes difficult to defend. Similarly, total operative time is also recorded and defense of a claim is difficult where the operation may appear to be "rushed" or performed "too quickly." A further factor that is scrutinized should a complication occur is the original indication for surgery and whether an adequate trial of appropriate medical therapy had been initially employed.

Complications related to surgery in general, not specific to frontal sinus operations, may also occur. Such events include anesthetic complications, postoperative wound infections, and pneumonias and will not be further discussed. In lengthy operations the use of prophylaxis against deep venous thrombosis and pulmonary embolism should be considered [3]. The remainder of this chapter will be devoted to particular complications which may occur with the variety of surgical approaches and operations that exist for the frontal sinus.

Transnasal Endoscopic Approaches to the Frontal Sinus

CSF Leaks

CSF leaks can be broadly divided into those leaks recognized at the time of surgery and those leaks diagnosed during the postoperative period. As a general rule, a CSF leak diagnosed intraoperatively should be repaired in the same surgical setting. An exception to this rule would be if the surgeon remained anatomically disoriented after recognition of the leak and attempts at surgical repair may risk a further complication, such as a brain parenchymal injury or an orbital insult. If there is uncertainty as to whether a small leak exists, a request to the anesthesiologist to produce a Valsalva maneuver when the procedure is performed under general anesthesia may be of help. Successful repair of the leak requires precise anatomical localization of the area of the defect – further dissection may be required to achieve this. Local intranasal tissue is generally used to repair the defect, although a variety of other tissue including fat from the ear lobule can be considered. The advantage of intranasal tissue is that no incision remote from the surgical site is required. Septal mucosa or turbinate tissue can be used. This material should be taken from the contralateral nasal cavity to reduce bleeding at the site of repair.

Intranasal flaps have also been employed [4]. The advantage of septal flaps is that they utilize vascularized tissue. This advantage is however more than offset by an increased difficulty of handling tethered flap tissue and the potential for retraction with healing. Nasal graft tissue should be inserted with the secretory surface towards the nose. While an underlay graft is often theoretically desirable, there is no practical demonstrated difference in success rates compared with onlay grafts. In repair of leaks recognized intraoperatively, a slurry of microfibrillar collagen can be used to reinforce the graft closure. Gelfoam is placed under this area and the nose is packed. The patient is placed at bed rest for 48 h and is restricted from activities likely to increase intracranial pressure for the ensuing 6 weeks. Antibiotics are only used while the packs are in the nose.

The principles of CSF leak repair are:

- Accurate pre-operative diagnosis
- Precise intraoperative localization of the leak site
- Meticulous surgery – a variety of surgical techniques enjoy similar success rates

The second broad category of CSF leaks are those where the diagnosis is made secondarily, after surgery. Patients most often complain of unilateral, clear rhinorrhea, but can also present with complications of CSF leakage such as meningitis. Even when the diagnosis of CSF leak seems clinically obvious, the identity of the leaking fluid should be confirmed by β-transferrin testing. This widely available test is reliable with few false positives [5]. The disadvantage for most practitioners is that the fluid must be sent to a central laboratory for diagnosis, delaying the time when the result is available. In the event that the patient is not leaking fluid during the office visit, the patient can be sent home with an appropriate container to collect the fluid. Some leaks are inducible by exercise, as it serves to increase intracranial pressure. A second test to complement the use of β-transferrin is a fine-cut coronal CT scan, which will localize any bony defects. A variety of other tests exist, which may be useful in selected circumstances. Intrathecal radioactive tracers can be useful in diagnosing intermittent leaks, as a result of the pooling effect that can occur in the frontal sinus. These leaks can be otherwise difficult to detect. A neurosurgical consultation is usually obtained in managing patients with a delayed diagnosis of CSF leak.

While the use of intrathecal fluorescein is not approved by the FDA, we have used it as a matter of routine in the intraoperative diagnosis and localization of CSF leaks. Specific consent for its use is obtained and a lumbar puncture, performed in our practice by a neurosurgeon, is performed immediately after induction of general anesthesia [6]. Ten cm^3 of CSF is removed, which is mixed with 0.25 cm^3 of 10% fluorescein, precisely measured in a tuberculin syringe. This is reinjected slowly in a timed 10-min sequence. Risks of intrathecal fluorescein injection, such as status epilepticus, have generally been associated with bolus injection and dosing errors. The fluorescein stains the CSF a remarkable green color, which allows confirmation of the leak and precise identification of the site. The next surgical step is to prepare the recipient site for the graft. This will likely involve further dissection and mucosal removal, which will enhance scarring and the security of the closure. A variety of graft materials have been described with no difference in success rates. With similar surgical "take" rates, the choice between different materials is based on other parameters, such as donor site morbidity, ease of surgical manipulation, and cost. We have most often preferred temporalis fascia and muscle. While an underlay graft is theoretically preferable, no difference exists in success rates when this technique is compared with an onlay procedure. Likewise, there is no statistically significant benefit in using a lumbar drain postoperatively. In situations where we have used a drain for intrathecal fluorescein administration at the start of surgery, we keep the drain in for about 3 days postoperatively. These patients with the drain are initially managed postoperatively on the neurosurgical floor. Nasal packing, separated from the repair by Gelfoam, remains in place for 5 days.

Orbital Complications

The proximity of the anterior ethmoidal artery to the posterior aspect of the frontal recess places it in special danger during transnasal approaches to the frontal sinus. In the event that the artery is damaged and significant bleeding occurs, this is best dealt with, in the first instance, by controlled suction and hemostatic packing. If bleeding persists, bipolar cautery can be used. One of the new combined suction bipolar cautery devices provides the best instrumentation in this situation. In general, monopolar cautery should be avoided on the skull base, particularly in close proximity to the orbit. Surgical manipulation adjacent to a bleeding anterior ethmoidal artery has the potential for further complications, as this is one of the areas where the skull base is weakest. Unexplained bleeding at the skull base may be suggestive of a concomitant CSF leak.

Damage resulting in transection of the anterior ethmoid artery, if the artery retracts, may produce the rapid onset of an orbital hematoma. The anterior ethmoidal artery also has an intracranial course and, while rare, intracranial bleeding requiring a craniotomy for control may occur. Orbital hematomas may occur more slowly from venous bleeding after breech of the lamina and periorbita [7]. These hematomas are often diagnosed postoperatively, and initial treatment begins with removal of any ipsilateral nasal packing. The more usual situation is a rapid-onset hematoma presenting with intraoperative proptosis. Surgery performed under local anesthesia with sedation affords the luxury of being able to assess the patient's vision. Subsequent treatment of the hematoma can be made based on the patient's vision. If the vision is normal and the circulation to the optic nerve, as assessed by fundoscopy, is not compromised, carefully selected patients can be closely monitored. Adjunctive treatment such as mannitol or steroids may decrease the intraorbital pressure. It should be emphasized however, that the single most important factor in managing these patients is close observation of their vision.

The principles of managing orbital hemorrhage and complications are:

- If a postoperative orbital hematoma develops, remove any ipsilateral nasal packing
- Firm pressure to the orbit for two minutes may help control active intraorbital hemorrhage
- When there is increased orbital pressure, lateral canthotomy and superior and inferior cantholysis may be beneficial
- With persistently increased orbital pressure, consider orbital decompression

As a practical matter, most frontal sinus operations are performed under general anesthesia. Vision cannot be assessed and decisions on hematoma management must be made as if the least favorable outcome is likely. Certainly, assistance from an ophthalmologist should be immediately sought. An ophthalmologist will likely examine the fundus, provide an estimate of proptosis, and measure the intraocular pressure. Intraocular pressure can be measured using a tonometer. As a generalization, an intraocular pressure of <30 mmHg suggests that the eye can be observed. An intraocular pressure of >40 mmHg may be associated with a poor vision result. Fundoscopy is used to assess blood flow to the optic nerve. In a 1980 study of central retinal artery occlusion and retinal tolerance time in laboratory monkeys, permanent ischemic damage to vision occurred at approximately 90 min [8].

In reality, immediate ophthalmological assistance may not be available or the ophthalmologist consulted may have limited expertise in orbital surgery. In these common circumstances, the patient relies on the judgment and surgical skills of the otolaryngologist. As initial treatment, firm four-finger pressure should be applied to the orbit for 2 min in an effort to control the hemorrhage with digital pressure. The pressure should be stopped if the globe becomes rock hard. This effort to stop the hemorrhage is important; otherwise further surgical steps simply provide a greater volume for the severed and retracted anterior ethmoidal artery to bleed into. A lateral canthotomy with upper and lower lid cantholysis should be performed [9]. This increases orbital volume and lowers the orbital pressure. This lowering of orbital pressure may allow bleeding to restart, and the eye requires close observation. If bleeding has stopped, "orbital massage," as described in some publications, to redistribute the intraorbital clot, has a high likelihood of restarting bleeding. After canthotomy and cantholysis, orbital decompression and exploration should be considered. Orbital decompression with removal of bone and subsequent periorbital incisions can be accomplished via a variety of approaches. These include external ethmoidectomy, endoscopic decompression [10], or via the newer transcaruncular approach [11]. The choice between these three techniques lies with the particular surgeon's experience and expertise.

29

Powered instrumentation is associated with special risks within the close confines of the frontal recess [12]. Powered instrumentation is, in fact, "suction-assisted" powered instrumentation, and adjacent tissue is sucked into the rapidly rotating powerful cutting blades. Treatment of the ensuing diplopia from inadvertent medial rectus resection is seldom successful. While restoration of fused vision in primary gaze may represent a surgical triumph in an individual patient, it is seldom of great clinical utility. The special impact of powered instrumentation is that an injury that might "only" have resulted in dural exposure or periorbital fat prolapse with conventional forceps dissection can rapidly turn into a catastrophe. An event that previously would have served simply as a salutary anatomical reminder to the surgeon with little chance of permanent significant sequelae is now a major complication. With conventional instrumentation, breech of the lamina and periorbita may produce only fat prolapse and, providing this is recognized and left alone, most of the remaining surgery can still be performed with little by way of lasting sequelae. With powered instrumentation, this tissue, together with whatever lies beneath, most often the medial rectus muscle, is sucked into and severed by the rotating blades in a fraction of a second (Fig. 29.1). Parenchymal brain injuries

and intracranial vascular damage may occur in situations which previously would have resulted in CSF leaks with a high likelihood of subsequent successful endoscopic repair. Powered instrumentation represents a remarkable advance in surgical technique. Its great power and efficiency of dissection need, however, to be treated with the utmost respect. Its associated suction, integral to its impressive soft tissue dissection capabilities, has opened up new realms of potentially devastating complications. No information exists as to whether powered instrumentation has increased the incidence of complications of sinus surgery. Unequivocally what it has done is to dramatically escalate the scale of injury.

Intranasal Modified Lothrop Procedure

Image-guided surgery has done much to increase the comfort of surgeons performing endoscopic-modified Lothrop procedures. Injuries to the orbit and dura may occur in this operation as in any endoscopic procedure. The use of powered dissectors and drills in close proximity to these vital structures calls for particular care and judgment on the part of the surgeon. Long-term patency rates and the potential for restenosis of the common frontal sinus/nasal opening have received a good deal of attention and are most appropriately dealt with in the chapter devoted to this operation. These issues need to be carefully reviewed with the patient as part of the informed consent for this procedure. What has received little attention is the potential for disrupted mucociliary clearance in the scar tissue that exists at the top of the nose and in the septal remnant. Particularly in dry climates, this can produce crusting in the vault of the nose with a sense of nasal fullness. Certain patients find these symptoms nearly as distressing as the symptoms that enticed them to have the intranasal modified Lothrop procedure in the first place.

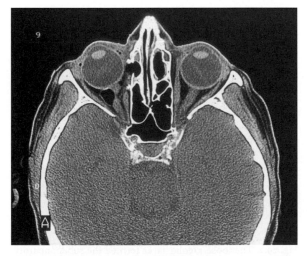

Fig. 29.1. Medial rectus injury during frontal recess exploration using powered instrumentation. Reproduced with permission from [12]

External Fronto-ethmoidectomy

One of the greatest problems with external fronto-ethmoidectomy occurs as a consequence of resection of the lamina papyracea. With lamina resection, orbital contents can prolapse medially, causing potential obstruction of the frontal recess. The external scar is subject to the vagaries of healing. Interrupting the linear incision with an inserted "v" adjacent to the medial canthus reduces the prominence of the scar by lessening the chance for webbing and by adding a degree of randomization of the surgical wound. Dissection at the junction of the roof and medial wall of the orbit can injure the trochlea of the superior oblique muscle. The trochlea comprises a U-shaped piece of fibrocartilage, closed above by fibrous tissue, which is attached to the fovea or spina trochlearis bone, just behind the orbital rim [13]. Interruption of the trochlea may result in postoperative diplopia.

Frontal Sinus Trephine

Misdirected attempts to enter a small frontal sinus may result in an intracranial entry. The procedure is performed through a stab incision, which usually, although not invariably, heals without a noticeable scar. In "above and below" approaches to the frontal sinus, a trephine is combined with an endoscopic approach to the frontal recess. This approach offers the benefit of irrigation in identifying the frontonasal drainage tract. When instrumentation for visualization is required, the trephine can be placed in the anterior wall of the frontal sinus. This can be placed in the eyebrow and slid up or in a brow skin crease with good cosmetic effect. A trephine through the anterior wall provides the potential to damage the supra-orbital nerve with associated numbness or paresthesia.

Osteoplastic Frontal Sinus Flap

Osteoplastic frontal sinus flap surgery can be achieved via a number of approaches. A gull wing or brow incision almost always results in a noticeable scar. Superior elevation of tissue off of the frontal bone will likely interrupt the supratrochlear and supraorbital nerves with predictable numbness. Frontal sinus fractures can often be profitably approached through an overlying laceration. Most osteoplastic flap frontal sinus surgeries are, however, approached via a coronal flap. The incision can be sited in a pretrichial location, or most commonly, behind the hairline. Some minor hair loss invariably occurs at the

site of the incision. This can be theoretically minimized by beveling of the incision to preserve hair follicles. Of more importance is the potential for visibility of the scar, which may occur with alopecia and advancing male pattern baldness. Numbness occurs over the scalp, posterior to the area of incision.

Elevation of the coronal flap requires a strategy to preserve the frontal branches of the facial nerve [14]. A loose areolar layer known as the subaponeurotic plane lies between the temporoparietal fascia and the deep temporal fascia. This loose tissue can be bluntly swept away to permit dissection directly on the surface of the deep temporal fascia (Fig. 29.2) [15]. This provides protection for the nerve, which travels on the undersurface of the temporoparietal fascia [15].

The potential for inadvertent intracranial entry exists when first entering the frontal sinus and raising the bone flap. This potential is minimized by careful preoperative planning. A surgical template can be fashioned from a nonmagnified plain frontal sinus Caldwell radiograph. Placement of a coin or similar object in the x-rayed field can verify that there is no magnification on the film. Special care must be taken to ensure that the template is able to sit properly at the superior orbital rim. Transillumination may also confirm the boundaries of the frontal sinus. More recently, image-guided surgery has provided another means by which to reduce the likelihood of inadvertent intracranial entry.

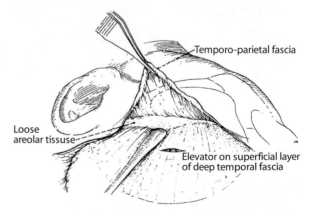

Fig. 29.2. The loose areolar layer termed the subaponeurotic fascia is bluntly swept away to permit dissection directly on the surface of the deep temporal fascia. Reproduced with permission from [15]

If frontal sinus obliteration, most often using abdominal fat, is planned, great care must be taken in removing and drilling all mucosa from the sinus. As a practical matter this can be very difficult or indeed impossible with certain anatomic sinus configurations. The danger of postoperative mucocele formation is ever present, and patients must be counseled regarding the need for long-term follow-up. Great care must also be taken to seal off the frontonasal communication. Contour defects may occur if viability of the bone flap is not completely maintained, and mesh or bone grafts may be used (particularly in revision cases) to restore a more aesthetic contour. The minor morbidity and potential for complications associated with obtaining an abdominal fat graft for sinus obliteration has led to a search for other more convenient substances. Hydroxyapatite enjoyed some preliminary enthusiasm; however, its use in the frontal sinus has been shown to be associated with the potential for infection and severe problems [16].

Conclusion

Frontal sinus surgery remains among the most challenging paranasal sinus surgeries to perform. Careful preoperative planning is required to reduce the potential for complications. Improvements in instrumentation have produced unquestioned advances in patient care. The remarkable dissecting capabilities of powered instrumentation, integral to some popular approaches to the frontal sinus, need to be treated with circumspection by experienced and inexperienced surgeons alike.

References

1. Cumberworth VL, Sudderick RM, Mackay IS (1994) Major complications of functional endoscopic sinus surgery. Clin Otolaryngol 19:248–253
2. Metson R (2003) Image-guided sinus surgery: Lessons learned from the first 1000 cases. Otolaryngol Head Neck Surg 128:8–13
3. Moreano EH, Hutchison JL, McCulloch TM, Graham SM, Funk GF, Hoffman HT (1998) Incidence of deep venous thrombosis and pulmonary embolism in otolaryngology-head and neck surgery. Otolaryngol Head Neck Surg 118:777–784
4. Yessenow RS, McCabe BF (1989) The osteo-mucoperiosteal flap in repair of cerebrospinal fluid rhinorrhea: a 20-year experience. Otolaryngol Head Neck Surg 101:555–558
5. Skedros DG, Cass SP, Hirsch BE, Kelly RH (1993) Sources of error in use of beta-2 transferrin analysis for diagnosing perilymphatic and cerebral spinal fluid leaks. Otolaryngol Head Neck Surg 109:861–864
6. Keerl R, Weber RK, Draf W, Wienke A, Schaefer SD (2004) Use of sodium fluorescein solution for detection of cerebrospinal fluid fistulas: an analysis of 420 administrations and reported complications in Europe and the United States. Laryngoscope 114:266–272.
7. Stankiewicz JA, Chow JM (1999) Two faces of orbital hematoma in intranasal (endoscopic) sinus surgery. Otolaryngol Head Neck Surg 120:841–847
8. Hayreh SS, Kolder HE, Weingeist TA (1980) Central retinal artery occlusion and retinal tolerance time. Ophthalmology 87:75–78
9. Nerad JA (2001) Oculoplastic surgery: the requisites in ophthalmology. Mosby, St. Louis, p 38
10. Graham SM, Carter KD (1999) Combined-approach orbital decompression for thyroid-related orbitopathy. Clin Otolaryngol 24:109–113
11. Graham SM, Thomas RD, Carter KD, Nerad JA (2002) The transcaruncular approach to the medial orbital wall. Laryngoscope 112:986–989
12. Graham SM, Nerad JA (2003) Orbital complications in endoscopic sinus surgery using powered instrumentation. Laryngoscope 113:874–878
13. Last RJ (1961) Wolff's anatomy of the eye and orbit. W.B. Saunders, Philadelphia and London, pp 236–237
14. Graham SM, Hoffman HT (2001) Extratemporal facial nerve injury: avoidance and pitfalls. In: Shelton C (Ed) Update on facial nerve disorders. Custom Printing, Inc, Rochester, MI, Chapter XXIII, pp 199–208
15. Stuzin JM, Wagstrom L, Kawamoto HK, Wolfe SA (1989) Anatomy of the frontal branch of the facial nerve: The significance of the temporal fat pad. Plast Reconstr Surg 83:265–271
16. Stankiewicz JA, Vaidy AM, Chow JM, Petruzzelli G (2002) Complications of hydroxyapatite use for transnasal closure of cerebrospinal fluid leaks. Am J Rhinol 16:337–341

Chapter 30

Open Approaches

Mark C. Weissler

Core Messages

- Open and endoscopic approaches are essentially ways of gaining exposure

- Choose the approach which can safely achieve the surgical objectives with the least morbidity

- There is still a role for open approaches to the paranasal sinuses

- Open approaches blend imperceptibly with other head and neck surgical skills necessary for the treatment of a variety of diseases, and form an important part of an overall surgical armamentarium

- Open and endoscopic approaches can complement one another

Contents

Introduction

Surgical intervention in diseases of the paranasal sinuses can change anatomy and drain infection. It does not intrinsically affect allergy, primary disease of the respiratory mucosa, the causes of nasal polyps, or other mucosal sensitivity to the environment. If one must operate on the paranasal sinuses, he or she should aim to accomplish the anatomic objectives and to do this in as safe a manner as possible. The underlying mucosal disease must then be addressed medically.

It is critical that the surgeon understand the underlying pathophysiology, know the relevant anatomy, set realistic surgical objectives, and then accomplish those objectives in as safe a manner as possible while causing the least morbidity. Whether this is to be accomplished endoscopically or via an open approach depends on the surgeon's experience and skill, the availability of necessary technology, and the specific disease entity being treated.

Historically the group of external sinus operations, e.g., external ethmoidectomy, Caldwell-Luc procedure, Lynch procedure, and osteoplastic frontal sinus obliteration have served as the basis for more complicated approaches to neoplasms, trauma, and other abnormalities of the craniofacial skeleton and skull base, and as a group of core operative skills from which to build.

Historical Perspectives

Dr. William Montgomery's 1979 textbook on *Surgery of the Upper Respiratory System* lists the following indications for sinus surgery, both external and intranasal: intracranial extension of infection, pain/purulence unresponsive to conservative therapy, necrosis with fistula formation, mucocele or pyocele, orbital cellulitis, and venous thrombosis [2]. Montgomery reviews the history of open procedures for chronic frontal sinusitis and attributes Riedel with the earliest modern day surgical approach in 1898 (Fig. 30.1). In Riedel's procedure, the anterior wall and floor of the sinus were removed along with an anterior ethmoidectomy and middle turbinectomy. In sinuses with a large anterior-posterior diameter, complete obliteration with the skin flap was not possible. Mosher modified the Riedel procedure by removing the posterior wall as well. In 1904 Killian modified this approach by leaving a 10-mm bridge of bone across the supraorbital rim, thus abrogating to some extent the cosmetic deformity. He also removed the anterior ethmoid cells and middle turbinate. Both of these procedures produced significant deformity in

30

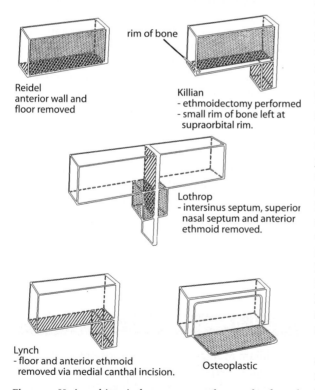

Reidel
anterior wall and
floor removed

Killian
- ethmoidectomy performed
- small rim of bone left at
  supraorbital rim.

rim of bone

Lothrop
- intersinus septum, superior
  nasal septum and anterior
  ethmoid removed.

Lynch
- floor and anterior ethmoid
  removed via medial canthal incision.

Osteoplastic

Fig. 30.1. Various historical open approaches to the frontal sinus

that the anterior wall of the frontal sinus was not reconstructed and the skin flaps were simply allowed to fall posteriorly into the former frontal sinus space. In 1914 Lothrop further modified the external approach by leaving the front wall intact, but removing the interfrontal sinus septum and upper nasal septum in addition to the anterior ethmoid and middle turbinate, creating a large inferior drainage fistula into the nose. This procedure worked best in patients with a deep frontal sinus in the anterior-posterior diameter. In 1920 Lynch combined removal of the floor of the frontal sinus and opening of the nasofrontal drainage system along with ethmoidectomy and middle turbinectomy with long-term stenting. This became the preferred procedure for some time, but was complicated by restenosis of the nasofrontal passage and mucocele/pyocele formation secondary to incomplete removal of the frontal sinus mucous membranes. The major alternative to such approaches was the osteoplastic frontal sinus obliteration, which originated in the late 19th century. The osteoplastic operation took its name from the fact that the anterior wall of the frontal sinus was opened as an inferior-based flap, fractured in the anterior roof of the orbit with intact periosteum over the superior orbital rim, resulting in a *vascularized* bone flap. The opened cavity was then obliterated with fat, which quickly became vascularized and prevented mucosal ingrowth. Montgomery performed experiments in cats showing that fat used to obliterate the frontal sinus survived long-term [3]. He stressed the *absolute importance* of removal of *both* the mucosal and inner cortical bone linings of the frontal sinus to insure successful vascular ingrowth and obliteration. Often today, when the frontal sinus is opened as part of a craniofacial approach with craniotomy, the anterior wall of the frontal sinus is taken as a free *nonvascularized* bone graft so that the periosteum can be utilized as part of a pericranial flap for relining of the floor of the anterior cranial fossa. To the best of my knowledge, no direct comparison of osteoplastic versus free bone graft techniques of opening the frontal sinus has ever been done.

Because of its relative inaccessibility and difficult exposure trans-nasally, the frontal sinus has been the most difficult to approach via endoscopic techniques. Special instrumentation and computerized intraoperative guidance is changing this today.

Modern Day Open Frontal Sinus Surgery

Intranasal Surgery

If chronic frontal sinusitis is due to problems within the nasal cavity, then septoplasty, intranasal ethmoidectomy, removal of the anterior aspect of the middle turbinate, and polypectomy may result in adequate frontal sinus drainage. External ethmoidectomy was traditionally the next step when chronic ethmoiditis was felt to be the root of frontal sinus problems. In 1979, Montgomery had this to say about intranasal approaches to the nasofrontal drainage system:

> ■ Intranasal probing and attempted enlargement or cannulization of the nasofrontal orifice are mentioned only to be condemned. Once the virginity of the nasofrontal passage is violated, scarring and stenosis are inevitable. If conservative intranasal surgery is not successful, then radical frontal sinus surgery is indicated.

Obviously times have changed, but the lessons remain valid. *Inadequate* intranasal attempts at opening the nasofrontal drainage system may well do more harm than good, and defining an adequate opening may be difficult and dependent on native anatomy. A congenitally narrow and shallow nasofrontal drainage system will be much more difficult to manipulate and alter in such a way as to maintain long-term postoperative patency than a wide system.

Trephination

The simplest open approach to the frontal sinus is trephination.

Indications for trephination include:

- ■ Acute painful frontal sinusitis unresponsive to conservative measures
- ■ Acute frontal sinusitis with impending complications
- ■ For frontal sinus exploration
- ■ Biopsy
- ■ As an adjunct to an endoscopic approach

When used adjunctively to an endoscopic approach, the trephination can help to assess adequate drainage and assist with guidance of the endoscopic approach either directly or by instilling colored saline into the sinus which can be followed endoscopically.

A trephination is performed through a stab incision in the superomedial aspect of the orbit. The incision is brought down through all layers including the periosteum to expose the floor of the frontal sinus (roof of the orbit). The periosteum is elevated with a Cottle elevator. It is best to perforate the bone with a small burr and to do this through the lamellar bone of the floor of the frontal sinus rather than the cancellous bone of the anterior wall, which has a marrow space. Contamination of the marrow space might lead to osteomyelitis. The sinus mucosa can be examined via the trephine with a small endoscope. Cultures are taken of the purulent material. The sinus is thoroughly irrigated with warm saline, and an angiocatheter is left in the sinus for irrigation with saline or antibiotics and decongestants. The angiocatheter is sewn to the skin of the medial orbit. At the time of surgery, endoscopic examination of the frontal recess can confirm patency of the nasofrontal drainage system, especially if the irrigant is colored with a small amount of methylene blue dye.

Postoperatively, the patient is treated with intravenous antibiotics and nasal decongestants. The initial choice of antibiotics is empiric and based on gram stain results, but once culture results are available, specific antibiotic therapy is instituted. The catheter in the frontal sinus is irrigated four times daily with saline or a dilute solution of antibiotics and decongestants such as 10 cc of gentamicin mixed as 80 mg in a liter of saline and 0.5 cc of 0.05% xylometazoline. When patency of the nasofrontal drainage system is

30

confirmed by free flow of irrigation solution into the nose, the catheter is removed. The small stab wound will heal by secondary intention.

The Lynch Procedure

> ■ This procedure has probably been the most commonly performed in the United States for the treatment of chronic frontal sinus disease.

It is performed via a medial canthal incision extended upward into the medial orbit. An external ethmoidectomy with resection of the anterior end of the middle turbinate is then performed. Classically, the entire floor of the frontal sinus was then removed along with all mucosa, and a stent was placed in the nasofrontal connection prior to closure. Much has been made in the literature over just what sort of stent should be used. Most commonly, a piece of polyvinyl chloride endotracheal tube or a piece of rolled silastic sheeting has been used. In more recent times, the mucosa of the sinus has not been stripped, but instead the drainage system is *reconstructed*. The main problem with this procedure has been restenosis of the nasofrontal drainage system. To avoid this, a variety of methods have been tried. The interfrontal sinus septum has been resected to allow drainage via the contralateral sinus, and various mucosal flaps have been laid in the area of the flap. Success rates of greater than 90% have been reported [1].

The procedure is performed under general anesthesia, with the patient in the supine position with the head of the bed slightly elevated. Pledgets or gauze strips impregnated with decongestant solution are placed in the nasal cavity. The eyelids are closed with tarsorrhaphy sutures placed at the lateral limbus of the iris. A gull-wing incision is made in the medial canthal area which is extended upward into the medial orbit. The incision is carried down through skin, subcutaneous tissue, and periosteum. The supratrochlear vessels are identified and cauterized or ligated and divided. The periosteum is retracted medially and laterally with stay sutures which are weighted with small hemostats and laid over gauze covering the eyes. The lacrimal sac is elevated out of the lacrimal fossa, identifying the anterior and posterior lacrimal crests. The medial canthal tendon is released by dissecting the periosteum from the medial orbital wall and retracting the orbital contents laterally with a Sewell retractor. The anterior ethmoid artery is identified and isolated, a medium size hemoclip is placed on the lateral (orbital) side, and the medial (nasal) side is then cauterized with a bipolar cautery and transected. The anterior ethmoid is entered via the lacrimal fossa, and the bone of the anterior lacrimal crest and a small portion of the nasal bone are removed with a Kerrison rongeur. The anterior ethmoid cells are removed along with the anterior portion of the lamina papyracea and the anterior tip of the middle turbinate. Entrance to the nasal cavity is confirmed by intranasal inspection and visualization of the nasal packing through the ethmoid. Next, the floor of frontal sinus is resected with the Kerrison rongeur, and the diseased mucosa is removed from the frontal sinus. Cultures should be taken as indicated by findings. Just how much bone and mucosa are removed remains controversial. Some would contend that all *irreversibly condemned* mucosa must be removed, along with most all of the frontal sinus floor. Others would argue that this predisposes to scarring and prolapse of orbital tissue into the frontonasal drainage system. Stenting also remains controversial with regard to what if any stenting material should be used. The most commonly used stents are rolled pieces of silastic sheeting and cut portions of polyvinyl chloride endotracheal tubes which are secured to the nasal septum for weeks to months postoperatively. The medial canthal wound is closed by first carefully reapproximating the periosteum and thereby repositioning the medial canthal tendon, and then closing the skin with either fine nylon or a fast-absorbing gut suture. Saline nasal irrigations are used postoperatively to cut down on crusting around the stent. Antibiotics are used as dictated by intraoperative findings and cultures.

The Osteoplastic Frontal Sinus Obliteration

The osteoplastic frontal sinus obliteration procedure remains an important part of the sinus surgeon's armamentarium. Although it can be carried out unilaterally, it is generally performed bilaterally (Figs. 30.2–30.4).

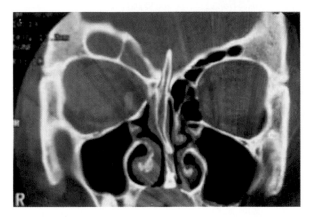

Fig. 30.2. Unilateral frontal sinus mucocele with congenitally narrow nasofrontal drainage system

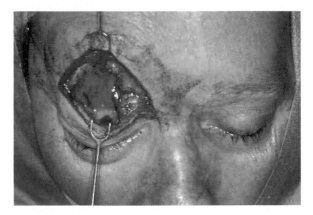

Fig. 30.3. Unilateral osteoplastic approach with mucocele unroofed

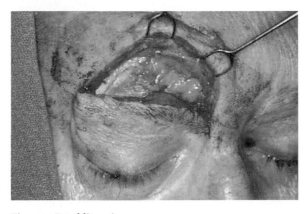

Fig. 30.4. Fat obliteration

The keys to success of the osteoplastic frontal sinus obliteration are:

- *Complete* removal of *all* frontal sinus mucosa
- Burring of the inner table of bone of the sinus cavity

Generally the sinus is obliterated with abdominal fat harvested from the left lower quadrant of the abdomen so as not to be confused in the future with an appendectomy incision. Montgomery has shown in cats, and personal experience corroborates, that fat can survive long-term within the sinus cavity.

Preoperatively, the patient has a Caldwell view x-ray taken from 6 feet away, and the frontal sinus is cut out of the film to be used as a template during surgery. Alternatively, one can use intraoperative CT guidance or transillumination to delineate the borders of the frontal sinus. A coronal flap is elevated in a plane *superficial* to the periosteum, down to the supraorbital rim. The supratrochlear and supraorbital nerves are spared and may be released from foramina as needed. Utilizing the template, or other method, the sinus is outlined and an oscillating or sagittal saw is used to cut the frontal bone slightly inside the limits shown by the template. There is no need to follow the exact lateral contours of the sinus. The saw blade should be greatly bevelled in toward the central sinus. At the supraorbital rims, the very thick bone must be completely transected, and a horizontal bony incision is made at the nasal root. A fine osteotome is inserted through the superior bony cut and used to divide the interfrontal sinus septum. The osteoplastic flap with vascularized periosteum adherent to its anterior wall is then fractured inferiorly through the roofs of the orbits. Next, all mucosa is painstakingly removed from the frontal sinus, and the lining cortical bone drilled with a cutting burr. Small 1–2-mm burrs can be helpful in removing mucosa from small extensions of the sinus. The intersinus septum is completely drilled away. This dissection extends down into the nasofrontal drainage system. The sinus is copiously irrigated with saline or bacitracin solution. Small pieces of fat or separately harvested temporalis muscle are used to obliterate the nasofrontal drainage system, and the frontal sinus is filled with *atraumatically* harvested abdominal fat. The flap is then returned to anatomic position and fixed in position with small wires or miniplates. The periosteum is closed with absorbable suture, and the coronal skin flap is closed in layers over closed suction drains which exit separate stab wound incisions laterally.

30

References

1. Amble FR, Kern EB, Neel B 3rd, Facer GW, McDonald TJ, Czaja JM (1996) Nasofrontal duct reconstruction with silicone rubber sheeting for inflammatory frontal sinus disease: Analysis of 164 cases. Laryngoscope 106:809–815
2. Montgomery WW: Surgery of the upper respiratory system, 2 vols. 2nd edn. Lea & Febiger, Philadelphia
3. Montgomery WW (1964) The fate of adipose implants in a bony cavity. Laryngoscope 74:816

Chapter 31

Osteoplastic Frontal Sinusotomy and Reconstruction of Frontal Defects

31

Ulrike Bockmühl

Core Messages

- Osteoplastic frontal sinusotomy provides wide exposure and safe access to the frontal sinus in the setting of complicated disease, trauma, and tumor

- In some cases, the anterior table of the frontal sinus may be disrupted requiring reconstruction. Options for reconstruction include alloplastic materials, pedicled calvarial bone grafts, and free calvarial bone grafts

- The calvarial bone graft provides excellent contouring with minimal morbidity to the graft donor site

Contents

Introduction

About 5% of all frontal sinus operations are performed via an external approach. Today, the osteoplastic flap procedure [10] is commonly performed for conditions of the frontal sinus that cannot be successfully treated endonasally [32, 33]. This approach permits an optimal view encompassing the entire frontal sinus, and allows complete microscopic removal of mucosa as well as obliteration of the frontal sinus with abdominal fat, as described by Tato and Bergaglio [30]. It overcomes the problems and complications of the external frontoethmoidectomy according to Jansen [13] and Ritter [25] or Lynch [18], which is an obsolete procedure in modern frontal sinus surgery.

Indications for the Frontal Osteoplastic Flap Procedure (or *Approach*) Are as Follows

- Recurrent chronic inflammation after previous endonasal or external operations (Type III drainage according to Draf [5,6] was technically impossible or failed)
- Laterally located muco-pyocele
- Major destruction of the anterior and/or posterior frontal sinus wall (e.g. severe fractures with dural disruption and/or involving the drainage pathways)
- Inflammatory complications after trauma (e.g. because of alloplastic material)
- Major benign tumors (e.g. osteoma)
- Aesthetic correction of the forehead contour (e.g. after removal of the anterior frontal sinus wall as done by the Riedel's operation [27] or in cases of pneumatosinus dilatans frontalis)

As the aesthetic forehead contour correction is one indication for the frontal osteoplastic flap approach, this technique will be described first, followed by demonstrating the surgical steps of anterior frontal sinus wall reconstruction, i.e. texture of the bony forehead region.

Regardless of frontal sinus pathology or surgery performed, preoperatively patients should undergo high-resolution CT scanning with primary axial slices (with 2-mm maximum thickness) and reconstruction in coronal as well as sagittal cuts. Additionally, MRI scanning is recommended.

Surgical Technique

Frontal Osteoplastic Flap Approach and Procedure

Depending on the extent of pathology and the degree of pneumatization, this operation demands great precision and may be time-consuming. Its success depends on numerous surgical steps and details that are specified in the following.

Surgery requires general anesthesia, with orotracheal intubation.

Patients appreciate it if shaving the hair can be avoided, as the coronal incision is used. The hair should be washed with disinfectant solution to avoid infection, the evening before operation.

The preferred incision for uni- and bilateral osteoplastic frontal sinus operations in individuals with a full head of hair is the bitemporal or coronal incision about 4–5 cm behind the hairline. The great advantage is an invisible scar, immediately after surgery. In patients with male pattern baldness, the incision is located more posteriorly in the hair-bearing corona.

Fifteen minutes before incision, local anesthesia of 10–20 ml of Xylocaine 1% with adrenaline (1:200000) is injected to reduce bleeding.

The coronal incision extends down as far as the periosteum. Using partly blunt, partly sharp dissection to the supraorbital ridge and over the root of the nose, the scalp flap is pulled caudally on both sides, leaving behind the periosteum and the bone, thus preserving the supraorbital and supratrochlear vas-

cular nerve bundles (Fig. 31.1). Special scalp clamps stop the remaining bleeding (Fig. 31.1).

Next, the template of the frontal sinus that was excised from the occipito-frontal plain X-ray and preserved in a disinfectant solution is carefully positioned on the root of the nose so that the borders of the frontal sinus can be estimated. The periosteum is incised 1.5 cm outside the template and elevated slightly, being pedicled caudally at the bone. Then the osteotomy is made at the marked line from the X-ray template using the oscillating saw angled at 30° directed towards the frontal sinus. In this way a surface that is as wide as possible is created for the later replacement of this bony lid. The bony incision reaches the supraorbital ridge on both sides. The fracture and elevation of the bony lid is done with a chisel. When opening the frontal sinus bilaterally, the intersinus septum must be separated from the anterior frontal sinus wall, i.e., with an angled chisel as well. The supraorbital ridge slightly anterior to the controlled fracture in the region of the frontal sinus floor is preserved, and the bony lid hinges on the periosteal flap.

The diseased tissue is then removed according to the pathological-anatomical findings. Fractures must be exposed to their full extent, repositioned and, if necessary, a dural lesion must be treated with duraplasty. In cases secondary to trauma or osteoma, where there is healthy frontal sinus mucosa, it must be decided whether the mucosa around the infundibulum is healthy enough to preserve the frontal sinus or whether obliteration should be carried out. If the sinus mucosa is preserved, a Type III median-drainage procedure [5, 6] can be performed easily from above with optimum exposure. Recently, this technique has been described in association with the "frontal sinus unobliteration procedure" by Javer et al. [14].

If obliteration is indicated, the frontal sinus mucosa must be removed completely and the inner layer of the bony walls must be drilled away under microscopic view (Fig. 31.1). Simple macroscopic stripping of the mucosa leads in a high percentage to inflammatory recurrences and mucoceles [4]. At the inner table of the anterior and posterior frontal sinus wall as well as for medial and lateral orbital roof, the cutting drill is the instrument of choice. It allows total removal of the mucosa leaving the bony vascular

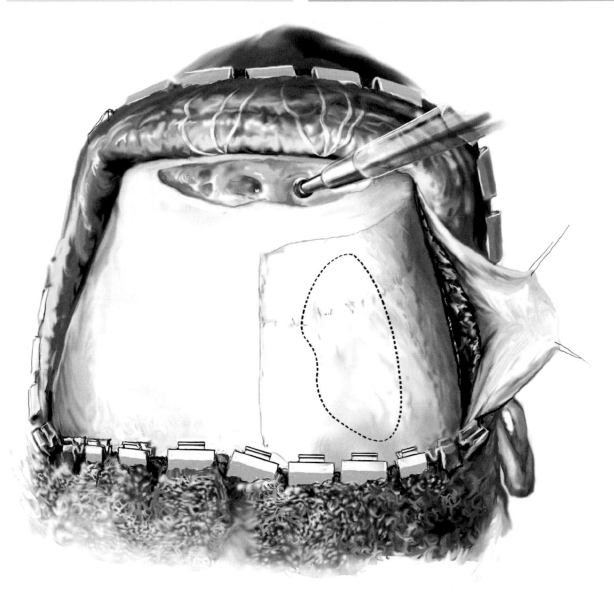

Fig. 31.1. Technique of the frontal sinus obliteration in case of missing anterior frontal sinus wall: Caudally pulled scalp and galea periosteal flap preserving supraorbital nerves. Complete removal of left frontal sinus mucosa and drillout of the posterior frontal sinus wall under microscopic view. Parietal donor calvarial bone site and shape are marked

channels open, which facilitates the revascularization of fat used for obliteration. In dangerous areas such as exposed dura and the central roof of the orbit, the frontal sinus mucosa can be removed safely using a diamond drill. As a principle: The larger the drill, the less the danger.

The mucosa in the region of the frontonasal ostium is inverted nasally, and the drainage opening is blocked with pinna conchal cartilage on one side covered by overlapping perichondrium and fixed with fibrin glue. The cartilage can be tightly sealed with fascia held within fibrin glue. Through this three-layered closure, the frontal sinus is securely isolated from the nasal cavity and the ethmoidal cells, respectively, and growth of mucosa into the sinus with the associated risk of mucocele formation is prevented (Fig. 31.2).

Next, abdominal fat is harvested either via a pre-existing scar or an incision around the navel. The abdominal fat is temporarily placed in isotonic saline solution and then placed by pieces into the frontal sinus holding together with fibrin glue, until the sinus cavity is completely filled.

Finally, the periosteal bone lid is replaced and wedged closed with a tap of the mallet, followed by suturing the periosteum. If the bone lid fractures during elevation, these bony fragments should be fixed together with absorbable threads, wire sutures, or miniplates.

At the end of the operation, the scalp flap is flipped back into place, two suction drains are inserted, and the coronal incision is closed with single-stitch sutures. The tube drains are removed not later than two days after surgery; otherwise removal is difficult and more painful.

The cranialization of the frontal sinus [3] with removal of the frontal sinus posterior table is a safe and reliable modification of the osteoplastic flap procedure. Its use is indicated in cases of comminuted fractures of the frontal sinus, severe posttraumatic edema of the frontal lobe, if an intracranial foreign body is present, or in cases with variable destruction of the posterior frontal sinus wall due to inflammation or a neoplastic process. In cases of frontal sinus extending far posterior at the frontal recess, removal of the posterior frontal sinus wall allows retraction of dura and eases complete removal of mucosa.

Reconstruction of the Bony Forehead Region

The initial part of the operation corresponds with the technique of the frontal osteoplastic flap procedure. Prior to reconstruction, residual frontal or ethmoid sinus disease, particularly any residual mucosa and mucoceles must be eliminated, and the three-layered closure must be performed as described above (Fig. 31.2). Cranial defects with open dura should be exposed extradurally, and if in doubt, dissection should be performed in conjunction with a neurosurgical team. If dead space is observed between the contracted scarred dura and the overlying bony surface, it can be obliterated with abdominal fat. Furthermore, it is essential to verify that adequate scalp and skin cover are available to resurface the more prominent reconstructed skull.

Many different grafts and implants have been used more or less successfully in craniofacial surgery to date. The most important ones together with their disadvantages are listed in Table 31.1.

In our hands, the autogenous calvarial bone has proven to be the most suitable material for anterior frontal sinus wall, i.e., bony forehead reconstruction [1, 28]. The most common harvesting site is the parietal region. Usually, the graft is taken more anteriorly and medially if a flat portion of bone is required, and more laterally and posteriorly if a curvilinear piece is needed.

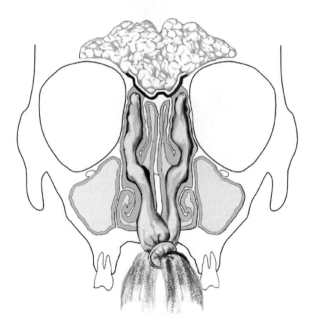

Fig. 31.2. Fat obliteration of the frontal sinuses and three-layer closure separating the frontal sinuses from the nasal and the ethmoid cavity. Nasal packing is carried out with Rhinotamps

31

Table 31.1. Recommended grafts and implants for reconstruction of the anterior frontal sinus wall, i.e. contouring the forehead region

Grafts		Disadvantages / Contraindications
Autogenous grafts		
a) Free bone graft		
Compact grafts	– Rib, scapula	Additional operating field, to small (rib), natural contour not sufficient [21]
Cancellous bone graft	– Iliac crest	Additional operating field, to small, high resorption rate [21]
Split bone	– Calvarial bone (inner and outer table)	
b) Free cartilage graft		
Rib cartilage		Additional operating field, to small, high resorption rate [21]
c) Pedicled autogenous graft		
Myo-osseous flap	– Calvarial bone pedicled at the temporalis muscle	Difficult technique, contour correction of temporal muscle defect necessary
Allogenic grafts		
Preserved cartilage or bone		Too small, high resorption rate [21]
Alloplastic materials		
Metal	– Titanium (plates or mesh filled with autogenous cancellous bone)	Expensive
Plastic	– Polymethylmethacrylate	Infection if in contact with paranasal sinuses [19]
	– Porous polyethylene	
Ceramic	– Hydroxyapatite, carbonated apatite	Resorption possible, causing hematoma, migration, conversion difficulties in wet fields, e.g. in contact with CSF or blood [8,26,29], expensive
Biocement	– Bioverit	Expensive

Three techniques exist for the transfer of calvarial bone grafts, and each has a separate set of indications:

■ Split-thickness calvarial graft

■ Single table calvarial graft

■ Calvarial bone flap

Split-thickness calvarial grafting involves removal of the outer table while leaving the inner layer in situ. Its disadvantage is the relatively small amount or size of bone that can be transferred. Briefly, the template placed over an appropriate donor site is outlined by a burr to the depth of the inner cortex (signaled by bleeding from the diploic space).

Calvarial bone flap involves transfer of donor calvaria on a muscle-facial-periosteal pedicle being vascularized bone as the main advantage. Of the three techniques, it is the most complicated and is reserved for the patient with soft-tissue recipient sites of poor quality, e.g. scars or defects due to tumor resection [20] or after radiotherapy.

Single table calvarial graft is the method we prefer and therefore will be described in detail. Before harvesting, the bony cranial defect margins are debrided until healthy margins of bleeding bone are identified.

To optimize the fit and curvature match of the donor bone to the recipient site, a malleable lead template of the entire forehead region is created preoperatively from an artificial skull. This template of Thermoplast is then sterilized overnight. Intraoperatively, it is trimmed to fit into the defect. The selection site of the donor bone is chosen based on availability and desired contour match. However, the parietal regions are preferred donor sites (Fig. 31.1). Importantly, a sagittal bar is maintained intact (approximately 2 cm lateral to the midline, respectively) to protect the sagittal sinus and to provide a stable skeletal reference for subsequent calvarial donor site reconstruction. With extremely large defects, a better recipient site match can be achieved by dividing the lead template in two, to isolate separate but well-matched skull donor sites.

After preparing a periosteal flap, a full thickness bone flap is harvested. Therefore, the template is outlined using the smallest cutting burr to allow access for the oscillating saw that is used until the diploic space is sawed through. The last inner bony layer is drilled off by a diamond burr under microscopic view. In this way the dura can be easily identified because of their color and vessels, and can be protected. Chisels are employed to remove the entire full-thickness calvaria. This donor bone is then split into two along the diploic interface between the inner and outer tables using a water-cooled oscillating saw and chisels (Fig. 31.3). The continuity of the calvarial do-

nor site is restored by replacing the inner table, while the outer table is used as the donor bone to fix the forehead defect (Fig. 31.4). Fine contouring can be carried out with the diamond burr. Once the outer table is perfectly fitted, the reconstruction is completed by rigidly fixing all bone grafts to the recipient site with titanium micro or mini plates (Fig. 31.5).

The final part of the operation corresponds with the technique of the frontal osteoplastic flap procedure as well.

Postoperative Care

The general principles of postoperative care include:

- Postoperative antibiotic coverage for 10 days
- Patient follow-up every 3 months for the first year to examine for instability, resorption, or infection of the reconstructed region
- Obtain CT (also MRI in cases of fat obliteration) scans 3 months after surgery to assess the bony and soft tissue as a baseline for further following
- In cases of doubt, bone scans using a technetium 99 m radioactive tracer can provide a crude measure of bone graft revascularization at the recipient as well as the donor site [1]

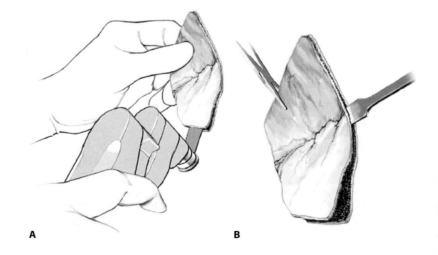

Fig. 31.3.
Splitting of harvested full thickness calvarial bone into inner and outer table using an oscillating saw (A) or chisels (B)

A   **B**

31

Fig. 31.4.
Condition at the end of the operation: Completely reconstructed anterior frontal sinus wall with the outer table giving an aesthetic forehead contour, and replaced inner table at the parietal donor site

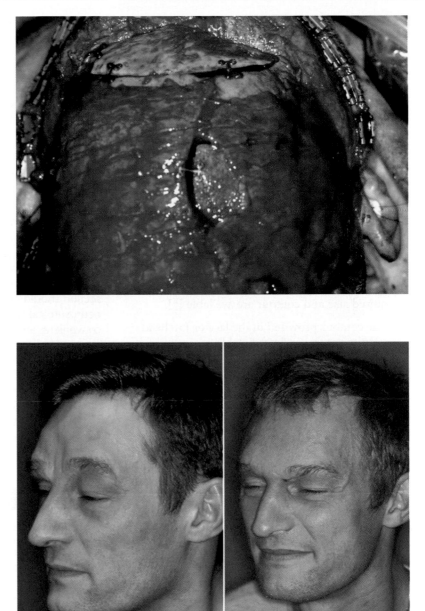

Fig. 31.5.
Patient in pre- and postoperative view after bony reconstruction of the anterior frontal sinus wall (as shown in Fig. 31.4) using calvarial split bone

Results and Complications

Calvaria was first employed in bone grafting (as part of a scalp osteocutaneous flap) by Müller [22] and by König [16] as early as 1890. However, its use was rarely reported until Tessier [31] described his experience with 234 calvarial grafts in 103 patients in 1982.

The calvaria offers several distinct advantages over other bones as donor sites:

■ It has been proven that graft volume survival is greater with membranous bone such as calvaria than endochondral bones like scapula, ilium, or rib [9,35].

■ The bone can be harvested through the same operative field, and grafts of almost any required size and contour are available [7].

■ The contour provided in the face or forehead is quite natural and predictable.

■ Calvarial bone can be used in potentially contaminated spaces, e.g. in contact with infected paranasal sinuses, in cases of facial trauma, under irradiated skins, as well as in cases with foreign body reaction against alloplastic materials [9].

■ The patient's discomfort is minimal.

Despite the low morbidity reported with the calvarial bone harvesting procedure, single significant donor site complications such as dural lacerations, sagittal sinus laceration, and intracerebral hematoma have been described [2, 11, 23, 34]. However, we have not seen any of these problems and neither have many others [1, 15, 24].

Besides the immediate complications during harvesting procedures, delayed complications are also possible. The most important one is infection, which has been reported to occur between 1.6 and 5.5% [12, 23]. Replacement or even extrusion of calvarial grafts has not been documented [1, 9, 20, 23, 31].

Four comprehensive studies reporting complex craniofacial reconstructions using calvarial grafts in 62, 44, 20, and 17 patients, respectively experienced excellent long-term aesthetic results without significant complications with harvesting or in placement of cranial bone [9, 17, 20, 23].

Conclusion

The most appropriate surgical approach to reconstruct the bony forehead region is the frontal osteoplastic flap approach. Prior to reconstruction, residual frontal or ethmoid sinus disease, particularly any residual mucosa and mucoceles must be eliminated, and a sufficient closure to the paranasal sinuses must be performed. Cranial defects with open dura should be exposed extradurally, and if in doubt, dissection should be performed in conjunction with a neurosurgical team. Calvarial bone is a very useful, convenient, and cost-effective graft in craniofacial reconstruction, particularly in repair of bony forehead defects. With the described harvesting technique, sufficient bone becomes available for large reconstructions, with minimum morbidity to the patient. The aesthetic results, even the long-term results with outer table calvarial grafts, are excellent.

References

1. Bockmühl U, Hendus J, Draf W (2004) Reconstruction of the forehead contour using split calvarial bone grafts. Unpublished data

2. Canella DM, Hopkin LN (1990) Superior sagittal sinus laceration complicating an autogenous calvarial bone graft harvest: Report of a case. J Oral Maxillofac Surg 48: 741–743

3. Donald PJ, Bernstein L (1978) Compound frontal sinus injuries with intracranial penetration. Laryngoscope 88: 225–232

4. Donald PJ, Ettin M (1986) The safety of frontal sinus fat obliteration when sinus walls are missing. Laryngoscope 96:190–193

5. Draf W (1991) Endonasal micro-endoscopic frontal sinus surgery: The Fulda concept. Operative Techniques Otolaryngol Head Neck Surg 2:234–240

6. Draf W, Weber R, Keerl R, Constantinidis J, Schick B, Saha A (2000) Endonasal and external micro-endoscopic sur-

31

gery of the frontal sinus. In: Stamm A, Draf W eds. Microendoscopic Surgery of the paranasal sinuses and the skull base. Springer, Berlin, New York 257–278

7. Elisevich K, Bite U (1991) En block forehead reconstruction with split-thickness cranial bone. Surg Neurol 35: 384–388

8. Friedman CD, Constantino PD, Snyderman CH, Chow LC, Takagi S (2000) Reconstruction of the frontal sinus and frontofacial skeleton with hydroxyapatite cement. J Biomed Meter Res 2: 428–432

9. Goodrich JT, Argamaso R, Hall CD (1992) Split-thickness bone grafts in complex craniofacial reconstructions. Pediatr Neurosurg 18: 195–201

10. Hardy JM, Montgomery WW (1976) Osteoplastic frontal sinusotomy: An analysis of 250 operations. Ann Otol Rhinol Laryngol 85: 523–532

11. Ilankovan V, Jackson IT (1992) Experience in the use of calvarial bone grafts in orbital reconstruction. Br J Oral Maxillofac Surg 30: 92–96

12. Jackson IT, Helden G, Marx R (1986) Skull bone grafts in maxillofacial and craniofacial surgery. J Oral Maxillofac Surg 44: 949–955

13. Jansen A (1894) Eröffnung der Nebenhöhlen der Nase bei chronischer Eiterung. Arch Laryng Rhinol(Berl) 135–157

14. Javer AR, Sillers MJ, Kuhn FA (2001) The frontal sinus unobliteration procedure. Otolaryngol Clin North Am 34: 193–210

15. Kellman RM (1994) Safe and dependable harvesting of large outer-table calvarial bone grafts. Arch Otolaryngol Head Neck Surg 120: 856–860

16. König F (1890) Der knöcherne Ersatz grosser Schädeldefekte. Zentralbl. Chir 17: 497

17. Kozak J, Voska P (1993) Reconstruction of the frontal region with skull bone grafts. Acta Chir Plast 35: 36–43

18. Lynch RC (1921) The technique of a radical frontal sinus operation which has given me the best results. Laryngoscope 31: 1–5

19. Maas CS, Merwin GE, Wilson J, Frey MD, Maves MD (1990) Comparison of biomaterials for facial bone augmentation. Arch Otolaryngol Head Neck Surg 116: 551–556

20. McCarthy JG, Zide BM (1984) The Spectrum of calvarial bone grafting: Introduction of vascularized calvarial bone flap. Plast Reconstr Surg 74: 10–18

21. Mohr C, Seifert V, Schettler D (1994) [Osteoplasty of osseous defects of the frontal bone and orbital roof –

Indications, technique and results]. Fortschr Kiefer Gesichtschir 39: 43–46

22. Müller W (1890) Zur Frage der temporären Schädelresektion anstelle der Trepanation. Zentralbl. Chir 17: 65

23. Powell NB, Riley RW (1987) Cranial bone grafting in facial aesthetic and reconstructive contouring. Arch Otolaryngol Head Neck Surg 113: 713–719

24. Psillakis JM, Nocchi VL, Zanini SA (1979) Repair of large defect of frontal bone with free graft of outer table of parietal bones. Plast Reconstr Surg 64: 827–830

25. Ritter G (1906) Eine neue Methode zur Erhaltung der vorderen Stirnhöhlenwand bei Radikaloperationen chronischer Stirnhöhleneiterungen. Dtsch Med Wochenschr 32: 1294–1296

26. Rosen G, Nachtigal D (1995) The use of hydroxyapatite for obliteration of the human frontal sinus. Laryngoscope 105: 553–555

27. Schenke H (1898) Über die Stirnhöhle und ihre Erkrankungen. Die Radikaloperation nach Riedel. Inauguraldissertation Friedrich-Schiller-Univ. Jena

28. Schick B, Hendus J, el Tahan A, Draf W (1998) [Reconstruction of the forehead region with tabula externa of the skull]. Laryngorhinootologie 77: 474–479

29. Schmitz JP, Hollinger JO, Milam SB (1999) Reconstruction of bone using calcium phosphate bone cements: A critical review. J Oral Maxillofac Surg 57: 1122–1126

30. Tato JM, Bergaglio OE (1949) Surgery of frontal sinus. Fat grafts: New technique. Otolaryngologica 3: 1

31. Tessier P (1982) Autogenous bone grafts taken from the calvarium for facial and cranial applications. Clin Plast Surg 9: 531–538

32. Weber R, Draf W, Kahle G, Kind M (1999) Obliteration of the frontal sinus--State of the art and reflections on new materials. Rhinology 37: 1–15

33. Weber R, Draf W, Keerl R, Kahle G, Schinzel S, Thomann S, Lawson W (2000) Osteoplastic frontal sinus surgery with fat obliteration: Technique and long-term results using magnetic resonance imaging in 82 operations. Laryngoscope 110: 1037–1044

34. Young VL, Schuster RH, Harris LW (1990) Intracerebral hematoma complicating split calvarial bone-graft harvesting. Plast Reconstr Surg 86: 763–765

35. Zins JE, Whitaker LA (1983) Membranous versus endochondral bone: Implications for craniofacial reconstruction. Plast Reconstr Surg 72: 778–784

Subject Index